Probiotic Bacteria

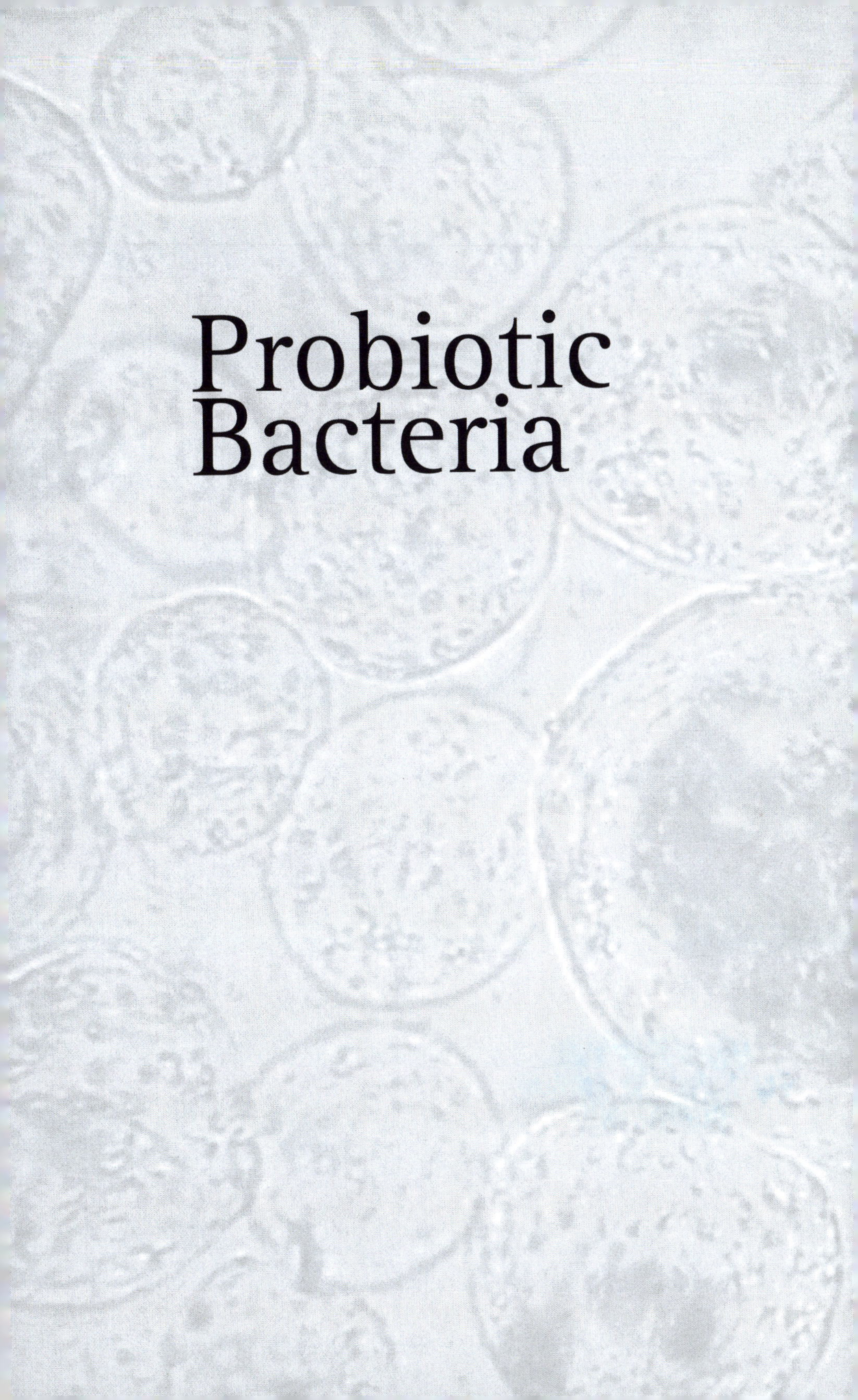

edited by
J. Paulo Sousa e Silva
Ana C. Freitas

Probiotic Bacteria

Fundamentals, Therapy, and Technological Aspects

Pan Stanford Publishing

Published by

Pan Stanford Publishing Pte. Ltd.
Penthouse Level, Suntec Tower 3
8 Temasek Boulevard
Singapore 038988

Email: editorial@panstanford.com
Web: www.panstanford.com

British Library Cataloguing-in-Publication Data
A catalogue record for this book is available from the British Library.

Probiotic Bacteria: Fundamentals, Therapy, and Technological Aspects

ISBN 978-981-4411-62-2 (Hardcover)
ISBN 978-981-4411-63-9 (eBook)

Printed in the USA

Contents

Foreword

It gives me immense pleasure to write a few words about the upcoming book *Probiotic Bacteria: Fundamentals, Therapy, and Technological Aspects* edited by Drs. J. Paulo Sousa e Silva and Ana Cristina Freitas. Probiotic organisms have been a subject of keen research for more than a century. Studies on probiotic organisms have come a long way from the era of Metchnikoff in the early 1900s, and our knowledge is being enhanced with each passing decade. Traditionally, probiotic organisms have been incorporated in fermented products like yogurt, however, as of recent times there are numerous probiotic products in the global market of varied types. The literature on probiotic organisms is vast and diverse and there is enough clinical evidence to support the health-enhancing potential of probiotic organisms.

This book is a unique compilation of technological aspects related to probiotic products, their benefits, and their therapeutic and physiological implications. The information is conveniently grouped under seven chapters. Chapter 1 details the fundamentals of probiotic bacteria. Chapter 2 covers the gastrointestinal physiology and its relevance to probiotic products. Chapter 3 deals with the various therapeutic roles of probiotics beyond gut-health. Chapter 4 gives an overview on the advances in probiotic food, with judicious insights into the technological and functional aspects. Chapter 5 provides a detailed analysis of several materials and techniques for immobilization and microencapsulation of probiotic bacteria. Chapter 6 is devoted to the development of probiotic dosage forms, and Chapter 7 focuses on the guidelines and regulation pertaining to the use of probiotic organisms.

In general, an attempt has been made to provide a comprehensive review on the fundamentals of probiotic organisms, along with their therapeutic and industrial aspects. The book is unique in presenting a dedicated section on the development of several dosage forms containing probiotic bacteria. The book provides a contemporary update and a holistic review of the topic, and is designed to augment related books in the market. The editorial team comprises individuals with noteworthy and remarkable experience in the field of probiotic organisms. It is anticipated that this book should be an indispensable resource for academicians, extension staff, and students working in the field of probiotic organisms and probiotic products. Also, the book should appeal to technologists and food scientists in the related industry.

Nagendra P. Shah
Professor of Food Science
School of Biological Sciences
The University of Hong Kong, Hong Kong

Preface

Probiotic organisms, according to the Food and Agriculture Organization (FAO) of the United Nations and the World Health Organization (WHO), are live microorganisms that when administered in adequate amounts could confer a health benefit on the host. Probiotics can play a major role in human health if they can be incorporated in food products or used as dosage forms. For this, a detailed knowledge of the microorganisms is required, which forms the basis of the selection and use of probiotics.

Probiotics may be useful in several functions, namely protection against pathogenic bacteria directly via displacement of these bacteria by competitive binding or growth inhibition, by antimicrobial compounds or pH reduction, or indirectly by neutralization or elimination of toxins from the intestine, improving gut barrier integrity by ameliorating epithelial and tissue integrity through low-dose NO synthesis, simulation of mucus production, or/and enhancing gut epithelial cell proliferation. In addition, probiotics have also been shown to have immunomodulation capacity, to inhibit endogenous carcinogen production, and to provide nutrients for enterocytes by short-chain fatty acid production. Such activities by a specific strain (or group) allow them to promote several health benefits, which enables assuring of different therapeutic applications, including alleviation of lactose intolerance, inhibition of *Helicobacter pylori* or other enteric pathogenic bacteria and enteric virus (particularly *Rotavirus*) with reduction of associated diarrhoea symptoms, prevention of inflammatory bowel disease, reduction of cholesterol level, treatment and prevention of allergy, reduction of the risk associated with mutagenicity and carcinogenicity, reduction and control of urogenital infections, improvement in liver and pancreas dysfunctions, promotion of oral health.

This book, organized in seven chapters, will help to understand what a probiotic is, how to isolate and assess the efficiency and safety of each strain, and to elucidate about health benefits and main mechanisms of action presenting the major current in *in vitro*, animal, and human studies supporting these properties.

Chapter 1 introduces the theme and summarizes the steps of launching probiotic products in the market. Chapter 2 presents an updated overview of the human intestinal microbial ecosystem from both endogenous and exogenous perspectives. At an endogenous level, the chapter covers the available knowledge on the dominant microbiota composition and stability, discusses the functional roles bacteria play in human health and well-being, and analyzes the consequences of homeostasis rupture among microbial balance as far as intestinal disorders are concerned. At the exogenous level, the chapter illustrates that target organisms are capable of modulating gut microbiota and of promoting different physiological roles. The chapter also gives perspectives on the use of probiotics in dietary management and disease risk reduction.

The main goal of Chapter 3 is to describe the relevant health potential of probiotics and current advances. The beneficial properties assigned to probiotics and the corresponding specific mechanisms of action that will support each of the subsequent therapeutic applications will be explored in this chapter.

Chapter 4 aims to provide a comprehensive overview on the advances in probiotic food, covering the technological issues, functionality aspects, and limitations of some foods as carriers of probiotics. This chapter is divided in two parts: the first part covers dairy products, fermented milks, and cheeses that constitute the major group of products that can carry and deliver probiotic bacteria; the second part covers non-dairy products where alternative functional foods with probiotics such as juices and other food carriers are presented and discussed.

To confer health benefits to the human host, probiotics must be kept alive until they reach their site of action. In Chapter 5 different approaches including immobilization and/or encapsulation of probiotics inside a protective material in order to increase the resistance of these sensitive microorganisms against adverse conditions have been revisited.

The probiotic strains intended to benefit health or treat illness may be incorporated into suitable dosage forms in which they can maintain their effectiveness. Therefore, Chapter 6 is concerned with dosage forms, such as oral powders, capsules, oral and vaginal tablets, vaginal suppositories, chewing gums, gels, eye drops, and pellets, that are used to administer probiotics. The definition of these dosage forms, their respective processes of manufacturing, and characterization tests are also addressed in this chapter.

In Chapter 7, which is the last chapter of the book, the global legal framework for probiotics is addressed. Generically, probiotics may be considered as a food, including food additives and dietary supplements, or as a drug. The chapter underlines the safety considerations and presents a comprehensive report on all necessary requirements related to them.

In summary, the book intends to provide a comprehensive overview of the fundamental concepts, mechanisms, therapeutic actions, technological aspects, and ongoing research related with probiotic bacteria. The book will be helpful for students and scientists from the food science and technology, pharmacy, and nutrition sciences fields; scientists working in the field of gastrointestinal disorders and other chronic diseases; companies who are designing and marketing new functional foods or nutraceuticals; as well as other public health professionals and clinicians. Furthermore, it provides important information for all readers interested in the relationship between food and health.

This scientific work was a team effort written by a group of scientists from the food and pharmaceutical research fields directly involved in the development of project PROBIOCAPS (PTDC/AGR-ALI/71051/2006; FCOMP-01-0124-FEDER-008792): Ana Gomes, Dina Rodrigues, Helena Amaral, Manuela Pintado, Paulo Costa, Sérgio Sousa, Teresa Rocha-Santos, and the editors of this book, and through individual research grants (SFRH/BD/77647/2011; SFRH/BPD/73781/2010; SFRH/BPD/65410/2009) by FCT. We would like to thank all these scientists for their contribution, and all others who, in different areas and skills, helped this project become a real success. We would also like to thank the reviewers for their professional advice and reviewing the chapters of this book.

J. Paulo Sousa e Silva
Ana C. Freitas
Winter 2013

Chapter 1

Probiotic Bacteria: From Science to Consumers' Benefit

Manuela M. Pintado,[a] Ana M. Gomes,[a] and Ana C. Freitas[b,c]
[a]*CBQF, Biotechnology School of Portuguese Catholic University, Rua Dr. António Bernardino Almeida, 4200-072 Porto, Portugal*
[b]*ISEIT/Viseu-Instituto Piaget, Estrada do Alto do Gaio, Galifonge, 3515-776 Lordosa, Viseu, Portugal*
[c]*CESAM & Department of Chemistry, University of Aveiro, 3810-193 Aveiro, Portugal*
mpintado@porto.ucp.p

Although there is still no official definition for probiotics, several authors have tried to define this concept throughout time. One of the most accepted and simplest definitions was that presented by an expert committee organized by the Food and Agriculture Organization (FAO) of the United Nations and the World Health Organization (WHO), which states: "Probiotic organisms are live microorganisms that when administered in adequate amounts confer a health benefit on the host" (FAO/WHO, 2001). Associated with probiotic organisms, prebiotics are defined as nondigestible food ingredients that benefit the host by selectively stimulating the growth and/or activity of one, or a limited number, of bacteria in

Probiotic Bacteria: Fundamentals, Therapy, and Technological Aspects
Edited by J. Paulo Sousa e Silva and Ana C. Freitas

ISBN 978-981-4411-62-2 (Hardcover), 978-981-4411-63-9 (eBook)
www.panstanford.com

the colon and thus improve host health (Gibson & Roberfroid, 1995). When we combine probiotic organisms and prebiotics in a product to obtain a presumably synergistic relationship, the term synbiotic is used.

Although any microorganism that would produce health benefits could be considered a probiotic, only some genera have proven to be probiotic. The genera of bacteria and fungi that have been employed for their probiotic properties are most commonly species of *Lactobacillus* and *Bifidobacterium* and species of the yeast genus *Saccharomyces*; other bacterial genera, such as *Streptococcus*, *Enterococcus*, and *Bacillus*, have also been studied. However, with regard to the genera *Enterococcus* and *Bacillus*, particular concerns have been raised concerning their safety properties (Hempel *et al.*, 2011). Some of these genera have been used as single cultures or in mixed formulations. In a very recent revision, Bengmark (2012) reported some probiotic starter cultures assumed with no identifiable adverse effects in clinical studies (e.g., no effect in terms of bacteria translocation, gastric colonization with enteric organisms, or septic morbidity, serum C reactive protein levels or mortality). This included isolated strains such as *Lactobacillus plantarum* 299v (Pro-Viva) or *L. rhamnosus* GG or multiple strains, Ecologic 641 (Winclove Bio Industries, Amsterdam, the Netherlands), a supplemented synbiotic composition consisting of six different strains of freeze-dried, viable bacteria: *L. acidophilus*, *L. casei*, *L. salivarius*, *Lactococcus lactis*, *Bifidobacterium bifidum*, and *B. lactis* along with corn-starch and maltodextrins, Trevis (Chr Hansen Biosystem, Denmark) with *L. acidophilus* La5, *B. lactis* Bb-12, *Streptococcus thermophilus*, and *L. bulgaricus* as well as VSL#3 (VSL Pharmaceuticals, Ft Lauderdale, Florida, USA) with four strains of *Lactobacillus* (*L. casei*, *L. plantarum*, *L. acidophilus*, and *L. delbrueckii* subsp. *bulgaricus*) along with three strains of *Bifidobacterium* (*B. longum*, *B. breve*, and *B. infantis*) and *S. salivarius* subsp. *thermophilus*.

Several health attributes have been ascribed to probiotics, which has increased commercial interest in exploiting different applications leading to the rapid growth and expansion of this market sector. From the selection of a probiotic strain to its incorporation in a final product, both in food matrices or pharmaceutical formulations, several steps must be accomplished if a safe and biological active product is to be achieved (Fig. 1.1).

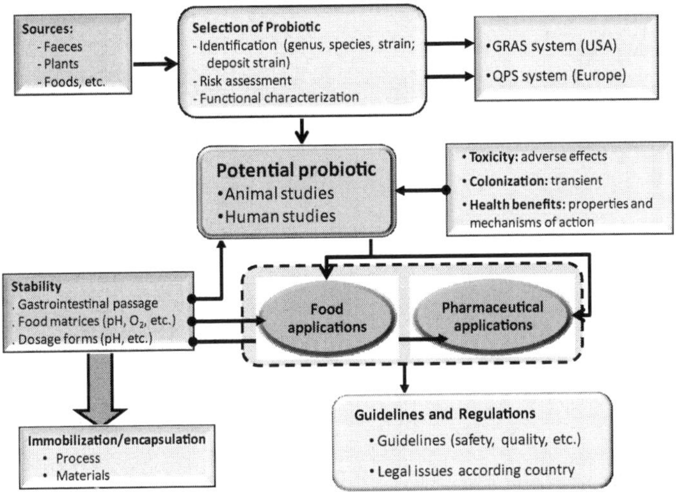

Figure 1.1 Schematic representation of the sequential steps required from probiotics selection to a final product be launched in the market.

Each potential probiotic strain isolated from a human, animal, plant, or food source, apart from its accurate identification, must be validated regarding safety issues according to guidelines defined by a system similar in concept and purpose at both US and European levels, denominated as GRAS (generally recognised as safe) or QPS (Qualified Presumption of Safety), respectively, permitting in both cases the identification of what is required to make an adequate safety assessment of a microorganism. In parallel, the probiotic must be submitted to functional characterization, as certain functionalities, namely, its survival through the gastrointestinal tract (GIT) (pH conditions, enzymes, and bile salts), and instead of help predict health benefits potential (production of antimicrobial compounds, activity upon cholesterol, and so on). These potential probiotics must be now tested through increasing complex systems from *in vitro* studies, to animal and finally human studies requiring, in general, double-blind, randomized, placebo-controlled human trials or other appropriate design with sample size and primary outcomes appropriate to determine if a strain/product is efficient. This efficacy is assured if probiotics colonize transiently the intestine, do not exhibit any adverse effect on the patient, and demonstrated one or more health benefits mediated by one or more mechanisms of actions to be associated with one or more of the therapeutic applications: (i) the prevention or treatment of infectious diseases, including viral, bacterial, or antibiotic-associated diarrhoea; (ii) relief of chronic bowel inflammatory diseases; (iii) immuno-modulation; (iv) lowering of serum cholesterol; (v) decreased risk of colon cancer; (vi) improvement of lactose digestion; (vii) reduction of allergies; and (viii) effect on intestinal microbiota (Saad *et al.*, 2013). However, some strains are not as stable as required to guarantee the passage throughout the GIT or to resist to the conditions and interactions when incorporated in the food or dosage forms. This reduced stability may be overcome by immobilization or encapsulation of probiotic strain using different encapsulation techniques and materials assuring the required protection for a certain environment and pre-determined period. The safe, functional, and stable probiotic may now be incorporated in a commercial product, either a food or a dosage form. However, launching of these products associated with health claims is regulated according to each country's legislative system and following strict guidelines. As an example, nutrition and health claims were harmonized at the European level to better protect consumers. EU regulation, EC No. 1924/2006, amended by the European Parliament and the Council of 15 January 2008 (EC No. 109/2008) establishes the necessary authorization procedures to ensure that the allegations contained on packages and in marketing of foodstuffs are clear, precise, and based on evidence accepted by the scientific community.

Despite the developed research performed in the last years, it should be emphasized that the effect of probiotics remains ambiguous and requires more investigations in order to be confirmed or validated. This fact may be not only due to action of these probiotics but also due to the lack of information about the pathogenesis of some diseases (Saad *et al.*, 2013). Although large investigation has been done on health benefits associated with probiotic bacteria as far as binomials strain-therapeutic application and strain-dose effects are concerned, experts still believe that the studies are not yet sufficient and information is still lacking. Such expert opinions have barred the possibility of European Food Safety Authority approval over 2012 of related health claims, limiting the use of probiotics with recognized health benefits at food industry level. So, in future, more studies, particularly well-designed, double-blind, randomized, placebo-controlled trials continue to be required.

In addition, a greater understanding of the mechanisms behind the action of probiotics on the gastrointestinal microbiota is required in order to better understand which probiotic is the most beneficial and how the genetic and bacterial profiles of the patient will influence treatment responsiveness.

References

Bengmark, S. (2013) Gut microbiota, immune development and function. *Pharmacol. Res.*, **69**(1), 87–113.

FAO/WHO (2001) Report on joint FAO/WHO expert consultation on evaluation of health and nutritional properties of probiotics in food including powder milk with live acid bacteria, Cordoba, Argentina.

Gibson, G.R. and Roberfroid, M.B. (1995) Dietary modulation of the human colonic microbiotia: introducing the concept of prebiotics. *J. Nutr.*, **125**, 1401–1412.

Hempel, S., Newberry, S. Ruelaz, A., Wang, Z. Miles, J.N.V., Suttorp, M.J., Johnsen, B., Shanman, R. Slusser, W., Fu, N., Smith, A., Roth, B., Polak, J., Motala, A., Perry, T. and Shekelle, P.G. (2012) Safety of probiotics to reduce risk and prevent or treat disease. *Evidence Report/Technology Assessment*, **200**, 1–94.

Saad, N., Delattre, C., Urdaci, M., Schmitter, J.M. and Bressollier, P. (2013) An overview of the last advances in probiotic and prebiotic field. *LWT - Food Sci.Technol.*, **50**, 1–16.

Chapter 2

Gastrointestinal Tract: Microflora and Transit Aspects

Ana M. Gomes,[a] **Manuela M. Pintado,**[a] **Ana C. Freitas,**[b,c] **and J. Paulo Sousa e Silva**[d]

[a]*CBQF, Biotechnology School of Portuguese Catholic University, Rua Dr. António Bernardino Almeida, 4200-072 Porto, Portugal*

[b]*CESAM & Department of Chemistry, University of Aveiro, 3810-193 Aveiro, Portugal*

[c]*ISEIT/Viseu-Instituto Piaget, Estrada do Alto do Gaio, Galifonge, 3515-776 Lordosa, Viseu, Portugal*

[d]*Faculty of Pharmacy, University of Porto, Rua de Jorge Viterbo Ferreira, 228, 4050-313 Porto, Portugal*

amgomes@porto.ucp.pt

2.1 Gastrointestinal Physiology

2.1.1 Introduction

Oral use is the most convenient way for administering probiotic products not only due to the easiness of the method but also to promote one of the main effects attributed to probiotics— improving intestinal microbial balance. Nevertheless, the upper gastrointestinal tract (GIT) is an adverse medium to probiotics; hence, there are

Probiotic Bacteria: Fundamentals, Therapy, and Technological Aspects
Edited by J. Paulo Sousa e Silva and Ana C. Freitas

ISBN 978-981-4411-62-2 (Hardcover), 978-981-4411-63-9 (eBook)
www.panstanford.com

many advantages in understanding the physiology of GIT in order to develop products containing probiotics. Many textbooks delve deeply into GIT anatomy and physiology, and for detailed descriptions, one may consult *Guyton and Hall Textbook of Medical Physiology* (2011).

Anatomically and physiologically, the digestive system is divided into the tubular GIT and accessory digestive organs (Fig. 2.1). The GIT is approximately 6 m in length and extends from the mouth to the anus. The organs of GIT comprise oral cavity, pharynx, esophagus, stomach, small intestine, and large intestine. The accessory digestive organs are the teeth, tongue, and salivary glands, liver, gallbladder, and pancreas.

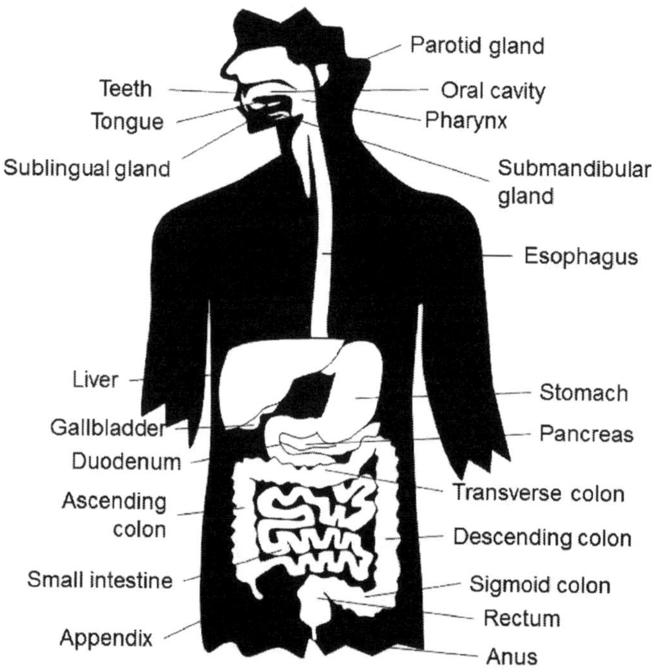

Figure 2.1 Anatomic structure of the human GIT and accessory digestive organs.

The GIT or alimentary canal wall is composed of four layers: from outer surface to the inner surface are the serosa, muscularis, submucosa, and mucosa. The mucosa is composed of a simple columnar epithelium separating the highly colonized intestinal lumen from the second, underlying layer, the lamina propria, and the muscularis mucosa. A mucus gel layer (composed predominantly of mucin glycoproteins) covers a large part of the GIT epithelium. The mucosa is the absorptive layer, maximizing nutrient absorption, but also has secretory and barrier function preventing the passage of strange luminal components (bacteria, food components), thus inhibiting pro-inflammatory host response (O'Hara *et al.*, 2006). Adjacent intestinal epithelial cells form tight junctions, which help maintain such selective impermeable barrier function (Bron *et al.*, 2011). Paneth cells and goblet cells also contribute to this function via innate immune defences. Paneth cells are responsible for the production of several antimicrobial compounds, including defensins and lysozyme, which prevent interaction between microorganisms and proliferative cells in the crypts, while goblet cells produce mucins, which confer to the epithelium its barrier effect by preventing direct contact from luminal microorganisms (Bevins and Salzman, 2011; Salzman, 2011). M cells or microfold cells founded in lymphoid tissue of ileum (Peyer's patches) are involved in the absorption of macromolecules, particularly protein antigens. The lamina propria is a special type of essentially sterile connective tissue that contains lymph nodules, which are involved in the protection against disease. The muscularis mucosa is responsible for the small folds in some parts of GIT.

2.1.2 GIT pH

Among other factors (transit time, bacteria metabolism, and chemical reactions) that might influence the performance of probiotic products, the pH is perhaps the most important due to general sensibility of probiotics to acidic conditions. According to Evans *et al.* (1988), the average pH in stomach is 1.8 and rises to 6.6 in the proximal intestine reaching 7.5 in the distal intestine, and then it decreases to 6.3 in right colon and it rises again, until it reaches 7.1 in left colon. The pH depends on prandial condition of individuals. Table 2.1 illustrates physiological pH in humans in the fasting and fed states (Gray and Dressman, 1996; Dressman *et al.*, 1998).

Apart from prandial condition, the pH in GIT is a function of many variables, including meal volume and content, and volume of secretions (Mudie *et al.*, 2010). It should be noted that the extrapolation of GIT pH data from healthy situations to pathological conditions must be made with precaution.

Table 2.1 Physiological pH in the GIT in the fasted and fed states

Gastrointestinal site	Fasting	Fed
Stomach	1.4–2.1	3.0–7.0
Duodenum	4.9–6.4	5.1–5.2
Jejunum	4.4–6.5	5.2–6.2
Ileum	6.5–8.0	6.8–8.0

Thus, it is not surprising that GIT pH varies between and within individuals.

2.1.3 Total Residence Time in the GIT

The residence time (transit time) of a probiotic product (e.g., dosage form or food) in the intestine is also a determinant of the viability of probiotics, as the exposure to the harsh conditions will depend substantially on gastric residence time.

The oesophageal residence time is usually short (in the order of seconds to minutes) and the small intestine residence time is relatively constant (3–4 h), but the gastric time varies widely (5 min to 2 h, although much longer times have been reported) according to factors such as volume, osmolality, pH, viscosity, and nature of ingested material or even emotional factors and age. Thus, the total residence time is dependent upon factors such as gastric emptying rate and flow rate, and can exhibit a significant intraindividual and interindividual variability (Mudie *et al.*, 2010).

2.1.4 Mouth and Oesophagus

During mastication or chewing, the contact of food and other products with oral mucosa is generally brief but sufficient to initiate the digestion of the starch by the saliva (salivary amylase). After this rapid passage through the mouth, the swallowed food is driven to the stomach by the peristaltic movements of oesophagus. The oesophagus is a muscular tube that connects pharynx to stomach and has a lumen pH between 5 and 6. The oesophageal transit time for dosage forms, liquids, or boluses of solids is approximately 10–20 s (Evans, 1993).

2.1.5 Stomach

Stomach has a J-shape with an approximate capacity of 1.5 l, but in a fasting state, it normally contains 20–30 ml of fluid (predominantly wet mucus). Stomach acts as a reservoir for food while it is mixed with acid, mucus, and pepsin in order to be released (as chime) into the duodenum at a controlled rate. The gastric emptying time may vary from few minutes to several hours, depending on the time of the last food ingestion, anxiety, position, and level of individual activity, among other factors.

During fasting, an interdigestive cycle of motility (migrating myoelectric complex, MMC) composed of four phases governs stomach activity. This cycle begins in the stomach and moves along the small intestine into the distal ileum. The Phase III of MMC (a burst of contractile activity of 5–15 min) opens the pylorus and clears the stomach. The ingestion of food stops the cycle.

The peristaltic movements appear 5–10 min after the intake of foods and remain until the gastric emptying, which lasts from 1 to several hours depending on the meal composition (Phillips, 1993). The hydrochloric acid secreted by parietal cells kills many bacteria and provides the pH for pepsin to begin protein digestion (Ganong, 2005).

2.1.6 Small Intestine

The small intestine (small bowel) extending from the pyloric sphincter of stomach to the ileocaecal valve has three distinct parts, namely, duodenum (20–30 cm), jejunum (approx. 2 m), and ileum (approx. 3 m). The main functions of this organ are the digestion of foods and the absorption of nutrients and other materials.

Several intestinal adaptations, which increase the surface area, favor absorption in small intestine. These adaptations are as follows:

- Folds of Kerckring—submucosal folds of several millimeters in depth
- Villi—finger-like projections of approx. 0.5 to 1.5 mm in length
- Microvilli—brush-like structures of approx. 1 μm in length

In the lumen of the small intestine, foods and other products are mixed with the bicarbonate (from Brunner's glands, located in duodenum), secretions of mucosal cells (mucus and enzymes), pancreatic juice (sodium bicarbonate and enzymes), and bile (bile acids, phospholipids, and bilirubin). The detergent property of bile confers a potent antimicrobial activity that hampers the survival of the microorganisms (including many probiotics) in the GIT. The small bowel constitutes a transition zone between stomach bacterial scarcity and highly populated colon.

2.1.7 Large Intestine

The large intestine (colon) stretches from the ileocecal valve to the anus and has two main functions:

- the absorption of water, sodium, and chloride ions
- the storage of feces

The colon is composed of the caecum, the ascending colon, the transverse colon, the descending colon, the sigmoid colon, and the rectum. The slower colon motility is responsible for transit times up to 60 h, which undoubtedly contributes to the tremendous number of microorganisms found in the colon.

The large intestine is colonized by about 10^{12} bacteria per gram of intestinal contents (about 35–50% of the volume content of the colon), which are responsible for several metabolic reactions.

These microorganisms may be in the lumen, at the mucus gel, or in the mucosal epithelial cells receptors (Berg, 1996; Madsen, 2001). The equilibrium of the microbial groups present in the GIT is essential for human health. *Bifidobacterium* and *Lactobacillus* species are the main strains with identified beneficial properties in the indigenous GIT microflora.

2.2 Gut Microflora: Human 'Virtual Organ'

2.2.1 Ecological Niches

The human GIT microbiota consists of about 10^{14} bacteria and up to an estimated 1000–1150 different bacterial species, whose collective genome (intestinal microbiome) consists of at least 100-fold more genes than the human genome (Qin *et al.*, 2010). These microbial communities are found in a diversity of environmental niches (digestive, urogenital, naso-bucal, and respiratory mucosal surfaces), yet, as previously mentioned, the large intestine is the most inhabited (average of 10^{11} bacteria per gram of stool). Although 55 divisions of bacteria have been described, only eight bacterial divisions have been identified so far in the GIT. Here, recent studies, involving culture-independent molecular microbiological techniques, have shown that the most abundant bacterial phyla found are the Gram-negative *Bacteroidetes* (include genera related to *Bacteroides* corresponding to 9–42% of total bacteria on average) and the Gram-positive, low guanine-cytosine (GC)% *Firmicutes* (composed of species belonging to the genera *Eubacterium, Clostridium, Ruminococcus, Butyrivibrio*); together, they may represent more than 90% of the phylogenetic groups present in the human gut, specifically in the distal part (Eckburg *et al.*, 2005; Lay *et al.*, 2005; Aureli *et al.*, 2011). Less abundant phyla, yet not less important in terms of host's health, include *Actinobacteria, Fusobacteria, Proteobacteria*, and *Verrucomicrobia* phyla. The dominant bacterial groups include *Clostridium coccoides-Eubacterium rectale* (often the most represented between 14 to 22% of total bacteria depending on the studies (Doré and Corthier, 2010), *Clostridium leptum* (including the species *Faecalibacterium prausnitzii, Ruminococcus albus*, and *R. flavefaciens* (at a dominance of 16–22% of total bacteria on average) (Lay *et al.*, 2005), *Bacteroides-Prevotella, Bifidobacterium* species, and *Atopobium* species (Diamant *et al.*, 2011). Among the occasionally found species are *Clostridium ramosum, Eubacterium cylindroides, Phascolarctobacterium, Verrucomicrobium, Sporomusa*, Selenomonas, or *Veillonella* (Doré and Corthier, 2010).

Each individual houses a unique collection of bacterial species (including the established core of at least 57 bacterial species considered common to all humans) that remain in a relatively complex equilibrium (within the same log-unit equivalent in terms of population) over time from day-to-day and even across years. Indeed, molecular ecology tools have shown that approximately 80% of an individual's fecal microbiota is individual-specific (Eckburg *et al.*, 2005). At the level of strains, stability is not as clear and will vary with individual (Doré and Corthier, 2010). Furthermore, species diversity for subdominant groups such as that of *Lactobacillus* is less stable than that of dominant groups (Vanhoutte *et al.*, 2004) and the colon shows better stability of communities than the ileum. Factors modulating ecological niches include transit time, pH, and quality and quantity of exogenous substances such as prebiotics or probiotics and endogenous mucins among others (Doré and

Corthier, 2010). Induction of durable alterations, especially among dominant bacterial groups, is not easy due to capacity of bacteria to resist change as well as resilience (capacity to recover original make-up following application of a stress)—two determinants responsible for maintenance of homeostasis (Doré and Corthier, 2010). Shifts in these ecological homeostatic niches (normobiosis) may either prompt specific disease-inducing activity (dysbiosis at metabolic, degenerative, or immune levels) or disease-protective activity (probiosis at similar levels of disease).

The well-established interindividual variability among microbial communities is related with either internal (genetic factors, age, gender, stress exposure, health status) or external factors. The latter include type of early exposure to microorganisms of maternal origin (faecal, vaginal, cutaneous and maternal milk (Doré and Corthier, 2010), lifestyle factors (Dicksved *et al.*, 2007), diet (Ley *et al.*, 2006), antibiotic therapy (Jernberg *et al.*, 2010), and even geographical influence—differences in the microbiota composition of healthy individuals from different locations have been reported (Mueller *et al.*, 2006; Fallani *et al.*, 2010). In fact, consideration of the highly individual gut microbial activity has been acknowledged as an important aspect of personalized nutrition strategies and is becoming a turning point among food industry innovation.

The diversity of the gut microbiota is relatively simple in infants but becomes more complex with increasing age, reaching a high degree of complexity in adults (Fanaro *et al.*, 2003). Human gut microbiota acquisition and development in the host may begin before birth (bacteria have been detected in amniotic fluid, umbilical cord and meconium (DiGiulio *et al.*, 2008; Koenig *et al.*, 2011), although in infants effective development occurs as a function of the first inoculi received from the environment, the mother's microbiota, the delivery mode, formula or breast-feeding, and subsequent weaning food practices and the use of antimicrobials (Fallani *et al.*, 2010). The existence of a fetal microbiome has clinical implications, with greater microbial diversity being associated with prematurity (DiGiulio *et al.*, 2008; Mshvildadze *et al.*, 2010).

The indigenous microflora of infants is dominated by one or a few genera, and among breast-fed infants, *Bifidobacterium* strains are dominant, and become established shortly after birth. Their proliferation is stimulated by specific nutrients, glycoprotein components of κ-casein in human colostrum and, to a lesser extent, breast-milk as well as bifidogenic bacteria in breast-milk (Martín *et al.*, 2004, 2009; Walker, 2010). Microbiota composition undergoes significant shifts as solid foods are introduced into the diet (Koenig *et al.*, 2011). The numerical proportion of bifidobacteria decreases with increasing age of the individual and eventually becomes the third most abundant genus (accounting for ca. 25% of the total adult gut flora), second to the genera *Bacteroides* and *Eubacterium* (Finegold *et al.*, 1983).

Undoubtedly, human gut microbiota may play an important buffer role between the host and the environment and several human microbiome projects are in progress in order to try and explore its relevance in health and disease. Two major projects, namely, the NIH Human Microbiome Project (HMP: http://commonfund.nih.gov/hmp/) in the United States and the Metagenomics of the Human Intestine (metaHIT: http://www. metahit.eu) project in Europe, are important contributions to this deciphering process.

2.2.2 Physiological Role of Gut Microflora

There is an increasing awareness of the role that intestinal microflora may play in human health. Tremendous progress has been made in this field and results indicate that it is likely that much of this impact is mediated through diet and the consumption of specific health-related foods. Growing evidence suggests that gut microbiota influence what the human host is able to extract from its diet, including energy (see Fig. 2.2).

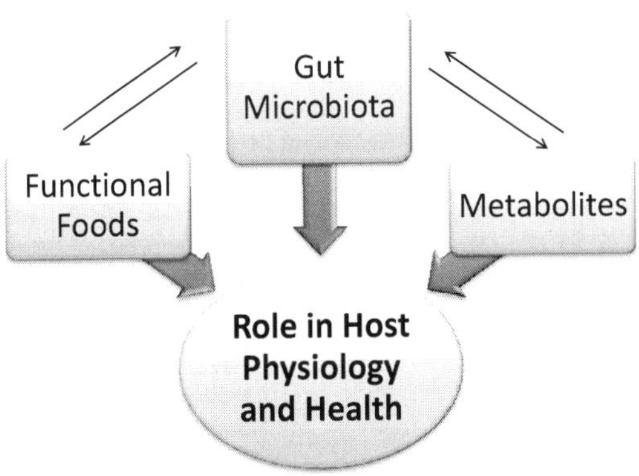

Figure 2.2 Possible interactions between gut microbiota-diet and generated metabolites therefrom toward beneficial functions in host physiology and health.

Considerable efforts have been made to better define the complex symbiotic role of the intestinal microbiota in host physiology and to discover the underlying mechanisms (Hörmannsperger and Haller, 2010; Bron *et al.* 2011). These have been associated with multiple functions, including (i) a metabolic function (including energy homeostasis, digestion and bioavailability of nutrients, supporting fat metabolism, fermentation of undigestible carbohydrates with concomitant production of short-chain fatty acids, SCFAs); (ii) a mucosal barrier function (including prevention of mucosal infections by pathogen invasion inhibition and maintenance of an intact intestinal barrier); and (iii) an immune modulatory function (including enteric nerve regulation and maintenance of intestinal epithelium homeostasis and regulation of the mucosal immune system by acting as an important source of stimulators (Preidis and Versalovic, 2009; Hörmannsperger and Haller, 2010; Holmes *et al.*, 2011).

2.2.2.1 Antagonistic mechanisms: barrier function

As previously mentioned, the intestinal epithelium constitutes an important primary line of defence composing a physical barrier that controls the transcellular and paracellular transit of exogenous substances and prevents the entry of most of luminal antigens. The commensal microbiota contribute to the "barrier effect" via participation in paracellular permeability regulation, mucin gene expression by goblet cells, and secretion of antimicrobial peptides (defensins and angiogenins) by intestinal Paneth cells.

Studies in germ-free animals have demonstrated that the normal functioning of intestinal epithelial cells is impaired in the absence of the intestinal microbiota. Intestinal epithelium expression of microbial recognition receptors, defensins, and antimicrobial peptides is reduced in germ-free animals (Bouskra *et al.*, 2008). A good overview on the very important role of antimicrobial peptides in the GIT and the existing dynamic interactions between the intestinal epithelial barrier and the commensal microbiota based on recent advances is available in the review by Muniz *et al.* (2012). Further studies have shown that a modulation of the gut microbiota through dietary supplementation with a prebiotic (i.e. oligofructose) increases epithelial barrier integrity by increasing the expression of tight junction proteins (i.e. zonulin ZO-1 and occludin), a mechanism that is dependent on the augmented secretion of the glucagon-like peptide-2 intestinal hormone (Cani *et al.*, 2009) (see Fig. 2.4).

2.2.2.2 Metabolic contribution

A growing body of evidence suggests that the gut microbiota impacts a wide range of host metabolic pathways influencing disease prevention and disease risk. Gut microbiota produce an almost limitless set of metabolites and their understanding may provide the key to unlocking many health-promoting functions of gut microbiota, including probiotics.

Intestinal microbiota act as a "metabolic organ" providing additional enzymes and regulating the expression of genes involved in the degradation of complex indigestible dietary carbohydrates and proteins, with subsequent generation of fermentation end-products (Falony *et al.*, 2006), cholesterol reduction, deconjugation and dehydroxylation of bile acids, production of vitamins (K and B group) and isoprenoids, metabolism of amino acids, and conversion of dietary polyphenolic compounds into their active form (van Duynhoven *et al.*, 2011). Indeed, the intact forms of dietary polyphenols have limited availability presenting low levels in plasma. A major part of the polyphenols persists in the colon, where the resident microbiota (e.g., *Escherichia coli*, *Bifidobacterium* sp., *Lactobacillus* sp., *Bacteroides* sp., *Eubacterium* sp.) produces metabolites that may suffer further metabolism upon enteric systemic circulation. For example, dietary flavonoids are normally present as poorly absorbed glycosides, which need to undergo enzymatic deglycosylation in the small intestine before being absorbed as aglycones (the nonsugar group) (Walle, 2004). Apart from microbial deglycosylation, the microbiota may also perform mild transformations such as dehydroxylation and demethylation and, in addition, catabolism of polyphenols into small fragments (see Fig. 2.3).

Apart from less active metabolites, bacterial metabolic conversion in the gut may also lead to metabolites with increased biological activity. For example, the pseudoestrogenic activity of prenylflavonoids from hops (Possemiers *et al.*, 2006), soy isoflavones, and lignans (Bowly *et al.*, 2003) is determined by intestinal bacterial activation followed by absorption of the microbial metabolites (van Duynhoven *et al.*, 2011), hence modifying host exposure to these components and their potential health effects.

Other studies have shown a beneficial impact of polyphenols on GIT microbiota profiles. Feeding wine polyphenols (57 mg/kg body weight by gavage for 10 days) to rats resulted in predominant fecal *Bacteroides, Lactobacillus,* and *Bifidobacterium* compared with the controls, which revealed predominant *Bacteroides, Clostridium,* and *Propionibacterium* (Dolara *et al.,* 2005). Parkar *et al.* (2008) demonstrated how several polyphenols, including caffeic acid, catechin, epicatehecin, coumaric acid, phloridzin, rutin, naringenin, daidzein, genistein, and quercetin, inhibited growth and adhesion of bacterial pathogens to human Caco-2 cells as well as enhanced the proliferation and adhesion of *Lactobacillus rhamnosus,* a probiotic strain. Further examples may be found in the recent review by Laparra and Sanz (2010) in which reciprocal interactions between intestinal microbiota and phytochemicals in food, and associated consequences toward human health are duly covered.

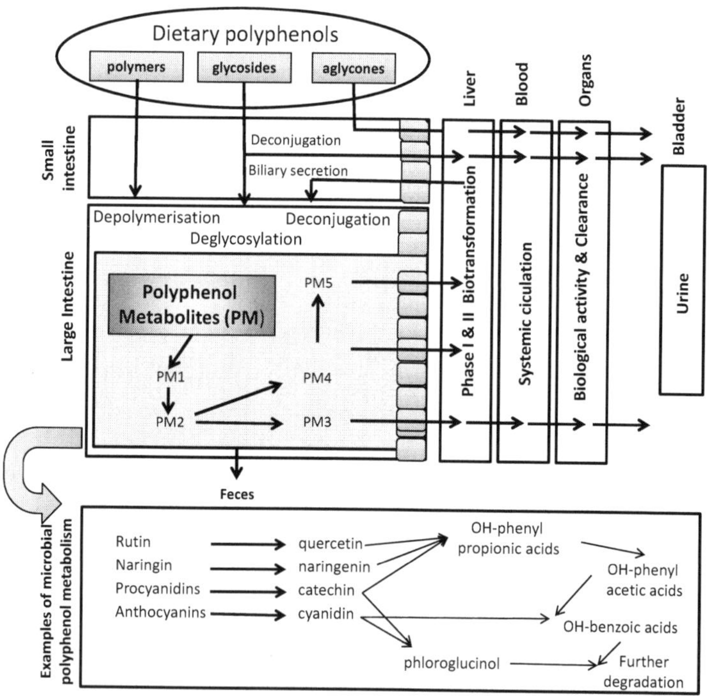

Figure 2.3 Representation of metabolic bioconversion of dietary polyphenols in the human-microbiota ecosystem. Adapted from van Duynhoven *et al.*, 2011, and Possemiers *et al.*, 2011.

The specific capacity of gut microbiota to use complex dietary carbohydrates may contribute to harvest energy from the diet, representing up to 10% of the daily energy supply (Falony *et al.*, 2006). Accordingly, comparisons between germ-free mice and mice colonized by the conventional distal gut microbiota revealed a host's increased ability to extract energy from the diet brought about by the microbiota; this energy was then stored in adipocytes, contributing to increased body weight (Bäckhed *et al.*, 2004; Turnbaugh *et al.*, 2008). Indeed, the obese microbiome was shown to extract more energy from the same amount of kilocalories than the lean microbiome (Turnbaugh *et al.*, 2008).

Commensal microbiota extract energy by direct fermentation of dietary carbohydrates, resistant to digestion, into short-chain fatty acids (SCFAs) (e.g., acetate, propionate, and butyrate), ethanol, and gases (e.g., carbon dioxide and hydrogen). In contrast, when proteins are fermented, the end products include toxic compounds such as amines and phenols (Tuohy *et al.*, 2006; Bernalier-Donadille, 2010).

The beneficial role of SCFAs in enterocyte growth and differentiation is well known; butyrate is preferentially metabolized and may also promote anti-inflammatory effects. Acetate may act as a precursor for lipid and cholesterol synthesis in the liver, whereas propionate may impact negatively thereon; indeed, propionate is a natural precursor for gluconeogenesis (Bernalier-Donadille, 2010). The role of SCFAs on food intake behavior and on energy intake is being targeted and available studies have been recently reviewed by Cani and Delzenne (2011). Here, it was proposed that SCFAs come directly into play following gut microbiota fermentation and may play a role in appetite regulation; modulation of plasma SCFAs was related to changes in gut peptides involved in appetite regulation.

Indeed, interactions between food, intestinal microbiota, and the host are fundamental to the maintenance of homeostasis in the ecosystem. Although many of the abovementioned roles may be beneficial for the host colonocytes, drawbacks are associated with the proneness to weight gain. Observations among microbiome capacity have been generated to uphold such statements. The expression of a monosaccharide transporter (Na^+/glucose cotransporter) has been induced in mono-colonized mice, leading to increased absorption of dietary monosaccharides and SCFAs, which in turn lead to *de novo* synthesis of lipids in the liver. Conventionalization of germ-free mice originates increased liver expression of acetyl-CoA carboxylase and fatty acid synthase, key enzymes in *de novo* fatty acid synthesis, as well as increased expression of the transcriptional factors carbohydrate response element binding protein and sterol regulatory element binding protein-1, both involved in hepatocyte lipogenic responses to insulin and glucose. In addition, levels of fasting-induced adipose factor (FIAF) in the gut are decreased by microbial colonization, which minimizes fat oxidation and promotes fat storage (Bäckhed *et al.*, 2004) (see Table 2.2). Additional evidence for such interrelationships between energy homeostasis and gut microbiota and metabolic functions are covered in a comprehensive review by Cani and Delzenne (2011). Several mechanisms are proposed herein on how gut microbiota control body weight and energy homeostasis including models on how gut microbiota may contribute to the onset of obesity and associated metabolic disorders (Fig. 2.4).

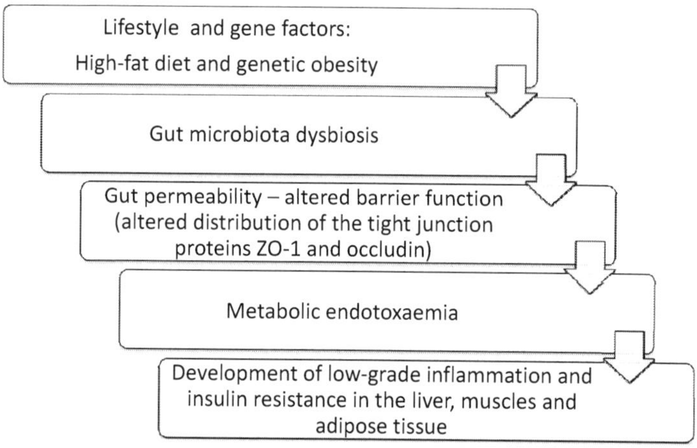

Figure 2.4 Possible mechanisms for describing how gut microbiota are involved in the onset of obesity and associated metabolic disorders. Adapted from Cani and Delzenne, 2011.

In summary, recent advances in cellular and molecular biology have provided solid evidence on the significant contribution of gut microbial metabolism to the presence of metabolites in the host (Wikoff *et al.*, 2009; Martin *et al.*, 2012). Metabolomic strategies have become an essential tool to decipher such gut microbiota–host metabolic interaction and impact on homeostasis and host health. A mass spectrometry based metabolomics strategy applied to germ-free mouse model systems has demonstrated the significant effect of the microbiome on blood metabolites (Wikoff *et al.*, 2009); numerous circulating molecules were determined to arise exclusively in the presence of gut microflora or significantly alter their concentration by its presence (Wikoff *et al.*, 2009). For example, production of the antioxidant indole-3-propionic acid (derived from tryptophan metabolism) was shown to be completely dependent on the presence of gut microbiota and could be established by colonization with the single bacterium *Clostridium sporogenes*. Martin *et al.* (2007) underlined the different bacterial modulation of the bile acid metabolism and enterohepatic cycle, with consequent effects on the absorption of dietary fat and concomitant to lipid accumulation in the livers of animals holding a nonadapted gut microbiota. With these studies, the authors showed the importance of maintaining a balanced and well-adapted gut microbiota to prevent onset of microbial-related metabolic disorders. Martin *et al.* (2012) further addresses nutritional approaches, in which the need for homeostatic balance is dependent on both the host and the nutritional modulation of the intestinal microbiota–host metabolic interactions.

2.2.2.3 Immunomodulation

The immune regulatory function of the intestinal microbiota consists of priming the mucosal immune system and maintenance of intestinal epithelium homeostasis. The intestinal microbiota may influence the content of lamina propria T cells, immunoglobulin A producing B cells, intraepithelial T cells, and serum immunoglobulin levels (Tlaskalová-Hogenová *et al.*, 2004). As already stated, studies in germ-free animals demonstrated impairment of immune function in the absence of the intestinal microbiota. Defective development of gut-associated lymphoid tissues, antibody production (i.e., sIgA), and maturation of isolated lymphoid follicles have been shown in germ-free animals, together with reduced Peyer's patches and mesenteric lymph node number and dimension (Bouskra *et al.*, 2008).

In this symbiotic relationship, it is also important that immune system adequately recognizes microbial components and establishes a state of tolerance towards them (Aureli *et al.*, 2011). According to Aureli *et al.* (2011), such tolerance of microbiota is mediated by complementary mechanisms, including (i) microbiota bacteria do not express virulence factors such as antigenic structures recognized by toll-like receptors on the surface of immune system cells or secondary to chemical modifications of pathogens-associated molecular patterns; or, (ii) several commensal bacteria are able to suppress inflammatory processes (e.g., downregulation of the activity of nuclear factor-kB responsible for inflammatory response via pro-inflammatory cytokine/chemokine and AMP production).

2.2.3 Balance between Detrimental/Beneficial Gut Microbiota and Intestinal Disorders

As previously stated, a strong ecological balance exists between the host and its gut microbiota, in terms of impact on health, yet consensus on the exact mechanisms by which microbes modulate disease onsets has not yet been achieved (Holmes *et al.*, 2011; Collado *et al.*, 2012).

In infants, recent findings have found associations between microbiome composition and two diseases prevalent among babies in neonatal intensive care units, namely, necrotizing enterocolitis and late-onset sepsis (Alexander *et al.*, 2011; Mai *et al.*, 2011). Furthermore, the implications of mode of delivery on gut colonization have also been shown in the context of disease wherein a wide range of immune-related diseases may be associated with cesarean section delivery (Neu and Rushing, 2011). Other recent evidence indicates associations between microbial ecology in children and the onset of type 1 diabetes (Vaarala *et al.*, 2008; Brown *et al.*, 2011). Collectively, these various lines of research may suggest that the early microbiome, from fetal development through childhood, can influence both short-term and long-term health.

Any disturbance of the abovementioned physiological functions may be intrinsically linked with alterations or maladaptations of gastointestinal microbiota and can consequently impair many of these homeostatic and physiological signals leading to varying states of disease, including allergy, inflammatory bowel disease (IBD), obesity, certain cancers, diabetes (Holmes *et al.*, 2011), celiac disease (CD), autism, cardiovascular disease as well as emergence of antibiotic-resistant strains as far as administration of antimicrobial agents is concerned (Jernberg *et al.*, 2010) (see Table 2.2). Restoration of this balance by increasing levels of *Bifidobacterium* either by food-based strategies (using prebiotics) or supplementation has been shown to reduce disease intensiveness in patients and to improve well-being in healthy volunteers. Associated mechanisms that underlie these effects will be visited in Chapter 3.

Table 2.2 Examples of disease models with modulation of gut microbiota

Disease	Model	Host–microbiome interaction	Reference
IBD	Human	Certain antibiotics improved the disease course of IBD patients, whereas several IBD animal models needed bacterial colonization for inflammation	Barnich *et al.*, 2007
	Human	IBD patients revealed reduced diversity of *Firmicutes* and *Bacteroidetes;* *E. coli* (example of mucous-invading bacteria) may be associated with disease-specific activity	Frank *et al.*, 2007
	Human	Bacterial species *Faecalibacterium prausnitzii*, if present in the mucosa-associated microbiota of the patient's ileum, is protective against postoperative recurrence of endoscopic signs of inflammation 6 months after surgical resection of the ileocecal region of the intestine	Sokol *et al.*, 2008
	Human	IBD patients revealed intestinal dysbiosis with a lower representation of the *Clostridium leptum* group among the *Firmicutes* phylum	Sokol *et al.*, 2009
	Human	The differential urinary signature of IBD from Crohn's disease and ulcerative colitis includes alteration of hippurate, 4-cresyl sulphate, and formate, all potential metabolites of gut microbial activity	Williams *et al.*, 2009
	Mouse	Induction of a transforming growth factor-β rich environment by indigenous *Clostridium* species promotes T regulatory cell accumulation in the colon and resistance to ulcerative colitis	Atarashi *et al.*, 2011

(Continued)

Table 2.2 (*Continued*)

Disease	Model	Host–microbiome interaction	Reference
Diabetes	Mouse	A dysfunction in the microbial responsive immune system can lead to autoimmunity and diabetes; nonobese diabetic mouse lacking the innate microbial-recognition immune system receptor MyD88 is resistant to type 1 diabetes	Wen *et al.*, 2008
	Human	Sequencing results revealed a bacterial composition of diabetic group different from that of the healthy group; *Bacteroides vulgatus*, *Bifidobacterium* genus, and *Clostridium leptum* subgroup have undergone changes of different degree in diabetic group; copy number of *Bifidobacterium* genus is significantly declining in diabetic group	Wu *et al.*, 2010
	Human	Amount of *Firmicutes* significantly reduced in diabetes type 2 patients compared with the control group. The ratio of *Bacteroidetes* to *Firmicutes* positively correlated with plasma glucose concentration but not with body mass index.	Larsen *et al.*, 2010
Obesity	Human	Aberrant compositional development of the gut microbiota precedes overweight; bifidobacterial numbers in fecal samples during infancy, assessed by fluorescent *in situ* hybridization (FISH) with flow cytometry, were higher in normal weight children (median: 2.19×10^9 cells/g) than in children developing overweight (1.20×10^9 cells/g); a greater number of *Staphylococcus aureus* were reported in overweight children; authors propose that *S. aureus* constitutes trigger for low-grade inflammation contributing to development of obesity.	Kalliomäki *et al.*, 2008

Disease	Model	Host–microbiome interaction	Reference
Obesity	Human	Significantly higher numbers of *Bacteroides* group in women with excessive weight gain upon pregnancy. Positive correlation between the number of *Bacteroides*, *Clostridium*, and *Staphylococcus* on the one hand, and the weight and BMI before pregnancy on the other hand. The *Bifidobacterium* genus was present at higher numbers in normal-weight than in overweight women and also in women with lower weight gain during pregnancy.	Collado *et al.*, 2008
	Mouse	Conventionalization of germ-free mice was shown to: promote body weight gain and fat mass development; promote a general increase in the activity of lipoprotein lipase (LPL), catalyzing the release of fatty acids and triacylglycerol from circulating lipoproteins in muscle, and adipose tissue. Such increase was proposed as a consequence of suppression of the FIAF in the gut. LPL activity is inhibited by FIAF; hence, lack of FIAF in conventionalized germ-free mice may lead to accumulation of lipids in the adipose tissue.	Bäckhed *et al.*, 2004
Cancer	Mouse	The use of probiotics, prebiotics, or synbiotics was able to protect against chemically induced colonic DNA damage in animal models	Tuohy *et al.*, 2005
	Rats	Rats inoculated with human flora and fed a diet containing lactulose compared with those fed a diet containing comparable amount of sucrose revealed colonoctyes with less DNA damage following oral treatment with dimethylhydrazine	Rowland *et al.*, 1996
	Mouse	Colitis-associated colorectal cancer can be reversed by colonization with normal gut microbiota	Uronis *et al.*, 2009

(*Continued*)

Table 2.2 (*Continued*)

Disease	Model	Host–microbiome interaction	Reference
CD	Human	Specific microbial TTGE profile and a significant higher biodiversity in CD pediatric patients' duodenal mucosa was noted; *Bacteroides vulgatus* and *E. coli* were detected more often in CD patients than in controls. No significant difference was found in the prevalence of *Bifidobacterium* spp. between CD patients and controls.	Schippa *et al.*, 2010
Autism	Human	Ten-fold higher numbers of *Clostridium* spp. in autistic children than in healthy individuals. Many *Clostridium* species may produce neurotoxins, which could contribute to the autism spectrum impaired GI symptoms	Sekirov *et al.*, 2010

2.3 Selection of Target Organisms

2.3.1 Probiotics and Their Effects Upon Gut Microbiota

As previously mentioned in Chapter 1, probiotics are live microorganisms, which when administered in adequate amounts, confer a health benefit on the host. Key aspects and requirements for probiotic strains and probiotic products have been the target of many reviews (Gobbetti *et al.*, 2010; Sanders and Marco, 2010; Sanders, 2011) and issues such as strain specificity of health effects, mechanisms of action, required dose for probiotic products, and safety considerations will be further detailed in the following chapters. In this chapter, an overview of their role in the GIT will be given.

The most common formulation of probiotics is as fresh fermentation products or as dried bacterial supplements, and their consumption has been associated with a variety of health benefits for the consumer either directly (interaction with host's mechanisms) or via modulation of intestinal microflora. Supplementation with probiotics is intended to either replace or reduce the number of potentially pathogenic bacteria in the intestine by enhancing the number of beneficial strains that are capable of fermenting carbohydrates and that have little proteolytic activity. Species of the microbial genera *Lactobacillus* and *Bifidobacterium* represent the great majority of marketed probiotics corresponding to 23 and five strains, respectively; other less representative strains include two *E. coli* and one strain each of *Bacillus*, *Streptococcus*, *Enterococcus*, and *Lactococcus* (Sanders, 2007; EFSA, 2010). Alternatively, prebiotics, which are known as nondigestible food ingredients, generally oligosaccharides, may modify the balance of the intestinal microbiota by stimulating the activity of these health beneficial bacteria, lactobacilli and bifidobacteria.

Probiotics may play a beneficial role on human health by interacting with the gut microbiome and impacting on host response (Aureli *et al.*, 2011; O'Flaherty and Klaenhammer *et al.*, 2011; van Baarlen *et al.*, 2011); it is less clear whether the observed human health benefits are actually mediated by the microbiome changes (Sanders, 2011). The mechanisms of action whereby probiotics may promote such health-promoting effects include competitive exclusion of pathogenic bacteria, either directly (inhibition or competition by probiotic strain) or indirectly (probiotic influence on endogenous commensal microbiota) (Corr *et al.*, 2009); strengthening of epithelial barrier function by modulating signaling pathways that may promote increased mucus production (Mack *et al.*, 2003), defensins generation (Schlee *et al.*, 2008) or tight junction function (Anderson *et al.*, 2010; Karczewski *et al.*, 2010), and apoptosis prevention (Yan *et al.*, 2007); modulation of the host immune system (O'Flaherty *et al.*, 2010). Noticeably, probiotic microorganisms do not act exclusively in the large intestine by affecting the intestinal flora but also mediate some of the abovementioned mechanisms (immunological modulation or provision of bioactive metabolites) in other organs. In particular, some of these interactions can be influenced by the *in situ* SCFA milieu, which may affect or even mediate some of the beneficial effects of probiotics.

Numerous studies report that probiotics can influence the nutritional status of mankind (Gobbetti *et al.*, 2010; Bhat and Bhat, 2011). A plethora of beneficial compounds may be generated directly from *in situ* secondary metabolism by probiotic bacteria or indirectly from overall production in food vectors. These may include bioactive peptides (Gobbetti *et al.*, 2010), water-soluble vitamins, including thiamine, nicotinic acid, folic acid, pyridoxine, biotin, and B_{12} (Lee *et al.*, 1999), oligosaccharides, organic acids (Bhat and Bhat, 2011), and polyunsaturated fatty acids such as conjugated linoleic acid (Rodrigues *et al.*, 2011; Rodriguez-Alcalá *et al.*, 2011). Furthermore, iron bioavailability may be increased by *L. acidophilus* and bile acids may be deconjugated by numerous lactobacilli.

An overall review of the mechanistic insights that many studies have provided concerning probiotics and their interactions with the composition and function of the intestinal mucosa via specific molecules (cell wall components such as peptidoglycan, teichoic acids or capsular polysaccharides, and immunomodulatory proteins) is given by Bron *et al.* (2012). In this review, the importance of human individuality is discussed as previously mentioned and the possibility of a personalized application of probiotics in the near future is proposed (Bron *et al.*, 2012). These mechanisms will be further probed in Chapter 3.

Criteria for rational use of probiotics will be given in Chapter 7, but in summary may include adequate identification and functional characterization of bacteria; administration of an appropriate quantity of bacteria (which is influenced by nature of strain employed, whether in combination with other strains of same or different species, and by the food/pharmaceutical matrix selected) and their enumeration; benefits for the host and their definition; and safety of use.

2.3.2 GIT *in vitro* Models for Selection

Use of probiotics as mediators of health and well-being or as therapeutic agents for the treatment of several GIT diseases has been suggested as a positive management strategy; nonetheless, their selection needs to be as target-oriented as possible as well as the food or supplement vector better appointed. In addition, the destiny of food compounds in the GIT, including probiotics, has a major impact on their nutritional quality or biological stability to reach specific targets in GIT. As previously discussed, gut microbiota and its metabolic capacity is among the factors that most influence how the host responds to nutrients/bioactive compounds. Furthermore, different microflora profiles, as a consequence of different pathologies, may necessarily implicate different host responses. Hence, there is currently a big challenge to develop reliable methods for providing important insights into digestion and the gut microbiota mode of action required toward maintenance/destruction of host health. Performance of these mechanistic studies *in vivo* is sometimes difficult not only due to sampling drawbacks but also due to ethical constraints. Due to such limitations, different *in vivo* animal models have been developed; the rat (Nyman *et al.*, 1986) and the pig (Glitso *et al.*, 2000) are the two main animals used in fermentation studies. Nevertheless, *in vivo* experiments are expensive and time-consuming; hence, different *in vitro* models simulating conditions in the human GIT are warranted. These model systems may potentially reduce the use of animals in testing new strains, products, and treatments. Several such models, of varying degrees of complexity, have been developed worldwide (Molly *et al.*, 1993; Nollet *et al.*, 1997; Gmeiner *et al.*, 2000; Spratt *et al.*, 2005). These *in vitro* models may be either upper intestinal models, which are used for removal of digestible components and for detection of changes in the nondigestible ones, or continuous, semi-continuous, or batch colon models, which elucidate the role of microbiota in the metabolism of all nondigestible parts of the diet. They provide a baseline for studying the micro-ecology of the gut, particularly changes induced after perturbation of flora by diet, drugs, or toxic chemicals; metabolic capacity of GIT microbiota and their effect on structural changes of food components (beyond that gained by chemical analysis alone) can also be assessed as a function of time. In addition, model systems enable assessment of a large number of samples over a short period of time. Nonetheless, systemic effects cannot be simulated by *in vitro* models, and as consequence of their predictive nature, studies with humans are ultimately required in order to be able to document health effects.

Most conventional methodologies have involved growing cells to be studied, centrifugating and ressuspending the cells in an acidic milieu, with or without washing, at pH values varying between 1.0 and 3.0 or incubating bacteria in a medium containing 0.3% oxgall bile, porcine bile, or bile salts (Jacobsen *et al.*, 1999). Currently, two types of simulators are available: those that simulate the human intestinal microbial ecosystem (*in vitro* colon models) and those that simulate the gastrointestinal physiological events (*in vitro* digestion models). A good example of the latter is the dynamic, computer-controlled model termed TNO GIT Model (TIM) that was developed by the Netherlands Organisation for Applied Scientific

Research TNO (Minekus *et al.*, 1995, 1999). It consists of four chambers to accurately replicate the dynamic *in vivo* conditions in the stomach and small intestine, such as the change of pH, bile salt concentrations, and chime transit, when food is being digested and absorbed. This model enables sampling at various times along the digestion process, which allows for a real-time assessment of the extent of release, dissolution, absorption, and bioconversion of food and its bioactive components under various conditions in the GIT (Gao *et al.*, 2006).

More appropriate for probiotic selection, the *in vitro* colon models maintain colonic microbiota, usually obtained from human feces from specific donors (according to the objectives of study), under strictly anaerobic conditions. The methods differ from each other in the structure of the fermentor, substrate-to-inoculum ratios, media, operating conditions, and sampling, which make comparison of results difficult (Aura *et al.*, 2005a). Culture media are variable and may be as simple as a mineral salt solution or as complex as a medium containing vitamins, hemin, SCFA, yeast extract and trypticase, a reducing agent, and different buffers. Cultures may be static or several mixing methods may be used: regular swirling, a shaking water bath, or periodic mixing (Aura *et al.*, 2005b).

Continuous and semi-continuous colon model systems are suitable for study of the colonic ecosystem and bacteriology (Allison *et al.*, 1989). Reproduction of conditions can be achieved in a multi-stage chemostat (Allison *et al.*, 1989). The foremost was a complex multi-compartmental simulator, the Simulator of the entire Human Gastrointestinal Microbial Ecosystem (SHIME; Molly *et al.*, 1993), which consisted of five reactors simulating the duodenum/jejunum, ileum, caecum and ascending colon, transverse colon, and descending colon, respectively. A sixth reactor was later added to simulate the stomach (Nollet *et al.*, 1997; Gmeiner *et al.*, 2000). This SHIME model was recently used to study the effects of two commercially available plant polysaccharide supplements on the structure, composition, and metabolism of an *in vitro* cultured colon microbial community (Marzorati *et al.*, 2010). Overall, results revealed that dietary supplements were selectively fermented along the entire colon, promoting a positive bifidogenic effect; the possibility of enhancing species belonging to *Bacteroidetes*, a phylum that has been associated with body weight management, was also discussed (Marzorati *et al.*, 2010).

At the University of Reading, an anaerobic three-stage continuous culture system was investigated in terms of carbohydrate metabolism and amino acid metabolism. Researchers demonstrated that carbohydrate breakdown and SCFA production occurred mainly in the first reactor, whereas amino acid fermentation producing branch-chain fatty acids occurred mainly in the second and third reactors corresponding to reactions occurring in the ascending, transverse, and descending colons *in vivo*, respectively (Macfarlane *et al.*, 1992; Macfarlane *et al.*, 1998; Probert *et al.*, 2004). Metabolic activities of gut microbiota and associated mechanisms have also been tested in this culture system. For example, the potential of the flavanol monomers (–)-epicatechin and (+)-epicatechin to positively influence the growth of specific bacterial groups, hence supporting gut health via a prebiotic effect, was shown with this model (Tzounis *et al.*, 2008). Another study used this model to demonstrate the impact of chain length on the selectivity of dextrans toward gut microflora, SCFAs, and gas production (Sarbini *et al.*, 2011).

A more robust development of a continuous *in vitro* model of the colon is the validated computer-controlled TIM-2 system, which simulates (ratio of microorganisms with composition and metabolic activity similar to that of the colon) the dynamic processes in the large intestine in a reproducible way (Minekus *et al.*, 1999) under both normal and impaired physiological conditions. The model uses a high-density complex microbiota and includes peristaltic mixing, water absorption, and absorption of fermentation products. The TIM-2 model system enables continuous monitoring and control of temperature, pH, peristaltic movements, absorption of water, and the fermentation products, as substrate is passed from one compartment to another through the model. The model has been validated in terms of metabolites produced, including SCFAs, branched-chain fatty acids, gases, ammonia, and phenolic compounds (Rehman *et al.*, 2012). It has been used for many applications in many different studies, including estimation of bioavailability of iron and phosphorous, survival of lactic acid bacteria (Minnekus *et al.*, 1995), bioconversion of flavonoids by the human colon microbiota (Gao *et al.*, 2006), prebiotic action of maize-based fibers with increased production of health-promoting metabolites and beneficial microbes (Maathuis *et al.*, 2009), or the protective effect of probiotics against antibiotic-associated disturbances (production of toxic metabolites or destruction of endogenous microbiota) of the intestinal metabolic homeostasis (Rehman *et al.*, 2012). An important aspect with regard to these continuous flow models is their requirement for high technical and scientific expertise and their high costs in terms of both hardware and running expenses.

The Enteromix tools include a small-scale, semi-continuous colon simulator. This model consists of four sequentially attached anaerobic vessels representing the ascending, transverse, descending, and distal colons, respectively. All fluid transfers and pH adjustments are computer controlled and they work with small amounts of substrate, as vessels have small working volumes (Mäkivuokko *et al.*, 2005). This model is considered a simple way of following adequately the temporal production of the microbial metabolites.

A simple reproducible batch system was setup and tested for its validity in a European interlaboratory study (Barry *et al.*, 1995). Fresh human feces were used as inoculum and mixed with a carbonate phosphate buffer supplemented with trace elements and urea. Five different carbohydrate sources were compared in five laboratories on three occasions in order to determine the pH, residual non-starch polysaccharide, and SCFA production during the *in vitro* fermentation. The optimal amount of carbohydrates was 10 g/l in a fecal suspension of 167 g/l. There was also a close correspondence between the *in vitro* data and an *in vivo* rat experiment using diets supplemented with the same sources of carbohydrate (Barry *et al.*, 1995). The model has since then been applied in many fermentation studies of nondigestible carbohydrates (Aura *et al.*, 2005a; Hanhineva *et al.*, 2012) or further developed for the study of phenolic compounds and their interaction with intestinal microbiota (Aura *et al.*, 2002, 2005b).

Other models include a dynamic model with two 1-l jacketed glass beakers representing the stomach and the duodenum (Mainville *et al.*, 2005), which has been used to test the survival of probiotic bacteria. Spratt *et al.* (2005) developed a model that realized some of the features not captured by the other models, by designing a system in which the flow could be modeled easily and which approached the more realistic features of dispersed plug flow; the model also intended to achieve substantial levels of mass transfer of water and fatty acids out of the flowing system across a growing biofilm. The system consisted of three membrane fermenters, each identical to the single stage reported previously joined in series by three sampling modules. Sumeri *et al.* (2008) designed an *in vitro* single bioreactor model that simulates food transit through the upper part of the GIT to enable us to evaluate the probiotic potential of food products. More recently, Mercuri *et al.* (2010) created the dynamic gastric model, which was the first dynamic *in vitro* model of the human stomach, and as such, it is able to mimic the digestive processes of the gastric compartment not only in terms of temporally varying enzymatic and acid secretions but also in terms of simulation of the mechanical forces exerted by the muscular tissue of the stomach, an important model for assessment of digestion and its impact on probiotics.

2.4 Conclusions

A balanced host–intestinal microbiota relationship is essential for intestinal homeostasis due to important roles in digestive, immune, and metabolic functions. Gut microbiota provides an array of functions for the host ranging from epithelial barrier function, through protection against infectious diseases to energy recovery from nutrients, generating SCFAs with different physiological roles. Different studies using advanced analytical strategies have highlighted the importance of modulation of intestinal microbiota toward the improvement of human health.

Specific dietary intervention programs involving food-based strategies or supplements, such as probiotics and prebiotics, are constantly being proposed as relevant solutions to be used in the management of microbiota-associated disorders. The use of probiotics in the treatment and prevention of gastrointestinal diseases has yielded important results, and in order to select the most adequate binomial strain-effect *in vitro*, gastrointestinal models are available for a first phase of development.

References

Alexander, V.N., Northrup, V. and Bizzarro, M.J. (2011). Antibiotic exposure in the newborn intensive care unit and the risk of necrotizing enterocolitis. *Journal of Pediatrics* **159**(3), 392–397.

Allison, C., Macfarlane, C. and Macfarlane, G.T. (1989). Studies on mixed populations of human intestinal bacteria grown in single-stage and multistage continuous culture systems. *Applied Environmental Microbiology* **55**, 672–678.

Anderson, R.C., Cookson, A.L., McNabb, W.C., Park, Z., McCann, M.J., Kelly, W.J., Roy, N.C. 2010. *Lactobacillus plantarum* MB452 enhances the function of the intestinal barrier by increasing the expression levels of genes involved in tight junction formation. *BMC Microbiology* **10**, 316.

Atarashi, K., Tanoue, T., Shima, T., Imaoka, A., Kuwahara, T., Momose, Y., Cheng, G., Yamasaki, S., Saito, T., Ohba, Y., *et al.* (2011). Induction of colonic regulatory T cells by indigenous *Clostridium* species. *Science* **331**, 337–341.

Aura, A.-M, Karppinen, S., Virtanen, H., Forssell, P., Heinonen, S.-M., Nurmi, T., Adlercreutz, H. and Poutanen, K. (2005a). Processing of rye bran influences both the fermentation of dietary fibre and the bioconversion of lignans by human faecal flora *in vitro*. *Journal of Science and Food Agriculture* **85**(12), 2085–2093.

Aura, A.-M., Martin-Lopez, P., O´Leary, K.A., Williamson, G., Oksman-Caldentey, K.-M., Poutanen, K. and Santos-Buelga, C. (2005b). *In vitro* metabolism of anthocyanins by human gut microflora. *European Journal of Nutrition* **44**, 133–142.

Aura, A.-M., O´Leary, K.A., Williamson, G., Ojala, M., Bailey, M., Puupponen-Pimiä, R., Nuutila, A.M., Oksman-Caldentey, K.-M. and Poutanen, K. (2002). Quercetin derivatives are deconjugated and converted to hydroxyphenylacetic acids but not methylated by human fecal flora *in vitro*. *Journal Agriculture Food Chemistry* **50**, 1725–1730.

Aureli, P., Capurso, L., Castellazzi, A.M., Clerici, M., Giovannini, M., Morelli, L., Poli, A., Pregliasco, F., Salvini, F. and Zuccotti, G.V. (2011). Probiotics and health: an evidence-based review. *Pharmacological Research* **63**, 366-376.

van Baarlen, P., Troost, F., van der Meer, C., Hooiveld, G., Boekschoten, M., Brummer, R.J. and Kleerebezem, M. (2011). Human mucosal *in vivo* transcriptome responses to three lactobacilli indicate how probiotics may modulate human cellular pathways. *Proceedings National Academy Science USA* **108**(suppl 1), 4562-4569.

Bäckhed, F., Ding, H-, Wang, T., Hooper, L.V., Koh, G.Y., Nagy, A., Semenkovich, C.F., Gordon, J.I. (2004). The gut microbiota as an environmental factor that regulates fat storage. *Proceedings National Academy Sciences USA* **101**, 15718–15723.

Barnich, N., Carvalho, F.A., Glasser, A-L., Darcha· C., Jantscheff, P., Allez, M., Peeters, H., Bommelaer, G., Desreumaux, P., Colombel J-F. and Darfeuille-Michaud, A. (2007). CEACAM6 acts as a receptor for adherent invasive *E. coli*, supporting ileal mucosa colonization in Crohn disease. *Journal Clinical Investigation* **117**, 1566–1574.

Barry, J.L., Hoebler, C., Macfarlane, G.T., Macfarlane, S., Mathers, J.C., Reed, K.A., Mortensen, P.B., Norgaard, I., Rowland, I.R. and Rumney, C.J. (1995). Estimation of the fermentability of dietary fibre *in vitro*: A European interlaboratory study. *British Journal of Nutrition* **74**, 303–322.

Berg, R.D. (1996). The indigenous gastrointestinal microflora. *Trends in Microbiology* **433**, 430-435.

Bernalier-Donadille, A. (2010). Fermentative metabolism by the human gut microbiota. *Gastroentérologie Clinique et Biologique* **34**, S16–S22.

Bevins, C.L. and Salzman, N. H. (2011). Paneth cells, antimicrobial peptides and maintenance of intestinal homeostasis. *Nature Reviews Microbiology* **9**, 356–368.

Bouskra, D., Brezillon, C., Berard, M., Werts, C., Varona, R., Boneca, I.G. and Eberl, G. (2008). Lymphoid tissue genesis induced by commensals through NOD1 regulates intestinal homeostasis. *Nature* **456**, 507–510.

Bowly, E., Adlercreutz, H. and Rowland, I. (2003). Metabolism of isoflavones and lignans by the gut microflora: a study in germ-free and human flora associated rats. *Food Chemistry Toxicology* **41**, 631–636.

Bron, P.A., Van Baarlen, P. and Kleerebezem, M. (2011). Emerging molecular insights into the interaction between probiotics and the host intestinal mucosa. *Nature Reviews Microbiology* **10**, 66–78.

Brown, C.T., Davis-Richardson, A.G., Giongo, A., Gano, K.A., Crabb, D.B., Mukherjee, N., Casella, G., Drew, J.C., Ilonen, J., Knip, M., Hyoty, H., Veijola, R., Simell, T., Simell, O., Neu, J., Wasserfall, C.H., Schatz, D., Atkinson, M.A. and Triplett, E.W. (2011). Gut microbiome metagenomics analysis suggests a functional model for the development of autoimmunity for type 1 diabetes. *PLoS One* **6**(10), e25792.

Cani, P.D., Possemiers, S., van de Wiele, T., Guiot, Y., Everard, A., Rottier, O., Geurts, L., Naslain, D., Neyrinck, A., Lambert, D.M., Muccioli, G.G. and Delzenne, N.M. (2009). Changes in gut microbiota control inflammation in obese mice through a mechanism involving GLP-2-driven improvement of gut permeability. *Gut* **58**, 1091–1103.

Cani, P.D. and Delzenne, N.M. (2011). The gut microbiome as therapeutic target. *Pharmacology & Therapeutics* **130**, 202–212.

Collado, M.C., Isolauri, E., Laitinen, K. and Salminen, S. (2008). Distinct composition of gut microbiota during pregnancy in overweight and normal-weight women. *American Journal Clinical Nutrition* **88**, 894–899.

Collado, M.C., Bäuerl, C. and Pérez-Martínez, G. (2012). Defining microbiota for developing new probiotics. *Microbial Ecology in Health and Disease* **23**, 18579.

Corr, S.C., Hill, C. and Gahan, C.G. (2009). Understanding the mechanisms by which probiotics inhibit gastrointestinal pathogens. *Advanced Food Nutrition Research* **56**, 1–15.

Diamant, M., Blaak, E.E. and de Vos, W.M. (2011). Do nutrient-gut-microbiota interactions play a role in human obesity, insulin resistance and type 2 diabetes? *Obesity Reviews* **12**, 272–281.

Dicksved, J., Floistrup, H., Bergstrom, A., Rosenquist, M., Pershagen, G., Scheynius, A., Roos, S., Alm, J.S., Engstrand, L. *et al.* (2007). Molecular fingerprinting of the fecal microbiota of children raised according to different lifestyles. *Applied Environmental Microbiology* **73**, 2284–2289.

DiGiulio, D.B., Romero, R., Amogan, H.P., Kusanovic, J.P., Bik, E.M., Gotsch, F., Kim, C.J., Erez, O., Edwin, S. and Relman, D.A. (2008). Microbial prevalence, diversity and abundance in amniotic fluid during preterm labor: a molecular and culture-based investigation. *PLoS One* **3**(8), e3056.

Dolara, P., Luceri, C., De Filippo, C., Femia, A.P., Giovannelli, L., Caderni, G., Cecchini, C., Silvi, S., Orpianesi, C., Cresci, A. (2005). Red wine polyphenols influence carcinogenesis, intestinal microflora, oxidative damage and gene expression profiles of colonic mucosa in F344 rats. *Mutation Research* **591**(1–2), 237–246.

Doré, J. and Corthier, G. (2010). The human intestinal microbiota. *Gastroentérologie Clinique et Biologique* **34**, Suppl. 1, S7–S15.

Dressman, J.B., Amidon, G.L., Peppas, C. and Shah, V.P. (1998). Dissolution testing as a prognostic tool for oral drug absorption: immediate release dosage forms. *Pharmaceutical Research* **15**, 11–22.

Duynhoven, J. van, Vaughan, E.E., Jacobs, D.M., Kemperman, R.A., Velzen, E.J.J. Van, Gross, G., Roger, L.C., Possemiers, S., Smilde, A.K., Doré, J., Westerhuis, J.A. and De Wiele, T. V. (2011). Metabolic fate of polyphenols in the human superorganism. *PNAS* **108**, 4531–4538.

Eckburg, P.B., Bik, E.M., Bernstein, C.N., Purdom, E., Dethlefsen, L., Sargent, M., Gill, S.R., Nelson, K.E. and Relman, D.A. (2005). Diversity of the human intestinal microbial flora. *Science* **308**, 1635–1638.

EFSA 2010. Scientific Opinion on the maintenance of the list of QPS biological agents intentionally added to food and feed (2010 update). *EFSA Journal* **8**(12), 1944, 56.

Evans, D.F., Pye, G., Bramley, R., Clark, A.G., Dyson, T.J. and Hardcastle, J.D. (1988). Measurement of gastrointestinal pH profiles in normal ambulant human subjects. *Gut* **29**, 1035–1041.

Evans, D. (1993). Gastrointestinal tract physiology ant its relevance to drug delivery. Current status on targeted drug delivery to the gastrointestinal tract, London, Capsugel Library.

Fallani, M., Young, D., Scott, J., Norin, E., Amarri, S., Adam, R., Aguilera, M., Khanna, S., Gil, A., Edwards, C., Doré, J. and other members of the INFABIO team. (2010). Intestinal microbiota of 6-week-old infants across Europe: geographic influence beyond delivery mode, breast-feeding, and antibiotics. *Journal Pediatrics Gastroenterology Nutrition* **51**, 77–84.

Falony, G., Vlachou, A., Verbrugghe, K. and De Vuyst, L. (2006). Crossfeeding between *Bifidobacterium longum* BB536 and acetate-converting, butyrate-producing colon bacteria during growth on oligofructose. *Applied Environmental Microbiology* **72**, 7835–7841.

Fanaro, S., Chierici, R., Guerrini, P. and Vigi, V. (2003). Intestinal microflora in early infancy: composition and development. *Acta Paediatrica* **91**, 48–55.

Finegold, S.M., Sutter, V.L. and Mathison, G.E. (1983). Normal indigenous flora. In: Human intestinal microflora in health and disease, pp. 3–31. Edited by D.J. Hengtes. New York, Academic Press.

Frank, D.N., St. Amand, A.L., Feldman, R.A., Boedeker, E.C., Harpaz, N., Pace, N.R. (2007). Molecular-phylogenetic characterization of microbial community imbalances in human inflammatory bowel diseases. *Proceedings National Academy Science U.S.A.* **104**, 13780–13785.

Gao, K., Xu, A.L., Krul, C., Venema, K., Liu, Y., Niu, Y.T., Lu, J., Bensoussan, L., Seeram, N.P., Heber, D. and Henning, S.M. (2006). Of the major phenolic acids formed during human microbial fermentation of tea, citrus, and soy flavonoid supplements, only 3, 4-dihydroxyphenylacetic acid has antiproliferative activity. *Journal of Nutrition* **136**, 52–57.

Ganong, W. (2005) Regulation of gastrointestinal function, *Review of Medical Physiology* Lange Medical Books/McGraw-Hill.Glitso, L.V., Mazur, W.M., Adlercreutz, H., Wähälä, K., Mäkelä, T., Sandström, B. and Bach Knudsen, K.E. (2000). Intestinal metabolism of rye lignans in pigs. *British Journal of Nutrition* **84**, 429-437.

Gmeiner, M., Kneifel, W., Kulbe, K.D., Wouters, R., De Boever, P., Nollet, L. and Verstraete, W. (2000). Influence of a synbiotic mixture consisting of *Lactobacillus acidophilus* 74-2 and a fructooligosaccharide preparation on the microbial ecology sustained in a simulation of the human intestinal microbial ecosystem (SHIME reactor). *Applied Microbiology and Biotechnology* **53**, 219–223.

Gobbetti, M., Cagno, R.D. and De Angelis, M. (2010). Functional microorganisms for functional food quality. *Critical Reviews in Food Science and Nutrition* **50**(8), 716–727.

Gray, V.A. and Dressman, J.B. (1996). Change of pH requirements for standard intestinal fluid. *TS Pharmacopeial Forum* **22**, 1943–1945.

Hall, J.E. (2011). Guyton and hall textbook of medical physiology. 12th edition, Saunders, Elsevier, Philadelphia, USA.

Hanhineva, K., Aura, A-M., Rogachev, I., Matero, S., Skov, T., Aharoni, A., Poutanen, K. and Mykkänen, H. (2012). *In vitro* microbiotic fermentation causes an extensive metabolite turnover of rye bran phytochemicals. PLoS One **7**(6), e39322.

Holmes, E., Li, J.V., Athanasiou, T., Ashrafian, H. and Nicholson, J.K. (2011). Understanding the role of gut microbiome–host metabolic signal disruption in health and disease. *Trends in Microbiology* **19**(7), 349–359.

Hörmannsperger, G. and Haller, D. (2010). Molecular crosstalk of probiotic bacteria with the intestinal immune system: clinical relevance in the context of inflammatory bowel disease. *International Journal of Medical Microbiology* **300**, 63–73.

Jacobsen, C.N., Nielsen, V.R., Hayford, A.E., Moller, P.L., Michaelsen, K.F. *et al.* (1999). Screening of probiotic activities of forty-seven strains of *Lactobacillus* spp. by *in vitro* techniques and evaluation of the colonization ability of five selected strains in humans. *Applied Environmental Microbiology* **65**, 4949–4956.

Jernberg, C., Löfmark, S., Edlund, C., Jansson, J.K. (2010). Long-term impacts of antibiotic exposure on the human intestinal microbiota. *Microbiology* **156**, 3216–3223.

Kalliomäki, M., Collado, M.C., Salminen, S., Isolauri, E. (2008). Early differences in fecal microbiota composition in children may predict overweight. *American Journal Clinical Nutrition* **87**, 534–538.

Karczewski, J., Troost, F.J., Konings, I., Dekker, J., Kleerebezem, M.K., Brummer, R.M., Wells, J.M. 2010. Regulation of human epithelial tight junction proteins by *Lactobacillus plantarum in vivo* and protective effects on the epithelial barrier. *American Journal Physiology Gastrointestinal Liver Physiology* **298**, G851–G859.

Koenig, J.E., Spor, A., Scalfone, N., Fricker, A.D., Stombaugh, J., Knight, R., Angenent, L.T. and Ley R.E. (2011). Microbes and Health Sackler

Colloquium: succession of microbial consortia in the developing infant gut microbiome. *Proceedings National Academy Sciences* **108**, 4578–4585.

Laparra, J.M. and Sanz, Y. (2010). Interactions of gut microbiota with functionalfood components and nutraceuticals. *Pharmacological Research* **61**, 219–225.

Larsen, N., Vogensen, F.K., van den Berg, F.W.J., Nielsen, D.S., Andreasen, A.S., Pedersen, B.K., Al-Soud, W.A., Sørensen, S.J., Hansen, L.H. and Jakobsen, M. (2010). Gut microbiota in human adults with type 2 diabetes differs from non-diabetic adults. *PLoS One* **5**, e9085.

Lay, C., Sutren, M., Rochet, V., Saunier, K., Doré, J. and Rigottier-Gois, L. (2005). Design and validation of 16S rRNA probes to enumerate members of the *Clostridium leptum* subgroup in human faecal microbiota. *Environmental Microbiology* **7**, 933–946.

Lee, Y.K., Nomoto, K., Salminen, S. and Gorbach, S.L. (1999). *Handbook of Probiotics*. New York, John Wiley & Sons.

Ley, R. E., Turnbaugh, P. J., Klein, S. and Gordon, J. I. (2006). Microbial ecology: human gut microbes associated with obesity. *Nature* **444**, 1022–1023.

Maathuis, A., Hoffman, A., Evans, A., Sanders, L., Venema, K. (2009). The effect of the undigested fraction of maize products on the activity and composition of the microbiota determined in a dynamic *in vitro* model of the human proximal large intestine. *Journal of the American College of Nutrition* **28** (6), 657–666.

Macfarlane, G.T., Gibson, G.R. and Cummings, J.H. (1992). Comparison of fermentation reactions in different regions of the human colon. *Journal of Applied Bacteriology* **72**, 57–64.

Macfarlane, G.T., Macfarlane, S. and Gibson, G.R. (1998). Validation of a three stage compound continuous culture system for investigating the effect of retention time on the ecology and metabolism of bacteria in the human colon. *Microbial Ecology* **35**, 180–187.

Mack, D.R., Ahrne, S., Hyde, L., Wei, S. and Hollingsworth, M.A. (2003). Extracellular MUC3 mucin secretion follows adherence of *Lactobacillus* strains to intestinal epithelial cells *in vitro*. *Gut* **52**, 827–833.

Madsen, K.L. (2001). The use of probiotics in gastrointestinal disease. *Canadian Journal Gastroenterology* **15**, 817–822.

Mai, V., Young, C.M., Ukhanova, M., Wang, X., Sun, Y., Casella, G., Theriaque, D., Li, N., Sharma, R., Hudak, M. and Neu, J. (2011). Fecal microbiota in premature infants prior to necrotizing enterocolitis. *PLoS One* **6(6)**, e20647.

Mainville, I., Arcand, Y. and Farnworth, E.R. (2005). A dynamic model that simulates the human upper gastrointestinal tract for the study of probiotics. *International Journal of Food Microbiology* **99**, 287–296.

Mäkivuokko, H., Nurmi, J., Nurminen, P., Stowell, J. and Rautonen, N. (2005). *In vitro* effects of polydextrose on colon fermentation and mucosal cyclooxygenase gene expression. *Nutrition Cancer* **52**(1), 94–104.

Martin, F.P., Dumas, M.E., Wang, Y., Legido-Quigley, C., Yap, I.K., Tang, H., Zirah, S., Murphy, G.M., Cloarec, O., Lindon, J.C., Sprenger, N., Fay, L.B., Kochhar, S., van,Bladeren, P., Holmes, E. and Nicholson, J.K. (2007). A top-down systems biology view of microbiome-mammalian metabolic interactions in a mouse model. *Molecular Systems Biology* **3**, 112: 1–16.

Martin, F-P.J., Collino, S., Rezzi, S. and Kochhar, S. (2012). Metabolomic applications to decipher gut microbial metabolic influence in health and disease. *Frontiers in Physiology* **3**, 1–11 (article 113).

Martín, R., Langa, S., Reviriego, C., Jiménez, E., Marín, M. L., Olivares, M., Boza, J., Jiménez, J., Fernández, L., Xaus, J., Rodríguez, J.M. (2004). The commensal microflora of human milk: new perspectives for food bacteriotherapy and probiotics. *Trends in Food Science and Technology* **15**, 121–127.

Martín, R., Jiménez, E., Heilig, H., Fernández, L., Marín, M.L., Zoetendal, E.G., Rodríguez, J.M. (2009). Isolation of bifidobacteria from breast milk and assessment of the bifidobacterial population by PCR-denaturing gradient gel electrophoresis and quantitative real-time PCR. *Applied and Environmental Microbiology* **75**, 965–969.

Marzorati, M., Verhelst, A., Luta, G., Sinnott, R., Verstraete, W., Van de Wiele, T. and Possemiers, S. (2010). *In vitro* modulation of the human gastrointestinal microbial community by plant-derived polysaccharide-rich dietary supplements. *International Journal of Food Microbiology* **139**, 168–176.

Mercuri, A. (2010). The dynamic gastric model: a new *in vitro* model for biorelevant dissolution and delivery assessment of oral dosage forms. *UKICRS Newsletter*, 28–30.

Minekus, M., Marteau, P., Havenaar, R. and Huis in 't Veld, J.H.J. (1995). A multi-compartmental dynamic computer-controlled model simulating the stomach and small intestine. *Alternatives to Laboratory Animals (ATLA)* **23**, 197–209.

Minekus, M., Smeets-Peeters, M., Bernalier, A., Marol-Bonnin, S., Havenaar, R., Marteau, P., Alric, M., Fonty, G. and Huis in´t Veld, J.H.J. (1999). A computer-controlled system to simulate conditions of the large intestine with peristaltic mixing, water absorption and absorption of fermentation products. *Applied Microbiology and Biotechnology* **53**, 108–114.

Molly,K., Vande Woestyne, M., Verstraete, W. (1993). Development of a 5-step multi-chamber reactor as a simulation of the human intestinal microbial ecosystem. *Applied Microbiology and Biotechnology* **39**, 254–258.

Mshvildadze, M., Neu, J., Shuster, J., Theriaque, D., Li, N. and Mai. V. (2010). Intestinal microbial ecology in premature infants assessed with non-culture-based techniques. *Journal of Pediatrics* **156**(1), 20–25.

Mudie, D.M., Amidon, G. L. and Amidon, G.E. (2010). Physiological parameters for oral delivery and *in vitro* testing. *Molecular Pharmaceutics* **7**, 1388–1405.

Mueller, S., Saunier, K., Hanisch, C. 2006. Differences in fecal microbiota in different European study populations in relation to age, gender, and country: a cross-sectional study. *Applied and Environmental Microbiology* **72**, 1027–1033.

Muniz, L.R., Knosp, C and Yeretssian, G. (2012) Intestinal antimicrobial peptides during homeostasis, infection, and disease. *Frontiers in Immunlogy* **3**, 1–13 (article 310).

Neu, J. and Rushing, J. (2011). Cesarean versus vaginal delivery: long-term infant outcomes and the hygiene hypothesis. *Clinics in Perinatology* **38(2)**, 321–331.

Nollet, L., Vande Velde, I. and Verstraete, W. (1997). Effect of the addition of *Peptostreptococcus productus* ATCC35244 on the gastro-intestinal microbiota and its activity, as simulated in an *in vitro* simulator of the human gastrointestinal tract. *Applied Microbiology and Biotechnology* **48**, 99–104.

Nyman, M., Asp, N.G., Cummings, J. and Wiggins, H. (1986). Fermentation of dietary fibre in the intestinal tract: comparison between man and rat. *British Journal of Nutrition* **55**(3), 487–496.

O'Flaherty, S. and Klaenhammer, T.R. (2011). The impact of omic technologies on the study of food microbes. *Annual Review of Food Science and Technology* **2**, 353–371.

O'Flaherty, S., Saulnier, D.M., Pot, B., Versalovic, J. (2010). How can probiotics and prebiotics impact mucosal immunity? *Gut Microbes* **1**, 293–300.

O'Hara, A.M., O'Regan, P., Fanning, A., O'Mahony, C., MacSharry, J., Lyons, A., Bienenstock, J., O'Mahony, L. and Shanahan, F. (2006). Functional modulation of human intestinal epithelial cell responses by

Bifidobacterium infantis and *Lactobacillus salivarius*. *Immunology* **118**, 202–215.

Parkar, S.G., Stevenson, D.E. and Skinner, M.A. (2008). The potential influence of fruit polyphenols on colonic microflora and human gut health. *International Journal of Food Microbiology* **124**, 295–298.

Phillips, S. (1993). Gastrointestinal physiology ant its relevance to trageted drug delivery. Current status on targeted drug delivery to the gastrointestinal tract, Short Hills (NJ), Capsugel Library.

Possemiers, S., Bolca, S., Grootaert, C., Heyerick, A., Decroos, K., Dhooge, W., De Keukeleire, D., Rabot, S., Verstraete, W. and van der Wiele, T. (2006). The prenylflavonoid isoxanthohumol from hops (Humulus lupulus l.) is activated into the potent phytoestrogen 8-prenylnaringenin *in vitro* and in the human intestine. *Journal Nutrition* **136**, 1862–1867.

Possemiers, S., Bolca, S., Verstraete, W. and Heyerick, A. (2011). The intestinal microbiome: A separate organ inside the body with the metabolic potential to influence the bioactivity of botanicals. *Fitoterapia* **82**, 53-66.

Preidis, G.A. and Versalovic, J. (2009) Targeting the human microbiome with antibiotics, probiotics and prebiotics: gastroenterology enters the metagenomics era. *Gastroenterology* **136**, 2015–2031.

Probert, H.M., Apajalahti, J.H., Rautonen, N., Stowell, J. and Gibson, G.R. (2004). Polydextrose, lactitol, and fructo-oligosaccharide fermentation by colonic bacteria in a three-stage continuous culture system. *Applied Environmental Microbiology* **70**(8), 4505–4511.

Qin, J., Li, R., Li, R., Raes, J., Arumugam, M., Burgdorf, K.S., *et al.* (2010). A human gut microbial gene catalogue established by metagenomic sequencing. *Nature* **464**, 59–65.

Rehman, A., Heinsen, F-A., Koenen, M.E., Venema, K., Knecht, H., Hellmig, S., Schreiber, S. and Ott, S.J. (2012). Effects of probiotics and antibiotics on the intestinal homeostasis in a computer controlled model of the large intestine. *BMC Microbiology* **12**, 47–56.

Rodrigues, D., Santos, C.H., Rocha-Santos, T.A.P., Gomes, A.M., Goodfellow, B.J., Freitas, A.C. (2011). Metabolic profiling of potential probiotic or synbiotic cheeses by NMR spectrometry. *Journal of Agriculture and Food Chemistry* **59**, 4955–4961

Rodriguez-Alcala, L.M., Braga, T., Gomes, A.M.P., Malcata, F.X. and Fontecha, J. (2011). Quantitative and qualitative determination of CLA produced by *Bifidobacterium* and LAB by combining spectrophotometric and Ag+-HPLC techniques. *Food Chemistry* **125**, 1373–1378.

Rowland, I.R., Bearne, C.A., Fischer, R. and Pool-Zobel, B.L. (1996). The effect of lactulose on DNA damage induced by DMH in the colon of human flora associated rats. *Nutrition Cancer* **26**, 37–47.

Salzman, N.H. (2011). Microbiota-immune system interaction: an uneasy alliance. *Current Opinion Microbiology* **14**, 99–105.

Sanders, M.E. (2007). Probiotics: strains matter. *Functional Food and Nutraceuticals.* June, 34–41.

Sanders, M.E. (2011). Impact of probiotics on colonizing microbiota of the gut. *Journal of Clinical Gastroenterology* **45(Suppl),** S115–S119.

Sanders, M.E. and Marco, M.L. (2010). Food formats for effective delivery of probiotics. *Annual Reviews on Food Science and Technology* **1**, 65–85.

Sarbini, S.R., Kolida, S., Naeye, T., Einerhand, A., Brison, Y., Remaud-Simeon, M., Monsan, P., Gibson, G.R. and Rastall, R.A. (2011). *In vitro* fermentation of linear and α-1,2-branched dextrans by the human fecal microbiota. *Applied and Environmental Microbiology,* **77**(15), 5307–5315.

Schippa, S., Iebba, V., Barbato, M., Nardo, G.D., Totino, V., Checchi, M.P., Longhi, C., Maiella, G., Cucchiara, S. and Conte, M.P. (2010). A distinctive 'microbial signature' in celiac pediatric patients. *BMC Microbiology* **10**, 175–184.

Schlee, M., Harder, J., Köten, B., Stange, E.F., Wehkamp, J. and Fellermann, K. (2008). Probiotic lactobacilli and VSL#3 induce enterocyte β-defensin 2. *Clinical Experimental Immunology* **151**, 528–535.

Sekirov, I., Russell, S.L., Antunes, L.C.M. and Finlay, B.B. (2010). Gut microbiota in health and disease. *Physiology Reviews* **90**, 859–904.

Sokol, H., Pigneur, B., Watterlot, L., Lakhdari, O., Bermúdez-Humarán, L.G., Gratadoux, J.J., *et al.* (2008). *Faecalibacterium prausnitzii* is an anti-inflammatory commensal bacterium identified by gut microbiota analysis of Crohn disease patients. *Proceedings National Academy Sciences U.S.A.* **105**, 16731–16736.

Sokol, H., Seksik, P. Furet, J.P., Firmesse, O., Nion-Larmurier, I., Beaugerie, L., *et al.* (2009). Low counts of *Faecalibacterium prausnitzii* in colitis microbiota. *Inflammatory Bowel Disease* **15**, 1183–1189.

Sousa, T., Paterson, R., Moore, V., Carlsson, A., Abrahamsson, B. and Basit, A.W. (2008). The gastrointestinal microbiota as a site for the biotransformation of drugs. *International Journal Pharmacology* **363**, 1–25.

Spratt, P., Nicolella, C. and Pyle, D.L. (2005). An engineering model of the human colon. *Food and Bioproducts Processing* **83**(2), 147–157.

Sumeri, I., Arike, L., Adamberg, K. and Paalme, T.(2008). Single bioreactor gastrointestinal tract simulator for study of survival of probiotic bacteria. *Applied Microbiology and Biotechnology* **80**, 317–324.

Tlaskalová-Hogenová, H., Stepánková, R., Hudcovic, T., Tucková, L., Cukrowska, B., Lodinová-Zádníková, R., *et al.* (2004). Comensal bacteria (normal microflora), mucosal immunity and chronic inflammatory and autoimmune diseases. *Immunology Letters* **93**, 97–108.

Tuohy, K.M., Hinton, D.J.S., Davies, S.J., Crabbe, M.J.C., Gibson, G.R. and Ames, J.M. (2006). Metabolism of maillard reaction products by the human gut microbiota—implications for health. *Molecular Nutrition Food Research* **50**, 847–857.

Tuohy, K.M., Rouzaud, G.C., Bruck, W.M., and Gibson, G.R. (2005). Modulation of the human gut microflora towards improved health using prebiotics-assessment of efficacy. *Current Pharmaceutical Design* **11**, 75–90.

Turnbaugh, P.J., Bäckhed, F., Fulton, L. and Gordon J.I. (2008). Diet-induced obesity is linked to marked but reversible alterations in the mouse distal gut microbiome. *Cell Host Microbe* **3**(4), 213–223.

Tzounis, X., Vulevic, J., Kuhnle, G.G.C., George, T., Leonczak, J., Gibson, G.R., KwikUribe, C. and Spencer, J.P.E. (2008). Flavanol monomer induced changes to the human faecal microflora. *British Journal of Nutrition* **99**, 782–792.

Uronis, J.M., Mühlbauer, M., Herfarth, H.H., Rubinas, T.C., Jones, G.S. and Jobin, C. (2009). Modulation of the intestinal microbiota alters colitis-associated colorectal cancer susceptibility. *PLoS ONE* **4**(6), e6026.

Vaarala, O., Atkinson, M.A. and Neu, J. (2008). The "perfect storm" for type 1 diabetes: The complex interplay between intestinal microbiota, gut permeability, and mucosal immunity. *Diabetes* **57**(10), 2555–2562.

Vanhoutte, T., Huys, G., Brandt, E. and Swings, J. (2004) Temporal stability analysis of the microbiota in human feces by denaturing gradient gel electrophoresis using universal and group-specific 16S rRNA gene primers. *FEMS Microbiology Ecology* **48**, 437–446.

Walker A. (2010). Breast milk as the gold standard for protective nutrients. *Journal of Pediatrics* **156**, S3–S7.

Walle, T. (2004). Absorption and metabolism of flavonoids. *Free Radical Biology and Medicine* **36**, 829–837.

Wen, L., *et al.* (2008). Innate immunity and intestinal microbiota in the development of Type 1 diabetes. *Nature* **455**, 1109–1113.

Wikoff, W.R., Anfora, A.T., Liu, J., Schultz, P.G., Lesley, S.A., Peters, E. C. and Siuzdak, G. (2009). Metabolomics analysis reveals large effects of gut microflora on mammalian blood metabolites. *Proceedings National Academy Sciences U.S.A.* **106**, 3698–3703.

Williams, H.R., Cox, I.J., Walker, D.G., North, B.V., Patel, V.M., Marshall, S.E., Jewell, D.P., Ghosh, S., Thomas, H. J., Teare, J.P., Jakobovits, S., Zeki, S., Welsh, K.I., Taylor-Robinson, S.D. and Orchard, T.R. (2009). Characterization of inflammatory bowel disease with urinary metabolic profiling. *American Journal Gastroenterology* **104**, 1435–1444.

Wu, X., Ma, C., Han, L., Nawaz, M., Gao, F., Zhang, X., Yu, P., Zhao, C., Li, L., Zhou, A., Wang, J., Moore; J.E., Millar, B.C. and Xu, J. (2010). Molecular characterisation of the faecal microbiota in patients with Type II Diabetes. *Current Microbiology* **61**, 69–78.

Yan, F., Cao, H., Cover, T.L., Whitehead, R., Washington, M.K. and Polk, D.B. (2007). Soluble proteins produced by probiotic bacteria regulate intestinal epithelial cell survival and growth. *Gastroenterology* **132**, 562–575.

Chapter 3

Probiotics and Their Therapeutic Role

Manuela M. Pintado,[a] Ana M. Gomes,[a] and Ana C. Freitas[b,c]
[a]*CBQF, Biotechnology School of Portuguese Catholic University, Rua Dr. António Bernardino Almeida, 4200-072 Porto, Portugal*
[b]*ISEIT/Viseu-Instituto Piaget, Estrada do Alto do Gaio, Galifonge, 3515-776 Lordosa, Viseu, Portugal*
[c]*CESAM & Department of Chemistry, University of Aveiro, 3810-193 Aveiro, Portugal*
mpintado@porto.ucp.p

3.1 Health Potential of Probiotics: Mechanisms of Action

Probiotics have been associated with many health-promoting effects, primarily focused on the gastrointestinal (GI) tract benefits through several modulating activities, but also demonstrating promising applications at other locations of the body, namely at respiratory and genital tract and subcutaneous tissue (Marco *et al.*, 2006). It is recognized that due to the numerous beneficial activities that can be assigned to probiotics, more than one mechanism of action is required to explain the effects of their activity that are generally explained by direct or indirect modification of the endogenous

Probiotic Bacteria: Fundamentals, Therapy, and Technological Aspects
Edited by J. Paulo Sousa e Silva and Ana C. Freitas

ISBN 978-981-4411-62-2 (Hardcover), 978-981-4411-63-9 (eBook)
www.panstanford.com

microbiota or the immune response. These beneficial properties are strain dependent, and although several properties may be attributed to a specific strain, the multiple activities are in general achieved by microorganism interaction either among them or with the host (Marteau and Shanahan, 2003).

Figure 3.1 summarizes the main mechanisms of action displayed by probiotic bacteria when in contact with gut mucosa. Concerning the improvement of endogenous microbiota, the colonization by probiotic bacteria involves, in first place, the adhesion of these bacteria to *in situ* cell receptors allowing for the competition for the sites of adhesion and for nutrients, reducing number of available receptors as well as accessible nutrients to be used by pathogenic bacteria. This adhesion is generally considered a pre-requisite for colonization that should not be permanent, but only transient colonization (Ouwehand *et al.*, 1999).

During their colonization and through their growth and metabolism, they can release antimicrobial substances, including bacteriocines—natural antimicrobial substances (generally of proteinaceous nature that can have a lipid or carbohydrate moiety) or organic acids (namely lactic and acetic acids, hydrogen peroxide, among others) that consequently decrease the local pH. These natural antimicrobials contribute toward *in situ* inhibition of pathogens. In addition, via immunological activation, they can also promote pathogen inhibition through induction of cytokine production or the increase *in situ* IgA secretion.

Apart from that, these beneficial microorganisms can also protect from toxins released *in situ,* generated from food digestion or by microorganisms, through the entrapment of toxins and consequent elimination from the gut. During their permanence in the gut, they can improve epithelial and tissue integrity and functionality, mainly through the production of low amounts of nitric oxide (NO) synthesis, enhancement of mucus production, improvement of gut epithelia cell proliferation, inhibition of carcinogenic substances production or elimination through detoxification, and generation of nutrients, namely production of short fatty acids and vitamins (Steidler, 2001). The mucus provides a barrier that protects the intestinal immune cells from the high level of antigens present in gut lumen and short-chain fatty acids (SCFAs) are the major source of energy for colonocytes and its deficiency has been suggested to promote colitis.

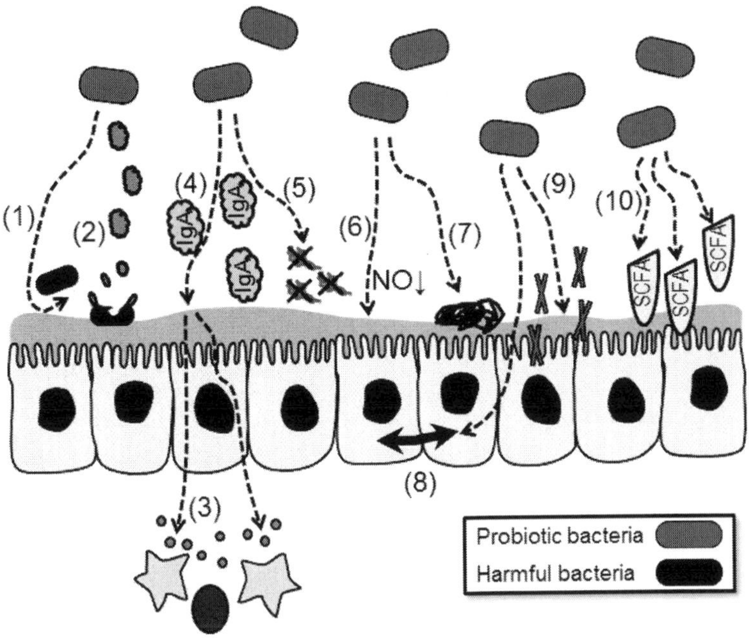

Figure 3.1 Summary of the main mechanisms of action associated with probiotic activity when in contact with gut mucosa. Probiotic strains can displace harmless bacteria by competitive binding (1) or killing/growth inhibition of pathogenic bacteria by antibacterial compounds or lowering of the pH (2). Probiotics have also proven immunomodulation ability by stimulation of the host immune cells such as the induction of cytokine production (3) or the increase in *in situ* IgA secretion (4). Probiotic bacteria still can neutralize toxins and eliminate them from the intestine (5). In addition, probiotics can influence epithelial and tissue integrity by low-dose NO synthesis (6), stimulation of mucus production (7), enhancing gut epithelial cell proliferation (8), inhibition of endogenous carcinogens production (9), and providing nutrients by SCFA production (10). This figure has been adapted from Steidler (2001).

Some probiotic bacteria develop positive *in situ* effects by strengthening the mucosal barrier by preventing and repairing mucosal damage, whether caused by pathogens, food antigens, or medicinal substances, and increase the pathogen-induced transepithelial resistance of the cell monolayer to induce mucin gene expression (Saxelin *et al.*, 2005).

In addition, the other relevant mechanism of action associated with the probiotics include their ability to modulate the immune system, which implies the activation of lymphoid cells of the gut-associated lymphoid tissue present in the lamina propria and sub-mucosa. These interactions with the lymphoid tissue may occur through the intact microorganism and its fragments [e.g., cell wall peptidoglycan, lipoteichoic acid (LTA) complexes, S-layer proteins, and unmethylated cytosine–phosphate–guanine (CpG) motifs of DNA, or metabolites produced *in situ* (Ouwehand *et al.*, 1999)]. The interaction of probiotics with host cells by adhesion might already activate a signaling cascade leading to immune modulation, or alternatively respond to the release of soluble factors (Oelschlaeger, 2010).

Our host's innate immune system discriminates signals from pathogens and from normal flora (commensals) by specific recognition receptors or Toll-like receptors (TLRs). Immune cells use specialized TLRs to detect different microbial components separately or simultaneously. The activation of different TLR triggers diverse host responses allowing for modulation of immune system (Marteau and Shanahan, 2003). The main immune responses mostly associated with infection events generally involve acquired immune system, including mainly B lymphocytes and sensitized T lymphocytes (Th1, Th2, and Th3), and the innate immune system, consisting mainly of macrophages and natural killer (NK) cells (Nomot, 2005). Dendritic cells (DCs), antigen-presenting cells that initiate *in situ* response in the intestinal mucosa and play a crucial immunoregulatory role in the balance of T helper cells Th1, Th2, and Th3 (Marteau *et al.*, 2002).

The immunomodulation role of probiotics is also explained (*Lactobacillus rhamnosus* commonly used as model) by the reduction of the production of the proinflammatory cytokines [tumor necrosis factor α (TNF-α) and interleukins 6 and 12 (IL-6 and IL-12)] by immature DCs and the production of IL-12 and IL-18 by mature DCs (Saxelin *et al.*, 2005).

Marco *et al.* (2006) described the main effects of probiotics on immune responses and intestinal barrier integrity identifying the bacterial and host effector molecules (see Fig. 3.2).

In first stage, DCs play a key role in initial bacterial recognition and, consequently, in influencing T-cell responses, favoring Th1,

Th2, or Th3 immune responses. This interaction was shown to be mediated in *Lactobacillus* by binding to the pattern-recognition receptor (PRR) DC-specific intercellular adhesion molecule 3-grabbing non-integrin (DC-SIGN). In particular, only those *Lactobacillus* strains able to interact with DC-SIGN were able to induce IL-10 producing and regulatory T-cell populations. On the contrary, intestinal and colonic epithelial cells (IECs and CECs) also demonstrated to be involved in bacterial recognition and immune modulation. Interaction of *Lactobacillus* GG (LGG) with Caco-2 IECs leads to reducing TNF α (TNF-α)-induced IL-8 production via the nuclear factor (NF)-kB signaling pathway. Other bacteria (namely the probiotic mixture VSL#3 consisting of eight different strains) showed to interact with CEC inhibiting the degradation of the NF-kB inhibitor I-kB. In addition, these may also occur after recognition of bacterial components (e.g., CpG DNA by TLR9 receptors). These effects positively affect the mucosa by reducing the intestinal inflammation. Probiotic also proved to reinforce the intestinal barrier through several mechanisms. A specific probiotic *Escherichia coli* (strain Nissle 1917) was shown to induce expression of the antimicrobial peptide β-defensin-2 (hBD2) via the NF-kB and activating protein 1 (AP-1) transcription factors. This activation of hBD2 production possibly leads to the enhancement of the intestinal mucosal barrier, and simultaneously justifies the antimicrobial activity upon pathogens in GI tract. Inhibition of pathogen can also be mediated by neutralizing attachment and growth by probiotic strains possessing mannose adhesins. On the contrary, the LTAs of probiotics have been identified as relevant in the modulation of specific immune responses and D-alanine substituents seem to be involved. The beneficial effect of probiotics at this level culminates on reduced levels of pro-inflammatory cytokines and higher levels of the anti-inflammatory cytokine IL-10 mediated by TLR2-mediated signaling.

In addition, specific heat shock proteins (Hsps) that regulate cytoskeletal integrity were produced after interaction of VSL#3 consortiums with IECs. Similarly, interaction of LGG with CECs also induced the production of Hsps via intracellular signaling with several mitogen-activated protein kinases (MAPKs). The final effect allows preventing apoptosis by the activation of IEC signal transduction pathway modulating the intestinal barrier function.

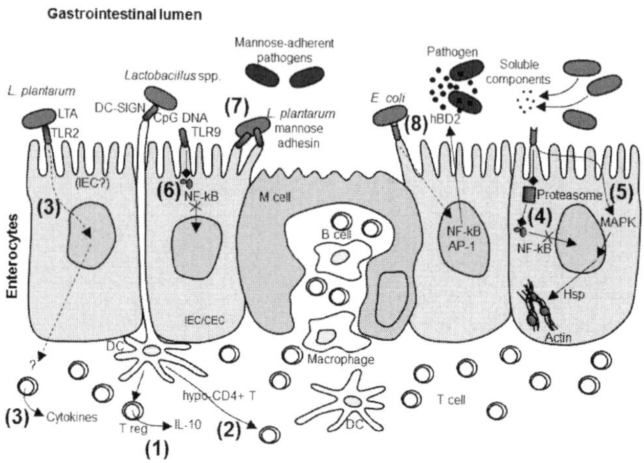

Figure 3.2 Illustration describing the main immune responses induced by probiotics and effects on intestinal barrier integrity. Some probiotic strains are able to promote IL-10 producing, regulatory T cells (Tregs) through DC-SIGN interaction (1). They can also induce hyporesponsive CD4+ T-cell populations after DC interaction (2). LTA composition is responsible for the differential modulation of cytokine production (3). Positive modulation of inflammatory responses by inactivation of the NF-kB signaling pathway is achieved through proteasome inhibition after IEC recognition of soluble probiotic components (4) or after recognition of bacterial motifs (e.g., CpG DNA by TLR9 receptors) (6). The induction of Hsps either via 4 or 5, stabilizing the actin cytoskeleton, would reinforce the mucosal barrier. Pathogen attachment and growth could be neutralized by strains possessing mannose adhesins (7) or by induction of hBD2 in IECs (8). M cell, an epithelial cell specialized in antigen uptake and transport. Reprinted from Marco *et al.* (2006), with permission from Elsevier.

During the subsequent sections, the beneficial properties assigned to the probiotics and the corresponding specific mechanisms of action that will support each of the subsequent therapy applications will be explored.

3.2 Alleviation of Lactose Intolerance

Lactose intolerance is a syndrome associated with the decrease of the intestinal β-galactosidase (β-gal or commonly known as lactase) activity to values lower than 10% of childhood levels. In general, the decline of this enzyme is a natural characteristic of the maturing intestine in the majority of the world's population, declining from the third year of life. However, this characteristic changes across the world population, and among Europeans, the incidence is between 7 and 20%, compared with 65–75% in Africans and 60–90% in people from Asia and the area around the Mediterranean (Ockeloen and Deckers-Kocken, 2012).

This enzyme lactase transforms lactose into glucose and galactose, which will be easily absorbed by mucosa to blood (Fig. 3.3).

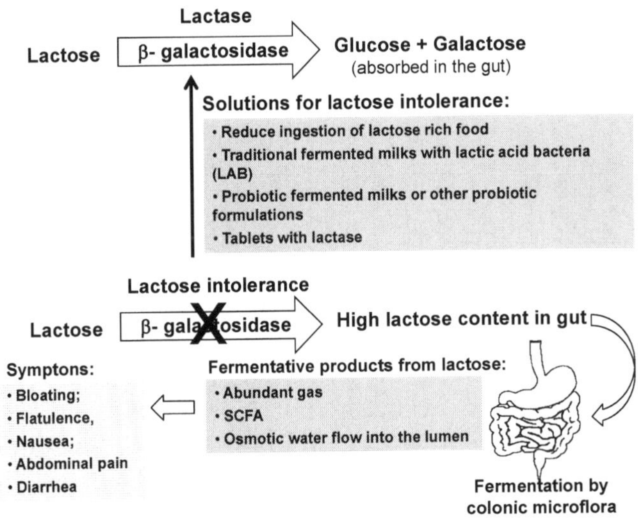

Figure 3.3 Schematic description of events associated with lactose intolerance and possible solutions to reduce lactose malabsorption clinical symptoms.

The lack or reduction of this enzyme (Fig. 3.3) leads to a high concentration of free lactose (not hydrolyzed) in the gut that is utilized by the local fermentative microflora resulting in abundant gas, short-chain organic acids, and an osmotic increase of the water flow into the lumen. These local events lead to characteristic lactose malabsorption clinical symptoms, including bloating, flatulence, nausea, abdominal pain, and diarrhea (Vasiljevic and Shah, 2008).

Lactose intolerance treatment implies the elimination or reduction of lactose ingestion, avoiding the consumption of food rich in lactose, in particular milk. However, fermented dairy products contain fermentative microorganism, which efficiently use lactose and reduce lactose contents. The marker for bacterial metabolism of lactose in the large bowel is the production of hydrogen in breath, and in individuals treated with fermented milk, there is lower hydrogen content than in group treated with nonfermented milk, indicating that lactose was metabolized (Mombelli and Gismondo, 2000). The advantage of fermented milks in lactose maldigesters is well established, and two mechanisms have been involved: digestion of lactose in the intestine by the lactase contained in the yoghurt bacteria, and slower GI transit time of yoghurt than milk (Marteau, 2001).

Probiotics can be beneficial in this condition, as lactobacilli produce lactase, which hydrolyses the lactose in dairy products as well as in gut when it is released within the intestinal lumen once these bacteria are lysed by bile secretions (Tuohy *et al.*, 2003).

Different factors appear to be responsible for a better tolerance of lactose in fermented milk, including starter culture, intracellular β-galactosidase expressed in these cultures, and most relevant the GI transit time. The common cultures used in milk fermentations, namely yoghurt, such as *Streptococcus thermophilus* and *L. bulgaricus* (but also other lactobacilli in fermented milk products), can alleviate symptoms of lactose intolerance by using lactose as an energy source during growth, allowing for the reduction of its content in fermented products as well as by providing bacterial lactase to the intestine and stomach (Singh *et al.*, 2011). After consumption of fermented products, the bacterial lactase may resist to GI conditions and arrive intact to terminal ileum, in which it contributes to lactose hydrolysis and improved lactose tolerance. Some clinical studies have been performed in patients with lactose intolerance. Ockeloen and Deckers–Kocken (2012) found that the abdominal pain was improved in 94% of children after 5 months using a lactose-restricted diet and/or probiotics and in 61% after 15 months. Nevertheless, these results were evident for short-term use, but not for long term.

However, some studies did not found direct relation for digestion and lactose tolerance, as even using fermented milks with different lactase activities, no corresponding tolerance to lactose was found. So, especially in this case, the higher viscosity of fermented product (mainly yoghurt) can slow the gastric emptying and consequently increase the time available to achieve the lactose digestion and improve lactose tolerance (Vasiljevic and Shah, 2008).

So, as final remark, the use of probiotic bacteria in lactose-intolerant patients may be a successful direction to reduce characteristic lactose malabsorption clinical symptoms, especially when incorporated in fermented milks, as lactose is reduced in dairy matrix by *in situ* fermentation and at same time in the gut by lactase that allows the efficient hydrolysis of lactose from other food sources.

3.3 Inhibition of *Helicobacter pylori* and Intestinal Pathogens

It has been reported that probiotics might be useful in the prevention and/or treatment of certain infections of the stomach and small and large intestines. The main agents involved include the *H.* pylori in the stomach and small intestine, and other intestinal pathogens, namely *Rotavirus, Salmonella, Campylobacter jejuni,* and *E. coli.* The main mechanisms reported, in general, include (Fig. 3.4) host–bacteria interaction mechanisms that include physical bacteria–epithelium interaction (adhesion to mucosal and epithelial cells, stimulation of mucus secretion, production of defensive molecules, reinforcement of gut barrier function), bacteria–immune system interaction that comprise modulation and regulation of immune responses, and also, bacteria–bacteria interaction, which consist of exclusion and inhibition of pathogens by prevention of adhesion, secretion of antimicrobial substances, competition for nutrients, and anti-toxin effects (Salminen *et al.*, 2010).

The role of probiotics and associated mechanism in GI tract infectious disease caused by each type of pathogen will be explored in the following section.

3.3.1 Inhibition of *Helicobacter pylori*

H. pylori was recognized for the first time in 1982 as *C. pyloridis.* This agent has been associated as a major agent with gastritis and peptic ulcer being also considered a risk factor for gastric adenocarcinoma or gastric mucosa associated lymphoid tissue (MALT) lymphoma. Although this microorganism has been found in a great number

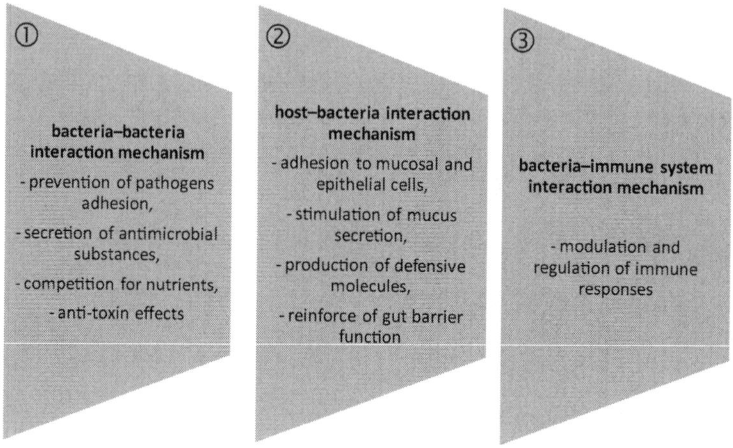

Figure 3.4 Main mechanisms of probiotic bacteria involved in the prevention and/or treatment of certain GI infections (based on Salminen *et al.*, 2010).

of population (70–90% in developing countries and 25–50% in developed countries), disease only occurs in a few percentage, as most of the carriers are asymptomatic (Hamilton-Miller, 2003).

The most common treatment of *H. pylori* infection includes one-week triple therapy, combining acid suppression with proton pump inhibitors and two antibiotics, among them the amoxicillin and clarithromycin are the most common. These solutions usually achieve high success rates, but have the disadvantage of the rapid development of antibiotic resistance associated with relevant side effects (Felley and Michetti, 2003), namely alterations to the intestinal microbiota.

As the *H. pylori* disease is located primarily on the gastric mucosa, a reduction of *H. pylori* by dietary measures might help to decrease the risk of developing *H. pylori* associated diseases.

In the last decade, the use of probiotics, mainly incorporated in food matrix, for the inhibition of *H. pylori* has been explored. Data obtained in both *in vitro* and *in vivo* report an inhibitory effect of probiotics upon *H. pylori* adhesion to gastric cells and reduction of viability.

In vitro studies have proposed that they could act through the production of organic acids and/or bacteriocins capable of inhibiting growth and its attachment to gastric epithelial cells. The first *in vitro* studies reported that *H. pylori* growth was inhibited by the secretion of lactic acid by the *Lactobacillus* tested *L. acidophilus* (Bhatia *et al.*, 1989). Later, Lorca *et al.* (2001) found that this strain possesses some specific properties, in particular, the secretion of a proteinaceous nature compound—an autolysin, released after cell lysis possibly involved in its anti-*H. pylori* activity. On the contrary, the probiotic strain *Bacillus subtilis* 3 has also been shown to inhibit the growth of *H. pylori* that was not related to pH or organic acid, but to two bacteriocines, one identified as amicoumacin A (Felley and Michetti, 2003). Two out of nine *L. reuteri* strains, JCM 1081 and TM 105, were able to bind to asialo-GM1 and sulphatide and to inhibit binding of *H. pylori* to both glycolipids, suggesting that selected *L. reuteri* strains could help to prevent infection in an early stage of colonization of the gastric mucosa by *H. pylori* (Felley and Micheti, 2003).

Several clinical trials have been performed and the most common markers used for control of positive effects include invasive tests such as endoscopy to observe the eradication of *H. pylori* in gastric mucosa or noninvasive test such as ^{13}C Urea breath test, in which the presence of *H. pylori* is directly proportional to the ^{13}C present in CO_2 liberated in breath resulting from hydrolysis of ingested ^{13}C Urea by urease produced by *H. pylori.* Another noninvasive method includes the determination of serum pepsinogens I (sPGI) and II (sPGII), serum gastrin-17 (sG-17), and IgG anti–*H. pylori* antibodies (IgG-Hp), markers that reflect both the morphological and functional status of the gastric mucosa (Myllyluoma *et al.*, 2007).

Some clinical trials produced conflicting evidence, especially when eradication was the main expected effect and *L. acidophilus* was found to be the only agent that showed this activity in published trials (Canducci *et al.*, 2002a). Part of these studies aimed to test the effect of several strains of probiotic bacteria (including *L. acidophilus, L. johnsonii* La1, *Bifidobacterium longum* BB536, *L. gasseri* OLL) alone on the treatment of *H. pylori* infections. The probiotic concentrations used in these studies range from 10^9 to 10^{10} cfu/ml and the trials duration range from 2 to 8 weeks of treatment. Although there is evidence in part of these studies that probiotics bacteria cleared *H. pylori*, or reduced the breath test values, indicating reduction of *H. pylori* density in gastric mucosa, the number of negative cases is much higher than the positive cases (see Table 3.1). Some studies also showed reduction of pepsinogen (Hamilton-Miller, 2003) or gastrin-17 (Myllyluoma *et al.*, 2007). Myllyluoma *et al.* (2007) also demonstrate that the probiotic combination of five bacteria (see Table 3.1) exerts a beneficial effect on gastric mucosa in *H. pylori* infected patients. Gotteland *et al.* (2008) also combine probiotics (*L. acidophilus* La1) with cranberry juice assuring 23% reduction of *H. pylori* against 14.9% when La1 was alone.

Table 3.1 Compilation of main regimen, number of patients, and main results obtained in clinical trials using probiotics alone in treatment of *H. pylori* infections

Study	Regimen	Number of patients	Main results
Hamilton-Miller, 2003	*L. acidophilus* 8×10^{10} for 8 weeks	20	Four patients cleared
	L. acidophilus NSA in "acidophilus milk" c. 5×10^{9} cfu/day for 8 weeks	14	Six patients cleared
	L. johnsonii La1 supernatant, 200 ml for 2 weeks	20	Breath test values reduced
	B. longum BB536 2.5×10^{10} cfu/day for 4 weeks in pasteurized yogurt	68	Breath test values reduced
	L. gasseri OLL 2716 c. 2×10^{9} cfu/day for 8 weeks in yogurt base	31	Breath test and pepsinogen values reduced
	Yogurt made with six "lactic acid" strains 7×10^{9} cfu/day for 30 days	27	Breath tests remained positive in 26/27
Myllyluoma *et al.*, 2007	*L. rhamnosus* GG (LGG), *L. rhamnosus* LC705, *P. freudenreichii* ssp. *shermanii* JS, and *B. lactis* Bb12, 2.5×10^{9} cfu/day for 8 weeks	13	Breath test and gastrin-17 reduced
Gotteland *et al.*, 2008	*L. acidophilus* La1 product (80 ml) daily with $>10^{7}$ cfu/ml for 3 weeks alone or combined with cranberry jus	295	Breath test values reduced and eradication of 14.9% for La1 and 22.9% when combined with cranberry juice

When probiotic bacteria was used as a supplement of *H. pylori* triple-therapy studies with *L. acidophilus* (Canducci *et al.*, 2002b) and *L. casei* subsp. *rhamnosus* (LGG) (Armuzzi, *et al.*, 2001), results showed a significant reduction in side effects incidence, with respect to placebo, in particular the reduction in the GI disorders in the course of antibiotic administration, but without significant differences in the eradication rate. Sabbi and Palumbo (2007) studied the effect of probiotics in combination with traditional treatment (omeprazole, clarithromycin, and amoxicillin) using 60 patients randomized into three groups: the first received LGG; the second received *Bacillus clausii*, and the third received placebo. The results showed that all patients exhibited eradication of *H. pylori*, and the incidence of side effects (nausea and abdominal pain) in patients treated with LGG and *Bacillus* was lower.

The main mechanisms by which the probiotics assure the aforementioned effects are not yet completely clarified. The most likely mechanism supporting the prevention of initiation of *H. pylori* infection by probiotics is the competition for binding sites. The adjunctive effect to antibiotic treatment has been explained as a direct additive antibacterial effect of inhibitory metabolites, on the antibiotic regime, complemented by a possible stimulation of the immune system (Hamilton-Miller, 2003).

Some studies were focused in the reduction of gastric ulcer through anti-inflammatory effect rather than other mechanisms. These findings suggested that LGG enhanced gastric ulcer healing via the attenuation of cell apoptosis to cell proliferation ratio and increase in angiogenesis. Some components may regulate these processes, namely ornithine decarboxylase (ODC) and B-cell lymphoma 2 (Bcl-2) protein expression, vascular endothelial growth factor (VEGF) expression and growth factor receptor (EGF receptor), and explain the healing action of LGG on gastric ulcer (Lam *et al.*, 2007).

As a final remark, it is important to point out that probiotics might be suggested as a new tool in the management of *H. pylori* colonization. However, due to the prevailing conflicting results, more studies are required in order to improve standardization for each new strain studied, namely, in dose, duration and conditions of regimen, and diet of the patient. Nonetheless, on the basis of consistent results, probiotics may have a place as adjunctive treatment in *H.*

pylori infections and possibly in prophylaxis, but cannot, as yet, be considered a valid alternative to conventional anti-*H. pylori* therapy.

3.3.2 Inhibition of Other Enteric Pathogenic Bacteria and Prevention and Reduction of Diarrhea Symptoms

Preservation of the intestinal ecological flora is important in preventing disease by controlling overgrowth of potentially pathogenic bacteria. Several studies have suggested that some probiotic strains could be used to prevent colonization of the GI tract by a large variety of pathogens. Although the underlying mechanism remains unclear, it could be due to organic acid production and associated pH reduction, depletion of nutrients, production of intestinal mucin, and inhibition of adhesion pathogen to the epithelium and of specific bacterial toxins, as well as to intrinsic activities of metabolites or to the synthesis of antimicrobial substances. In addition, adherence of probiotics to intestinal epithelial cells ensuring temporary colonization of the gut is probably one of most important functionalities for their beneficial health effect upon intestinal pathogen. Although the last mechanism is referred as one of the principal mechanism of action, most beneficial effects are thought to be by immunomodulation with an interaction with TLRs and intracellular pathways, activation of macrophages and NK cells and gut lymphoid tissue, and enhance in immunoglobulins and specific cytokines (Forestier *et al.*, 2001; Salvatore *et al.*, 2007).

Saccharomyces boulardii, a yeast used for a long time in diarrhea, is one of the well-studied probiotics and results have proved several mechanisms, namely neutralization of bacterial toxins, stimulation of host immune response, influence of inflammatory pathways (by nuclear factor-B, microtubule-associated protein kinase), enhancement of the maturation of brush border enzymes (lactase, sucrase, maltase, and aminopeptidase) and increase of glucose carriers in the enterocyte membrane via a 54-kDa protease, and the liberation of prolamine and soluble factors (Salvatore *et al.*, 2007).

Enteropathogenic microorganisms such as enterotoxigenic *E. coli*, *Shigellae*, and *Salmonella* are the main causes of acute diarrhea in travelers accounting for about 80% of the cases in which a pathogen was identified. This acute diarrhea is quite common and may occur in 10–60% of travelers; however, depending on the capacity of hydration and electrolytes reposition, usually it is a shelf-limited disease (Sullivan and Nord, 2002).

Culture cells have been used to prove the efficacy of probiotic bacteria inhibiting the adhesion of pathogen bacteria to gut cells. Using intestinal Caco-2 cell line, Forestier *et al.* (2001) reported the inhibitory effects of *L. casei* subsp. *rhamnosus* strain (Lcr35) on the adherence of three pathogens, enteropathogenic *E. coli* (EPEC), enterotoxigenic *E. coli* (ETEC), and *Klebsiella pneumonia*. Results indicated that for all bacteria, there was a decrease in the number of adhering pathogens. In addition, the supernatant obtained by LCR35 growth showed inhibition (but not bactericidal effect) upon nine human pathogenic bacteria, namely ETEC, EPEC, *K. pneumoniae, Shigella flexneri, Salmonella typhimurium, Enterobacter cloacae, Pseudomonas aeruginosa, Enterococcus faecalis,* and *Clostridium difficile.* Other probiotic strains and their combinations were also able to significantly inhibit the adhesion of *B. vulgatus, C. difficile, S. aureus,* and *C. sakazakii* (Salminen *et al.*, 2010). *L. acidophilus* and *L. reuteri* cell-free supernatants also prove to inhibit protozoan parasites of the genus *Cryptosporidium*, a leading cause of diarrhea in domestic livestock and humans worldwide (Glass *et al.*, 2004). The *L. acidophilus* and *L. reuteri* cultures reduced the infectivity of bovine C. *parvum* and *C. hominis* in a cell culture by 21–42% and 30–35%, respectively, as well as reduced oocyst viability 40–80% and oocyst infectivity up to 95%. Authors hypothesized that production of antimicrobial compounds may be a mechanism by which *L. acidophilus* and *L. reuteri* adversely affect bovine *C. parvum* and *C. hominis.*

It is important to highlight that this antimicrobial activity is probiotic strain dependent and the pathogen target is also quite variable. Tuomola *et al.* (1999) showed that the probiotic strains LGG and *L. rhamnosus* LC-705 slightly reduced S-fimbria mediated adhesion of *E. coli*, while adhesion of *S. typhimurium* was significantly inhibited by probiotic *L. johnsonii* LJ1 and *L. casei* Shirota.

An *in vitro* study in a reactor showed that two probiotics, *L. plantarum* 0407 and *B. bifidum* Bb12, combined with prebiotics (oligofructose and xylo-oligosaccharides) under batch conditions inhibit *E. coli* and *C. jejuni*, but only *C. jejuni* was inhibited under continuous conditions. Results suggested that the effect of acetate and lactate was responsible for antimicrobial activity, rather than the low culture pH (Fooks and Gibson, 2003).

Concerning the clinical trial studies, no effect of probiotics (or slight) to prevent traveler's diarrhea has been demonstrated, and in some studies, the clinical effects have been considered as minimal. However, in some cases, a significant reduction was observed, namely a reduction of clinical effects of 71% compared with 43% in the placebo group, but in this study, the placebo group showed a diarrhea abnormally high. The effect of drinking LGG strain was investigated in 820 travelers who traveled to two regions in Turkey. The effect of LGG was not significant in the combined results of the two regions, but the incidence of diarrhea was significantly decreased in travelers to one region (Nomoto, 2005). Others studies did not show enough evidence, namely in a placebo-controlled study on children, a group with invasive pathogens (*Salmonella, Shigella, Campylobacter, Yersinia,* or *Entameba*) did not reveal benefits on duration of diarrhea between children receiving LGG or placebo (Sullivan and Nord, 2002).

The most frequent side effect of antimicrobial therapy is antibiotic-associated diarrhea with relevant prevalence (5–25%). The antimicrobial treatment alters the ecological balance of the normal microflora, which can result in diarrhea and emergence of pathogens such as *C. difficile* (Sullivan and Nord, 2002). There are only two standard antibiotic treatments for *C. difficile* infection; the vancomycin and metronidazole and resistance to metronidazole has been increasing (McFarland, 2009). Probiotics may be used as an adjunctive therapy (given parallel with standard antibiotics vancomycin or metronidazole) for *C. difficile* infections, as several strains produce proteases that directly degrade *C. difficile* toxins or increase the immune response to *C. difficile* toxins A and B. Clinical trials combining probiotics with standard antibiotics have shown, in general, a significant reduction in the risk of *C. difficile* infections. Wullt *et al.* (2003) during a clinical trial compared the use of probiotic *L. plantarum* 299v (5×10^{10} cfu/day) combined with metronidazole with metronidazole alone during 38 days in the treatment of *C. difficile* infection. Results showed that the frequency of CDI relapses in probiotic group was four of 11 cases (36%) against six of nine cases (67%); however, due to the small size of the group (20 adults finished the study), the data collected could not prove to be of any statistical significance. On the other side, McFarland and Elmer (1997) mentioned a study using larger size group; they observed that the combination therapy of standard antibiotics (vancomycin or metronidazole) together with *S. boulardii* was shown to be effective in a placebo-controlled clinical trial of 124 with *C. difficile* infections. The recurrence of disease was found to be 26% in the yeast-treated group and significantly higher (45%, $P < 0.05$) in placebo group. Other studies have proven efficiency or lack significant differences as reported by McFarland (2009) during a complete revision, recommended for the reason that more research is required using efficient randomized controlled trials of sufficient size to detect significant differences and using different types of probiotics.

In fact, there is some evidence that different probiotics exert specific effects on diarrhea for specific pathogenic bacteria, but more studies on the mechanisms of action, particularly in clinical situations, are also required. In addition, to reduce contradictory results, studies must be more conscious with strain specificity, dose, and timing of supplementation.

3.3.3 Inhibition of Enteric Virus: Rotavirus

The major viral agents involved in human diarrhea include rotaviruses, caliciviruses (noroviruses and sapoviruses), enteric adenoviruses, and astroviruses. Among these, rotaviruses are one of the most important enteric virus, as it is responsible for about one-third of the cases of severe diarrhea in childhood in both developed and developing countries, accounting for 600,000 deaths in children under 5 years of age annually, almost exclusively in developing countries where they die especially due to the lack of dehydration (Colbére-Garapin *et al.*, 2007). Clinically, the intestinal mucosa is partially compromised and the GI normal microflora is disturbed, leading to diarrhea. The first episode is osmotic diarrhea and the second is associated with bacterial overgrowth. The common treatment includes oral rehydration, but several studies have reported that combinations with probiotic microorganisms shorten the duration of diarrhea (Sullivan and Nord, 2002).

It is well recognized that certain probiotics, such as LGG, *L. casei* Shirota, *L. reuteri*, *B. lactis* Bb-12, and a number of other probiotic strains, are effective against rotavirus by shortening the recovery time from diarrhea approximately by 1–1.5 days, reducing the shedding of rotaviruses or increasing the production of rotavirus-specific antibodies (Salminen *et al.*, 2010).

The main mechanisms against viral infection ascribed to probiotics have been reported as follows (Colbére-Garapin *et al.*, 2007):

Interference with a viral cycle at several levels, by specific or nonspecific mechanisms. Extracellular, they can inhibit the adsorption of virus, involving steric hindrance, or improve the barrier effects of mucus, glycocalyx, and intercellular junctions. If the virus adsorbs onto probiotics, it is not available to interact with eukaryote cell and fails to infect it.

Probiotics could also block viral attachment by competitive inhibition if they are able to bind viral receptors at the surface of intestinal cells. Probiotic binding to molecules adjacent to viral receptors could also confer some protection to cells.

Clinical trial studies using probiotics to prevent or reduce symptoms during diarrhea caused by rotavirus have demonstrated, in general, significant positive results. Nomoto (2005) and Salvatore *et al.* (2007) report several positive results during a complete revision. In general, these effects are positive demonstrating a reduction of the duration of viral diarrhea and significantly reduced rotavirus shedding as well as higher level of antirotavirus immunoglobulin A (see Table 3.2). Although some studies showed prevention of rotavirus diarrhea, few negative results were also reported; *L. paracasei* strain ST11 did not reduce the volume of fecal matter output in rotavirus infection but improved the outcome of non-rotavirus diarrhea in children from Bangladesh (Colbére-Garapin *et al.*, 2007).

Table 3.2 Positive effects (reduction of symptoms or prevention) of probiotic bacteria upon rotavirus diarrhea (compilation of clinical trials by Nomoto, 2005, and Salvatore *et al.*, 2007) observed in clinical trials

Probiotic strain	Patients	Main results
L. casei GG (2×10^{11} twice daily for 5 days)	71 children	Reduced significantly the duration of hospitalization in rotavirus diarrhea (1.4 versus 2.4 days)
L. casei GG (5×10^{9} cfu/g twice daily for 5 days)	123 hospitalized children (33% with rotavirus and 21% with bacterial diarrhea)	Reduced the duration of viral diarrhea (2.7 versus 3.7 days) versus 75% at 48 h

Probiotic strain	Patients	Main results
L. reuteri in different doses (10^7 and 10^{10} cfu/g once a day for 5 days).	66 hospitalized children	The probiotic shortened the duration of diarrhea with a dose-dependent effect (2.5 d in the placebo group versus 1.9 and 1.5 d in the *L. reuteri* groups, respectively)
LGG (3×10^9 cfu/g twice daily for a maximum of 6 days)	—	Reduction of the duration of diarrhea in outpatient children and significantly reduced rotavirus shedding
L. acidophilus LB [Lacteol Fort (Houdan, France), containing heat-killed lactobacilli, 10^{10} cfu/ 5 doses]	73 children with acute diarrhea (50% rotavirus positive)	Reduction in duration (43 versus 57 h in placebo)
Mixture of three *L. rhamnosus* strains (573L/1, 573L/2, and 573L/3) at a dose of 1.2×10^{10} cfu, twice daily, for 5 days	87 Polish children with infectious diarrhea	Significantly shortened the duration of rotavirus diarrhea (76 ± 35 versus 115 ± 67 h in placebo), but not of diarrhea of other aetiology
Formula supplemented with *B. bifidum* (1.9×10^9/g) and *S.* thermophilus (0.14×10^8/g)	55 hospitalized infants	Decrease in the number of the episodes of diarrhea (7 versus 31% of placebo), rotavirus shedding, and overall infections
L. reuteri SD 2222 strain (10^{10}–10^{11} CFU) for 5 days	Patients aged 6–36 months (75% were infected with rotavirus)	Shortened the duration of watery diarrhea, compared with the placebo group

(*Continued*)

Table 3.2 *(Continued)*

Probiotic strain	Patients	Main results
The test group was divided into powdered milk group, B. Bb12-supplemented powdered milk group, and B. Bb12 and *S. thermophilus*-supplemented powdered milk group	175 nursery school children aged 6–36 months in Thailand	The antibody titer (anti-rotavirus IgA - index of rotaviral infection) increased 4 times or more in 30.4% of the individuals in the control group who ingested powdered milk alone. No significant increase in the group that ingested *B.* Bb12 alone or with *S. thermophilus*.
Maternal milk or 10^{10} CFU LGG during hospital stay compared with artificial milk	220 patients aged 1–18 months	The incidence of rotaviral infection was significantly lower in patients fed maternal milk than in patients fed artificial milk, but daily preventive administration of probiotic did not decrease the incidence.
L. casei GG (1×10^{10} cfu twice daily for 5 days)	39 children with rotavirus enteritis	Significantly increased humoral immune response—a specific increase in immunoglobulins (G, A, and M) during the acute infection and a subsequent higher level of antirotavirus immunoglobulin A

Promising results from *in vitro* and *in vivo* studies have been obtained with probiotics on rotaviral infection, but further studies are required, in particular in the prevention of infection.

3.4 Prevention of Inflammatory Bowel Disease

Inflammatory bowel disease (IBD) is a chronic and recurrent inflammation generally affecting the colon or the small intestine.

This disease includes ulcerative colitis and Crohn's disease. The etiology of IBD remains unclear, but there is some evidence that the immune system reacts abnormally toward the endogenous microflora (Sullivan, and Nord, 2002). Whereas ulcerative colitis and Crohn's disease are both included in the term IBD, these conditions can be quite distinct, with different pathogenesis, inflammatory profiles, symptoms, and treatment strategies. Crohn's disease is predominantly a Th1-driven immune response, characterized initially by increased IL-12 expression, followed by interferon (IFN)-γ and tumor necrosis factor (TNF)-α. In contrast, ulcerative colitis has been associated with a Th2 immune response, leading to increased production of pro-inflammatory cytokines including IL-5 (Geier *et al.*, 2007).

Epithelial and immune cells of the intestinal mucosa recognize specific bacterial molecules via TLR and nucleotide-binding oligomerization domain (NOD) proteins such as receptors (NLR), and this interaction modulates the inflammatory response (activation of the NF-κB pathway) (Marteau *et al.*, 2009). Although NOD acts in a similar fashion to TLRs, NOD is present intracellularly, in the cytoplasm, as opposed to TLRs, which are located at the cell surface or in vesicles.

In the healthy gut, there is a symbiotic relationship between the host and the commensal bacteria in which contact leads to the downregulation of inflammatory genes, inhibiting the immune response of the gut to other pathogens. However, in the case of IBD, genetically predisposed individuals appear to lose the normal tolerance to commensal bacteria, leading to an elevated inflammatory response (Geier *et al.*, 2007).

Outstandingly, the first genetic polymorphisms found to be associated with a higher risk of IBD concern genes coding for NLRs (NOD2-CARD15) and TLRs (TLR4) [2]. The genetically determined modulation of defensin secretion is also significantly related with IBD. In addition, significant alteration of the intestinal microbiota has been frequently observed in patients with IBD, including instability of prevailing microbiota, reduction in biodiversity of Firmicutes, increased concentration of *Enterobacteriaceae*, and higher concentrations of bacteria in the mucus layer at the mucosal surface (Marteau *et al.*, 2009)

The number of agents used for treatment of IBD has increased, including corticosteroids, 5-aminosalicylic acid, immunosuppressives, elemental diets, antibiotics, and biological solutions (Fiocchi, 2006). So, it is thus coherent to try treatments that could modify intestinal microbiota in patients with IBD, including probiotics.

There are many different preparations of probiotics of which LGG, *L. johnsonii* LA1, *E. coli* Nissle 197, and VSL#3 (a combination of *S. thermophilus, B. breve, B. longum, B. infantis, L. acidophilus, L. plantarum, L. casei,* and *L. bulgaricus*), *L. reuteri,* and *L. salivarius* have been studied in IBD either in animal studies or in clinical trials. Several animal studies have been performed using different models of colitis and different probiotic bacteria. Pagninia and Cominelli (2006) extensively review these studies, which are summarized in Table 3.3.

Table 3.3 Summary of the published studies on probiotic bacteria utilization in animal models of IBD

Probiotic	Main results	Possible mechanism
L. reuteri	Improvement	—
LGG VSL#3	Improvement	Sulfhydryl compounds
L. salivarius	Improvement K reduction	Flora modification
L. plantarum	Improvement and prevention	Preventing downregulation of pro-inflammatory cytokines
B. infantis and *L. salivarius*	Prevention	Downregulation of Th1 pro-inflammatory cytokines
VSL#3	Improvement	Decrease barrier permeability
VSL#3	Improvement	TLR-9 mediated anti-inflammatory effect of DNA
VSL#3	Improvement of recurrent colitis	IL-10 dependent induction of regulatory cells
LcS	Improvement	Downregulation of pro-inflammatory cytokines (IL-6)

Source: Adapted from Pagninia and Cominelli (2006)

Concerning the clinical trials, several studies have been done in different forms of IBD, including pouchitis, ulcerative colitis, and Crohn's disease.

Pouchitis is more frequent when pouch-ileoanal anastomosis has been performed for IBD than for other forms of colonic diseases, and is associated with an imbalance of microbiota, and the antibiotics metronidazole and quinolone have proven efficacy (Marteau *et al.*, 2009). Two randomized, double-blind placebo controlled trials of VSL#3 in adult patients with ulcerative colitis after ileal pouch-anal anastomosis demonstrated a significant decrease in the incidence of pouchitis in the VSL#3 treated groups during a 1-year follow-up (Noble *et al.*, 2008); however, some other studies showed reduced evidence of positive effects on pouchitis, requiring more clinical studies to demonstrate the real feasibility of probiotic application in this condition.

Regarding the ulcerative colitis, three randomized, double-blind, placebo-controlled trials have shown that *E. coli* Nissle 1917 (ECN), commercialized in Germany (Mutafl or; Ardeypharm GmbH, Herdecke, Germany), was as effective as low doses of mesalazine to prevent relapse of ulcerative colitis; however, the efficacy of other probiotics in this condition is lower (Marteau *et al.*, 2009).

In contrast to pouchitis and ulcerative colitis, randomized controlled trials on the use of probiotics in Crohn's disease have been negative. One of the few positive results in Crohn's disease has been obtained in a small (n = 32) randomized controlled trial with the probiotic yeast *S. boulardii* versus mesalamine for preventing relapse in inactive disease (Cabré and Gassull, 2007).

The mechanism of action that supports the probiotic positive effects on IBD is still unclear. However, it is becoming apparent that the different probiotic bacteria act through multiple and concurrent pathways rather than by a single, common mechanism. The main possible mechanisms of action of probiotic bacteria include antagonism against pathogens, suppression of pro-inflammatory mediators, and induction of protective factors, namely mucosal trophism, intestinal permeability, and regulatory cytokines (Pagnini and Cominelli, 2006). In addition, they seem to enhance epithelial cell proliferation, inhibit apoptosis, and provide metabolic energy for enterocytes. Some studies with live and dead LGG showed attenuation of TNF-α-induced IL-8 production, often observed in human IBD. In addition, the bacterial DNA from VSL#3 was able to decrease IL-8 secretion, delay NF-κB activation, and stabilize IκB levels (Geier *et al.*, 2007). Fiocchi (2006) highlights the modulation of host immune response in IBD by probiotics assuming the changes of DC phenotype and function, modulation of NF-κB and AP-1 pathways, modulation of innate immunity through TLR engagement by CpG-DNA motifs, altered cytokine release, induction of Tregs, modulation of apoptosis, and induction of PPR-γ.

Probiotics and prebiotics may offer a new therapeutic option for the treatment of IBD; however, more double-blind, randomized, placebo-controlled trials are required. In addition, a greater understanding of the mechanisms behind their action on the GI microbiota is required in order to determine which probiotic is the most beneficial and how the genetic and bacterial profiles of the patient will influence treatment responsiveness.

3.5 Hypocholesterolemic Effect

Cholesterol-lowering effects of probiotics have been a target extensively studied in the last years and are well documented. Ooi and Liong (2010) recently published a review focused on this subject taking into account the *in vivo* and *in vitro* findings. Animal and human models have been used to evaluate the effect of probiotics on serum lipid profiles including cholesterol (Figueroa-González *et al.*, 2011). Several mechanisms have been indicated as responsible for the lowering effect by probiotics; probiotics that modulate hypocholesterolemic effects as proposed by several authors have been summarized in Fig. 3.5. In the review by Chen *et al.* (2011), several cholesterol-lowering functional foods are listed as well as their active ingredients and respective action mechanism; probiotic (lactobacilli and bifidobacteria) fermented dairy products are included in which hydrolysis of conjugated bile acids is indicated as the mechanism responsible for lowering cholesterol in serum blood.

Although much evidence exists of hypocholesterolemic potential effect of several probiotic strains on animals or humans (Baroutkoub *et al.*, 2010; Fazeli *et al.*, 2010; Jeun *et al.*, 2010; Ooi *et al.*, 2010; Shin *et al.*, 2010) with positive effects in lowering cholesterol with improvement of lipid profiles, this achievement is not absent of controversy. Studies refuting the hypocholesterolemic effect have been published by Hatakka *et al.* (2008b), Simmons *et al.* (2006), and Lewis and Burmeister (2005) with *L. rhamnosus* and *Propionibacterium freudenreichii* ssp *shermanii* (2×10^{10} cfu of each

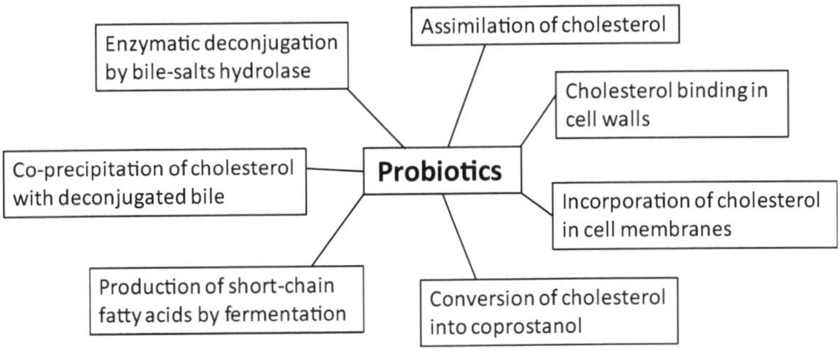

Figure 3.5 Proposed mechanisms by which probiotic bacteria can modulate hypocholesterolemic effects. Adapted from Lye *et al.* (2010) and Ooi and Liong (2010).

strain in two capsules daily) for 4 weeks in 38 men, *L. fermentum* (2 × 10^9 cfu/capsule, four capsules daily) for 10 weeks in 46 individuals, and with *L. acidophilus* (3 × 10^{10} cfu in two capsules; six capsules daily) for 6 weeks in 80 volunteers with high cholesterol. The authors did not find significant changes in the blood lipid profile. However, according to Guo *et al.* (2011) who performed a meta-analysis of 13 randomized controlled trials with 485 participants with high to normal cholesterol levels, they concluded that a diet enriched with probiotics decreases the total and low-density lipoprotein (LDL) cholesterol levels in plasma. Despite the strong evidences from the literature that probiotics could be used as an alternative way to drugs to low cholesterol in humans, more clinical evidence is still needed to totally assure this desirable effect, as it is known that the risk of heart attack in people with hypercholesterolemia is much higher than those who have normal blood lipid profiles (Ooi and Liong, 2010). More information is also needed about effective dosage of probiotics to exert potential hypocholesterolemic effect as well as to understand the underlying mechanisms of probiotics to reduce cholesterol levels in blood (Figueroa-González *et al.*, 2011). According to Ooi and Liong (2010), the probiotic dosage to be effective to exhibit hypocholesterolemic effects is strain specific. In the near future, better knowledge about dosage and associated mechanisms will allow better formulation to combat hypercholesterolemia. Interesting results have also been published with prebiotics (e.g., inulin) and symbiotic products to reduce cholesterol (Ooi *et al.*, 2010).

3.6 Treatment and Prevention of Allergy

During the last decades, an increasing prevalence of allergies could be observed in westernized countries. It is uncertain that genetics are the primary causative factor due to the quickness with which allergic disease has progressed. So, other factors are thought to be involved, namely the loss of microbial burden resulting from the more aseptic environment, a decrease in family size, a lack of physical exercise, and a change in nutrition. The "hygiene hypothesis" has been used as a base to explain the possible relation between microbial burden and allergy, assuming that children with hygienic backgrounds and a limited exposure to antigens from bacteria have a greater predisposition to suffer from allergies (Chalk and Chalk, 2003).

Allergies are associated with the generation of Th2-type cytokines, including IL-4, IL-5, and IL-13, which promote IgE production and eosinophilia. Initial signals to release IL-4, and thereby IgE and atopy, and IL-5 generated eosinophilic inflammation may originate from components of the innate immune system and structural components of bacteria (Isolauri, 2004). The intestinal mucosa and the mucosa-associated immune system are the primary local of allergen contact and stimulation of immune responsiveness, and are dependent on gut permeability. Antigens cross at the junctions between epithelial cells and activate our immune systems, forming antigen–antibody complexes. Antigen–antibody reactions can produce oxidants that lead to inflammation at distant sites in the body. In addition, areas of intestinal mucosa with reduced integrity are frequently brought about by local inflammation (Chalk and Chalk, 2003).

The original conception of infectious diseases providing protection from atopic disease by causing immune deviation in the form of TH1-driving signals that downregulate atopic TH2 responsiveness is explained by three relevant facts (Fig. 3.6).

First, the role of the indigenous intestinal microbiota might compensate the induced stimulus caused by infections in providing maturational signals to the infant's immune system.

Second, the role of the innate immune system and anti-inflammatory adaptive responses produced by TGF-β secreting TH3 cells and IL-10 secreting TR1 cells is beneficial. These intestinal Tregs through suppressive mechanisms can control inflammation of both TH1 and TH2 types and are thus implicated in protection against both atopic and autoimmune disease.

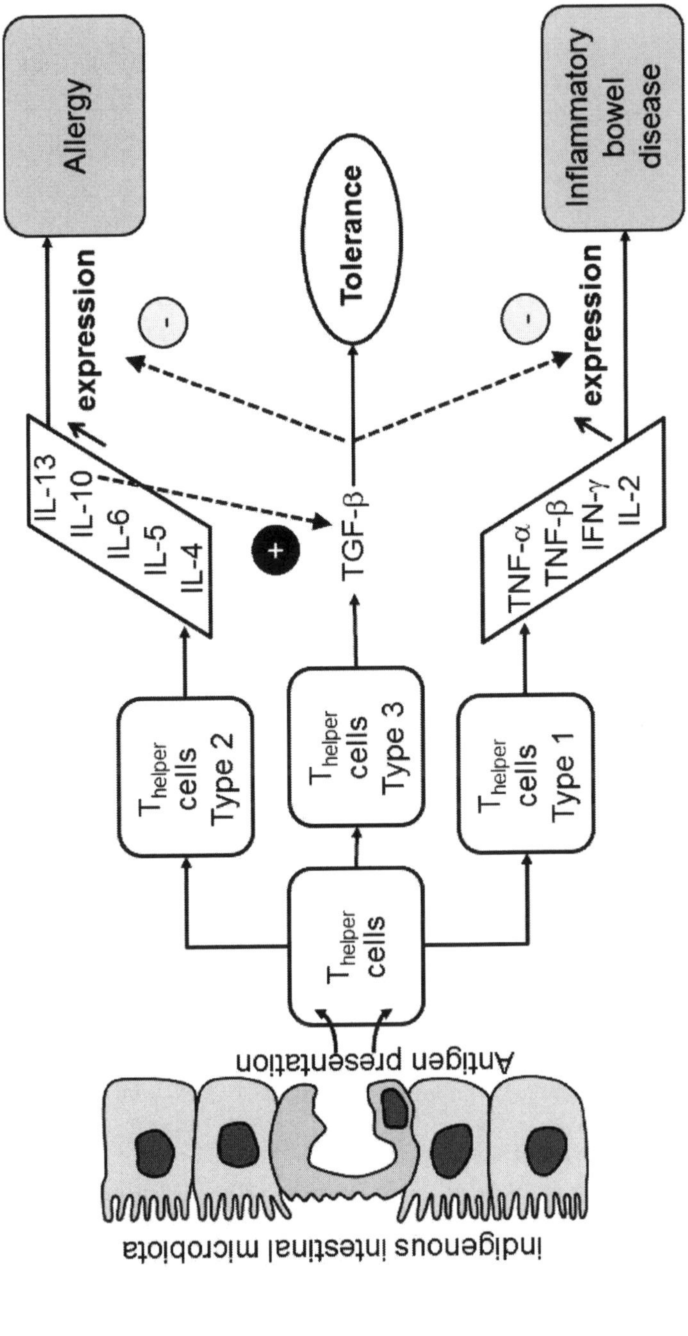

Figure 3.6 Anti-inflammatory role of the immune regulation and enhancement of gut barrier by probiotics. Adapted from Rautava *et al.* (2004).

Third, the development of proper and adequate immune competence as a result of contact with microbes might be essential not only in establishing a nonatopic immune responder phenotype but also in protection against infectious and autoimmune disease (Rautava *et al.*, 2005).

In fact, specific gut microbes may exert an immunosuppressive function by inhibition of the transcription factor NF-kB pathway (see Fig. 3.2). In addition, specific probiotic strains have been shown to counter allergy by the generation of IL-10 and TGF-β. The main effect results in the suppression in proliferation of Th cells and reduced secretion of pro-inflammatory cytokines, with control of IgE responses and reduced allergic inflammation in the gut (Isolauri, 2004). However, Viljanen *et al.* (2005) demonstrated that in LGG treated infants with IgE-associated atopic eczema–dermatitis syndrome, there was stimulation of the intestinal immune response and induction of low-grade inflammation [concomitantly increased IL-6 and C-reactive protein (CRP) levels] that might paradoxically alleviate allergic symptoms.

These evidences support the use of probiotics in supporting immunologic maturation and reducing the risk of disease (namely atopic and autoimmune; see Section 3.5) during immunological system development.

Most clinical studies explore the role of probiotics in the treatment of allergic disease, namely food allergy and atopic dermatitis. Studies in older individuals with established respiratory disease have failed to show any improvement except for a larger study that showed that probiotics can improve quality of life in patients with allergic rhinitis (Prescott *et al.*, 2007). Taylor *et al.* (2007) determined whether early probiotic supplementation prevents allergic disease in high-risk infants by using a group of infants whose mothers had a history of allergy (n = 231) and had received *L. acidophilus*. Although from the 178 infants who completed the supplementation period, the probiotic group has shown significantly higher rates of *Lactobacillus* colonization; they did not reduce the risk of AD in high-risk infants. However, the presence of *Lactobacillus* at 6 months of age was associated with an increased risk of subsequent cow's milk sensitization, which deserves to be investigated in further studies.

Recently, Ly *et al.* (2011) reviewed the efficacy of probiotic application in allergy. They reported a study of 132 infants with a family history of atopic, and the treatment with *L. rhamnosus* strain GG before and after birth split the risk of eczema [95% confidence interval (CI) for relative risk, 0.3–0.8] but not that of allergen sensitization. In a large and recent study of 925 mother–infant pairs, prenatal administration of probiotics (containing four bacterial strains) during the last month of gestation and postnatal administration of probiotics and prebiotics from birth to age 6 months resulted in short-lived changes in the neonatal gut flora and diminished the incidence of atopic eczema (but had no effect on other atopic ailments or allergic sensitization) at age 2 years. In general, these studies demonstrate an increased production of cytokines by Treg cells (IL-10 and TGF-β) associated with a reduced severity of atopic dermatitis in a small number of infants.

Concerning prevention of allergy, no study showed significant evidences to recommend probiotics. Regardless of all of the immunomodulatory effects described in experimental models, so far, none of these studies has shown any clear effect on preventive sensitization or any allergic disease other than eczema (Prescott and Bjorkste, 2007), which alerts us to the needs of further systematic studies. However, the study (Van Overtvelt *et al.*, 2010) of 11 lactic acid bacteria as an adjuvant for sublingual allergy vaccines has been performed as a promising application, in which they compared immunomodulatory properties of 11 strains as well as their capacity to enhance sublingual immunotherapy efficacy in a murine asthma model, proving that probiotics acting as a Th1/possibly Treg, but not Th1 adjuvant, potentiate tolerance induction via the sublingual route.

3.7 Reduction of the Risk Associated with Mutagenicity and Carcinogenicity

Colorectal cancers (CRCs) are a significant cause of mortality in Western countries. The disease development from normal epithelium to the acquisition of the malignant phenotype is accompanied by several biochemical and genetic alterations. It is known that a high level of carcinogenic substances is released into the intestine through the diet. Some carcinogens are formed in the colon, as intestinal microbiota is capable of hydrolyzing glycosidic linkages (occurring naturally in foods or formed in the liver and excreted via the bile) by producing β-glucosidase, β-glucuronidase, and β-galactosidase, leading to the release of potentially carcinogenic compounds (Hatakka *et al.*, 2008a). So, it is evident that diet and nutrition and the intestinal flora are key factors in modulating colon cancer onset and progression. As described in previous subchapters, it is evident that probiotics may modulate the activities of the intestinal microflora via different mechanisms, and some of them may also contribute to explain anticarcinogenic activity of probiotics. They seem to exert different effects along the various steps of carcinogenesis, in general summarized as antigenotoxicity, inhibition of the colic enzymes activity, controlling the growth of potentially harmful bacteria, interaction with colonocytes, and stimulation of the immune system and production of physiological active metabolites (Boutron-Ruault, 2007).

Several results strengthen the hypothesis of an antiproliferative effect of probiotics on the GI mucosa, in particular by affecting polyamine biosynthesis. Polyamines and their metabolizing enzymes are closely linked to neoplastic proliferation; so, any solution that reduces these components could be an efficient way of CRC chemoprevention and chemotherapy. This relation among cell proliferation, polyamines, and probiotics activity could be regulated by different elements, including (1) the specific metabolic activities of the probiotic strains, (2) different survival times in the lumen, (3) the period of administration, and (4) the proliferative behavior of different segments of GI mucosa (Linsalata and Russo, 2008).

In 2006, Capurso and collaborators analyzed existing data from *in vitro* models and animal and human (epidemiological and interventional) studies concerning the CRC. From the identified 29 animal studies aiming to establish the effect of probiotics administration on the incidence of CRC and/or of precursor lesions, most studies employed lactobacilli or bifidobacteria. In general, all studies had positive results (except three studies), and when prebiotics were also evaluated, relating the synergistic effect of such combination. In addition, the preventive effect on the CRC seems more important when they were administered before, and not after the carcinogen formation.

On the basis of the very few human epidemiological studies specifically designed to analyze the effect of probiotics on CRC incidence, it was possible to observe several important confounding factors, such as role of fibers, mixture with other dairy products, and presence of vitamin D. In general, the epidemiological studies have failed identifying significant effects of probiotic fermented milks against CRC. On the contrary, some interventional studies have suggested reduction of biomarkers for CRC risk, but others did not observed significant differences in the development of new CRC following administration of either fibers or probiotics in patients (Capurso *et al.*, 2006).

A very recent study (Stein *et al.*, 2012) demonstrated that the combined effect of probiotics and prebiotics on CRC is in fact positive, whereas isolated probiotics do not make enough evidence of cancer-preventive effect. The study demonstrated that wheat aleurone through the modulation of markers of primary chemoprevention may possibly have a cancer-preventive potential, which could be partially favored by the addition of the probiotics LGG and *Bifidobacterium* Bb12.

In general, the main mechanisms exhibited by probiotic bacteria toward the cancer inhibition can be explained by a group of activities that maybe dependent on the type of probiotic strain. Ouwehand *et al.* (1999) earlier described the possible mechanisms of probiotics on the inhibition of cancer (see Fig. 3.7).

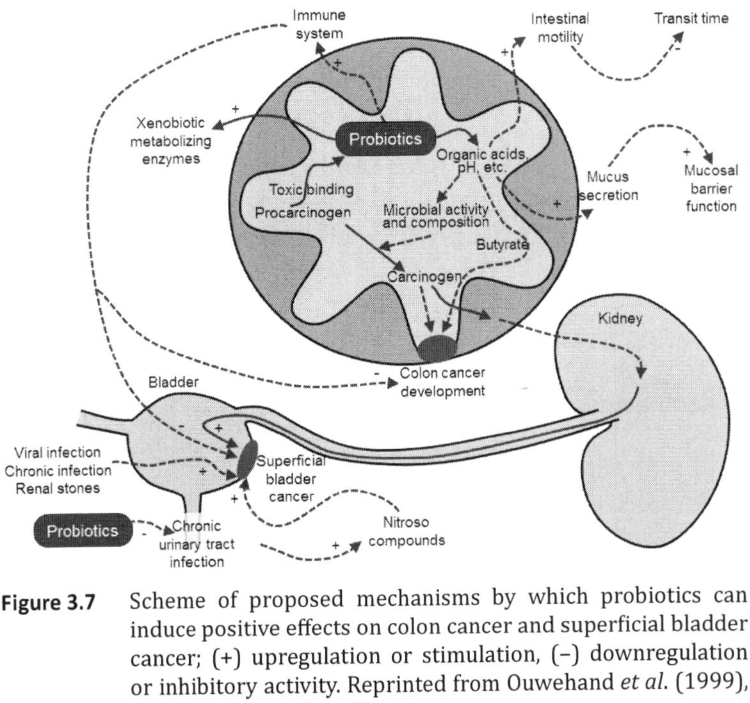

Figure 3.7 Scheme of proposed mechanisms by which probiotics can induce positive effects on colon cancer and superficial bladder cancer; (+) upregulation or stimulation, (–) downregulation or inhibitory activity. Reprinted from Ouwehand *et al.* (1999), with permission from Elsevier.

Such mechanisms include an alteration of the metabolic activities of intestinal microflora; an alteration of physicochemical conditions in the colon; the binding and degradation through enzymes of potential carcinogens; quantitative and/or qualitative modifications in the intestinal microflora implicated in producing carcinogen(s) and promoters (e.g., bile acid metabolizing bacteria); the production of antitumorigenic or antimutagenic compounds; an increase of the host's immune response; and effects on host physiology (Rafter, 2003). Specific strains of probiotic bacteria are able to downregulate intestinal microbial enzyme activities, leading to a decrease in the activity of carcinogen-activating microbial enzymes. This activity may be exerted in the colon, the urinary tract, and the bladder. The studies do not always find a reduction in the same enzymes, although findings with β-glucuronidase and nitroreductase are most consistently positive. Hatakka *et al.* (2008a) potentially demonstrated carcinogenic bacterial activity in human colon in a randomized, double-blind, placebo-controlled study including 38 healthy men with treatment periods of 4 weeks with *L. rhamnosus* LC705 together with *P. freudenreichii* ssp. *shermanii* JS (2×10^{10} cfu of each strain daily). The results showed an increase in the fecal counts of lactobacilli and propionibacteria and a decrease in the activity of β-glucosidase (10%) and urease (13%) enzymes; however, a decrease in β-glucosidase activity was related to the increasing counts of propionibacteria. It is also known that colon carcinogenesis involves a cytotoxic response on the colonic epithelium exerted by environmental compounds such as bile acids in the aqueous phase of the stools (soluble bile acids), followed by an increased proliferation of cells in the intestine. Administration of probiotics resulted in a lower concentration of soluble bile acids in feces and change of pH, which were related to tumor reduction. The probiotics may physically bind the bile salts, using the hydrolase active, *L. reuteri*, showed to control cell toxicity in the presence of bile salts (Commane *et al.*, 2005).

Mutagenic compounds, commonly released through the diet, namely 3-amino-1,4-dimethyl-5H-pyrido[4,3-b]indole (Trp-P-1, 2), can be bound to the intestinal and lactic acid bacteria *in vitro*, and some lactobacilli have also been shown to degrade nitrosamines. This binding or degradation correlated well with the reduction in mutagenicity observed after exposure to the bacterial strains (Rafter, 2003).

Simultaneously, the production of beneficial compounds such as SCFA (e.g., butyric acid) may improve mucosal nutrition and integrity. Another established mechanism to exert an antitumor effect includes their antimutagenic properties and ability to modulate immune parameters by increasing specific and nonspecific mechanisms, including T-cell, NK cell, and macrophage activity, which are important in delaying cancer development (Ouwehand *et al.*, 1999). On the contrary, it has been demonstrated to also induce the production of several cytokines, resulting in an inhibition of tumor growth. Concerning the bladder tumor, as viral infections have been suggested to play some role in bladder cancer, the antiviral properties of IFN-χ and TNF-α may be important.

Little evidence has been found in the application of probiotics on other cancers. LeBlanc *et al.* (2005) demonstrated the immune-regulatory capacity of milk fermented by *L. helveticus* R389 on the immune response in mammary glands in presence of a local breast tumor. Positive effects included increased IgA and CD4-positive cells, increased IL-10, and decreased IL-6 in mammary glands.

Nackerdien (2008) described that probiotics may be employed to reduce treatment side effects in breast cancer; probiotic adjuvant regimens may provide natural alternatives to pharmaceutical antiemetic therapy, currently being used in conjunction with the chemotherapy of this cancer. In addition, as pathogenic gut microbes have been associated with extra-intestinal tumor development in the breast, probiotics could be also involved in the preventive occurrence of these tumors as intestinal pathogen inhibitors. Using *L. casei* Shirota in superficial bladder cancer reduced recurrence of this tumor (Ouwehand *et al.*, 1999).

So, an effort must thus be made to identify the strains with the most prominent antitumoral characteristics and it will require a greater understanding of the mechanisms involved before we can fully justify their use as cancer prophylactics in humans. In addition, clinical investigators should design clinical studies using well-defined bacterial strains in predefined quantities and with appropriately chosen characteristics to elucidate the discrepant result existing between experimental and epidemiological evidences.

3.8 Effect on Urogenital Infections

Use of *Lactobacillus*-containing probiotics has been proposed to restore commensal vaginal flora for the treatment and prophylaxis of bacterial urogenital infections. In fact, the microbiota that covers epithelial cells in a healthy female genital tract lacks infectious pathogens but contains high populations of lactobacilli. However, this equilibrium can be affected by several factors, including hormonal concentrations, sexual activity, oral contraceptive use, glycogen content, vaginal pH, steroid therapy, immunosuppression, and diseases. So, dysfunction of normal microbial ecosystem, in particular decrease in lactobacilli, may lead to bacterial urogenital infections (Hoesl and Altwein, 2005).

Several *in vitro* and animal studies have proven that probiotic bacteria must accomplish at least two criteria: assure colonization of vaginal mucosa and possess inhibitory ability against urogenital pathogens. So, on the basis of this fact, three main *Lactobacillus* strains, namely *L.* rhamnosus GR-1, *L.* fermentum RC-14, and *L. crispatus* CTV-05, possess optimal properties to be effective as probiotic therapeutics against infections in the urogenital tract (Hoesl and Altwein, 2005). Mutaflor is a possible alternative probiotic in which the active agent is Nissle 1917 (a commensal *E. coli* strain that eradicates pathogenic bacteria from the GI tract), which may have the potential to prevent recurrent urinary tract infections (UTIs), as it adversely affected the growth of 34 of the 43 uropathogen isolates (Storm *et al.*, 2011).

The efficacy of *L. rhamnosus* GR-1 and *L. fermentum* RC-14 was evaluated in several clinical pilot studies. In 1995, a randomized, double-blind clinical trial showed that *L. rhamnosus* GR-1 and *L. fermentum* B-54 significantly reduce UTI rates (from 6 per year to 1.9 per year) when administered vaginally once weekly (Hoesl and Altwein, 2005).

Another study of 10 women and in a randomized, placebo-controlled trial of 64 women, daily oral intake of strains *L. rhamnosus* GR-1 and *L. fermentum* RC-14 resulted in a restoration of a normal vaginal flora in patients with asymptomatic bacteria vaginosis, and a significant depletion of yeast and coliforms. Direct application of lactobacilli into the vagina would be more efficient to reduce the associated symptomatology (Reid and Burton, 2002).

A prospective clinical pilot study was performed to confirm the safety and effectiveness of *Lactobacillus* vaginal suppositories against the recurrence of bacterial UTI. The strain used was *L. crispatus* GAI 98322, and in this study, a significant reduction in the number of recurrences was noted, without any adverse complication. The main mechanisms involved were believed to be its ability to produce hydrogen peroxide and to bind to vaginal epithelial cells (Uehara *et al.*, 2006).

In general, clinical trials use *Lactobacillus* doses at least 1.0×10^8 cfu per solid dosage formulation (oral capsule, intravaginal capsule, vaginal suppository, or vaginal tampon), at least 1.0×10^8 cfu/ml milk or yogurt, and 4.0×10^{10} cfu/100 ml cranberry–lingon berry juice administered for at least 5 days, involving at least 28 days of follow-up (Barrons and Tassone, 2008).

Although no significant *in vivo* evidence of mechanisms of action exists, data suggest that to be multifactorial and complex, it must involve (1) the ability to produce antimicrobial compounds such as lactic acid, bacteriocins, hydrogen peroxide; (2) the competitive exclusion of genitourinary pathogens; (3) the ability to produce a biosurfactant and collagen-binding proteins, which block pathogen adhesion that inhibits the adhesion of uropathogens to surfaces; and (4) the nonspecific augmentation of the innate immune system (Hoesl and Altwein, 2005; Uehara *et al.*, 2006).

Most of clinical trials were insufficient to show a treatment effect and failed to validate the dosing strategy by quantifying local bacterial colonization. So, future randomized controlled trials of the use of lactobacilli in bacterial genitourinary infections in women should be adequately implemented to detect treatment effects (Barrons and Tassone, 2008).

3.9 Benefits for the Healthy Function of the Liver and Pancreas

The relation between the positive effects of probiotics and liver health is not direct, but rather it seems to be more based on prevention; probiotic microflora can avoid the production or increase the uptake of compounds such as lipopolysacchrides (LPS) in the gut, which could leave to reductions in low-grade inflammation (Gratz *et al.*, 2010). According to the review by Jonkers and Stockbrügger (2007), the application of probiotic therapy in liver and pancreatitis diseases is promising and its positive effects are related with modulation of gut microbiota and the immune system being strain specific. Although mechanisms by which probiotics could be related to hepatic fat metabolism remain unclear, it seems that hepatic metabolism is influenced by the presence of probiotics in gut microflora, modulating intestinal barrier function. According to Gratz *et al.* (2010), the understanding of these mechanisms is of utmost importance in the future, because a set of liver disorders (low-grade inflammation, hepatic fat infiltration, hepatitis, and so on) will probably become more prevalent due to high-fat diets and increasing obesity; nonalcoholic fatty liver disease is one of the most common liver disease in some countries, the incidence of which has risen in patients suffering from obesity and type II diabetes. Probiotic therapy (lactobacilli and bifidobacteria) and/or prebiotic therapy (which increase bifidobacteria incidence in gut microflora) modulating the gut microflora could counterpart the negative effects of Gram-negative bacteria or pathogens, which are responsible for hepatic oxidative stress related to ethanol production and/or LPS (Cani and Delzenne, 2009). Similar positive effects in alcoholic liver disease or in patients with liver cirrhosis have been reported (Cani *et al.*, 2007; Zhao *et al.*, 2004). The levels of lactobacilli, bifidobacteria, and enterococci are reduced in alcoholics through probiotic therapy that is capable of improving liver function parameters such as alanine aminotransferase and aspartate aminotransferase (Kirpich *et al.*, 2008). Although more controlled trials are needed, it appears that the microflora is an important cofactor in the aetiology of chronic liver disease, and that probiotics might have a therapeutic role (Gratz *et al.*, 2010).

Bacterial translocation, due to factors such as bacterial overgrowth, disturbed intestinal motility or mucosal barrier, overproduction of proinflammatory cytokines, and so on, is one of the major causes of infectious complications in severe acute pancreatitis patients, which may be prevented by probiotics (Jonkers and Stockbrügger, 2007). However, Zhang *et al.* (2010), who performed a meta-analysis of use of probiotics, prebiotics, and symbiotics in acute pancreatitis patients, reported that neither showed a significant effect on this type of patients but reduced their length of stay in hospital. Kumar *et al.* (2011) also observed a positive effect of probiotic-fermented milk combined with chlorophyllin on gene expressions and genotoxicity during aflatoxin B1 induced hepatocellular carcinoma. The studies demonstrated an enhanced protective potential of probiotic-fermented milk with LGG and *L. casei* strain shirota combined with chlorophyllin (potent antimutagen) in hepatic cells during carcinogenesis induced by aflatoxin B1.

3.10 Oral Health: Promoting Properties

Oral applications have been tested in particular in the prevention of caries. On the contrary, the effect of probiotics on improving oral diseases such as gingivitis, periodontitis, and halitosis has been less explored. A possible danger is that these groups of organisms are acid producers and implicated in dental caries. Nevertheless, one potentially useful strain of *L. paracasei* retains its coaggregation activity with *S. mutans* when killed. There are some proofs that probiotic organisms, such as *L. reuteri*, can reduce the numbers of *S. mutans* in the mouth, but whether this would result in reduced levels of caries remains to be demonstrated (Wade, 2010). Recently, Bosch *et al.* (2011) summarized the clinical trials aimed to evaluate the effect of probiotics on oral health. They reported 12 clinical trials using probiotic strains in caries prevention, in which the main marker was *S. mutans*, mainly responsible for this disease. Most of the studies report a significant evident reduction of these bacteria after probiotic application. The main carrier of probiotic bacteria include food products, mainly dairy products—milk, yoghurt, ice cream, and cheese—as well as tablets, capsules, rinsing solution, chewing gums, medical device, and straw. The dose ranged between 9×10^8 and 1.4×10^{12} cfu/day. The main probiotics used were LGG, *L. reuteri*, *Bifidobacterium* DN-173 010, *B. lactis* Bb-12, and *L. paracasei*. Another study reported that including probiotics reduced the prevalence of oral *Candida*, in particular, in the elderly. Evidence of halitosis reduction was also reported with two bacteria: *S. salivarius* K12 and *Weissella cibaria*. *L. reuteri* has been also tested for gingivitis reduction on the basis of reduction of gingivitis and plaque in patients, and improvement of bleeding on probing and reduction of pro-inflammatory cytokines. *L. salivarius* WB 21 was successfully tested in periodontitis as well as ProBiora (a probiotic mouthwash) and *B. subtilis*.

Mechanisms of probiotic action within the oral cavity can possibly be by direct interactions within dental plaque, including the disruption of plaque biofilm formation through competition for binding sites on host tissues and other bacteria, and competition for nutrients as well as antimicrobial compounds (organic acids, hydrogen peroxide, low-molecular-weight antimicrobial compounds, bacteriocins, and adhesion inhibitors) that inhibit oral bacteria, which may also have a significant role.

Indirect probiotic actions within the oral cavity, including the modulation of aspects of both innate and specific immune function, were also reported (Allakera and Douglas, 2009).

3.11 Other Therapeutic Applications

Other therapeutic applications with limited studies have been described for probiotics. Effects of the probiotic *B. infantis* in the maternal separation model of depression showed that probiotic treatment resulted in normalization of the immune response, reversal of behavioral deficits, and restoration of basal noradrenaline concentrations in the brainstem. These findings point to a more influential role for bifidobacteria in neural function and suggest that probiotics may have broader therapeutic applications (Desbonnet *et al.*, 2010).

Forsyth *et al.* (2010) showed that LGG treatment ameliorates alcohol-induced intestinal oxidative stress, gut leakiness, and liver injury in a rat model of alcoholic steatohepatitis. This improvement was associated with reduced markers of intestinal and liver oxidative stress and inflammation and preserved gut barrier function.

Many probiotic organisms, including *L. rhamnosus* GR-1, have shown a significant promise in supporting the immune function of people living with HIV, as people infected with HIV often suffer from significant disturbances in nutritional status. In a review, Wilson *et al.* (2008) provided evidence that probiotics were supportive in modulating aspects of gut physiology, barrier integrity, and immune function. Probiotic use is a supportive adjunct therapy, worthy of consideration and further research in persons infected with HIV. Hemsworth *et al.* (2011) tested a micronutrient-supplemented probiotic yogurt for people living with HIV, which had very good acceptability and may be applied as a supportive adjunct therapy.

Another interesting application was studied by So *et al.* (2008) to elucidate whether *L. casei* affects the induction of oral tolerance in experimental rheumatoid arthritis. This study provides evidence that *L. casei* could potentiate antigen-specific oral tolerance and suppress Th1-type immune responses of arthritic inflammation. Other specific applications have been reported, but the results did not produce significant evidence, and more studies must be implemented in order to further explore more interesting applications.

3.12 Conclusions

The different mechanisms of action explored in this chapter may lead to relevant health benefits, namely in infection defence, prevention of cancer, in stabilizing or reconstituting the physiological balance between the intestinal microbiota and its host, and influencing immunological processes at different locations. However, it must be highlighted that one probiotic cannot exhibit all activities at the same time, at least not to that extent that it could be used for the prevention or cure of all mentioned kinds of disease. The overall effect attributed to a certain probiotic strain depends on the metabolic properties, the kind of surface molecules expressed, and components to be secreted with probiotic actions (Oelschlaeger, 2010).

The studies analyzed during this chapter will increase our knowledge concerning the functional attributes of known probiotics and facilitate probiotic product improvements.

The capability to control and envisage probiotic-based effects will permit both industry and the consumer to choose, based on science, the probiotics with well-known health benefits. These multidisciplinary efforts to develop more probiotics to be delivered through medication or food additives will increase available solutions to fight old and new diseases.

References

Allakera, R.P. and Douglas, I. (2009) Novel anti-microbial therapies for dental plaque-related diseases. *Int. J. Antimic. Agents,* **33**, 8–13.

Armuzzi, A., Cremonini, F., Ometti V., Bartolozzi, F., Canducci, F., Candelli, M., *et al.* (2001) Effect of *Lactobacillus* GG supplementation on antibiotic-associated gastrointestinal side effects during *Helicobacter pylori* eradication therapy: a pilot study. *Digestion*, **63**, 1–7.

Baroutkoub, A., Mehdi, R.Z., Beglarian, R., Hassan, J., Zahra, S., Mohammad, M. S. and Hadi, E.M. (2010) Effects of probiotic yoghurt consumption on the serum cholesterol levels in hypercholestromic cases in Shiraz Southern Iran. *Sci. Res. Essays,* **5**, 2206–2209.

Barrons, R. and Tassone, D. (2008) Use of *Lactobacillus* probiotics for bacterial genitourinary infections in women: a review. *Clin. Ther.*, **30**, 453–468.

Bhatia, S.J., Kochar, N., Abraham, P., Nair, N.G. and Mehta, A.P. (1989) *Lactobacillus acidophilus* inhibits growth of *Campylobacter pylori in vitro*. *J. Clin. Microbial.*, **27**, 2328–2330.

Bosch, M., Nart, J., Audivert, S, Bonachera, M.A.,Alemany, A.S, Fuentes, M.C and Jordi C. (2011). Isolation and characterization of probiotic strains for improving oral health. *Arch. Oral Biol.*, **57**, 539–549.

Boutron-Ruault, M.C. (2007) Probiotics and colorectal cancer. *Nutrition Clinique et Métabolisme*, **21**, 85–88.

Canducci, F, Cremonini, F., Armuzzi, A., Di Caro, S., Gabrielli, M., Santarelli, L., Nista. E., Lupascu, A., De Martini, D. and Gasbarrini, A. (2002a) Probiotics and *H. pylori* eradication. *Digest. Liver Dis.*, **34**, S81–S83.

Canducci, F., Armuzzi, A., Cremonini, F., Cammarota, G., Bartolozzi, F., Pola, P., *et al.* (2002b) A lyophilized and inactivated culture of *Lactobacillus acidophilus* increases *Helicobacter pylori* eradication rates. *Aliment Pharmacol Ther.*, **14,** 1625–1629.

Cabré, E. and Gassull, M.A. (2007) Probiotics for preventing relapse or recurrence in Crohn's disease involving the ileum: are there reasons for failure? *J. Crohn's Colitis*, **1**, 47–52.

Cani, P.D. and Delzenne, N.M. (2009) The role of the gut microbiota in energy metabolism and metabolic disease. *Curr. Pharm. Des.*, **15**, 1546–1558.

Cani, P.D., Neyrinck, A.M., Fava, F., Knauf, C., Burcelin, R.G., Tuohy, K.M., Gibson, G.R. and Delzenne, N.M. (2007) Selective increases of bifidobacteria in gut microflora improve high-fat-dietinduced diabetes in mice through a mechanism associated with endotoxaemia. *Diabetologia*, **50**, 2374–2383.

Capurso, G., Marignani, M. and Fave, G.D. (2006) Probiotics and the incidence of colorectal cancer: when evidence is not evident. *Digest. Liver Dis.*, **38**, Suppl. 2, S277–S282.

Chalk, C.S. and Chalk, A.J. (2003) Probiotics and allergy: current understanding and application for the PCCP (Primary Care Chiropractic Physician). *J. Chiropractic Med.*, **3**, 131–133.

Chen, Z., Ma K.Y., Liang Y., Peng C. and Zuo Y. (2011) Role and classification of cholesterol-lowering functional foods. *J. Functional Foods*, **3**, 61–69.

Colbére-Garapin, F., Martin-Latil, S., Blondel, B., Mousson, L., Pelletier, I., Autret, A., Francois, A., Niborski, V., Grompone, G., Catonnet, G., and van de Moer, A. (2007) Prevention and treatment of enteric viral infections: possible benefits of probiotic bacteria. *Microbes Infect.*, **9**, 1623–1631.

Commane, D., Hughe, R., Shortt, C. and Rowland, I. (2005) The potential mechanisms involved in the anti-carcinogenic action of probiotics. *Mutation Res.*, **591**, 276–289.

Desbonnet, L., Garrett, L., Clarke, G., Kiely, B., Cryana, J.F. and Dinana, T.G. (2010) Effects of the probiotic *Bifidobacterium infantis* in the maternal separation model of depression. *Neuroscience,* **170,** 1179–1188.

Fazeli, H., Moshtaghian, J., Mirlohi, M. and Shirzadi, M. (2010) Reduction in serum lipid parameters by incorporation of a native strain of Lactobacillus plantarum A7 in mice. *Iranian J. Diabetes Lipid Disord.,* **9**, 1–7.

Felley, C. and Michetti, P. (2003) Probiotics and *Helicobacter pylori. Best Practice Res.Clin. Gastroent.,* **17**, 785–791.

Figueroa-González, I., Cruz-Guerrero A. and Quijano G. (2011) The benefits of probiotics on human health. *J. Microbial. Biochem. Technol.,* **S1**:003.

Fiocchi, C. (2006) Probiotics in inflammatory bowel disease: yet another mechanism of action? *Gastroenterology,* **131**, 2009–2011.

Fooks L.J. and Gibson, G.R. (2003) Mixed culture fermentation studies on the effects of synbiotics on the human intestinal pathogens *Campylobacter jejuni* and *Escherichia coli. Anaerobe,* **9**, 231–242.

Forestier, C., De Champs, C., Vatoux, C. and Joly, B. (2001) Probiotic activities of *Lactobacillus casei rhamnosus*: *in vitro* adherence to intestinal cells and antimicrobial properties. *Res. Microbiol.* **152**, 167–173.

Forsytha, C. B., Farhadia, A. Jakate, S.M., Tanga, Y. Shaikha, M. and Keshavarziana, A. (2010) *Lactobacillus* GG treatment ameliorates alcohol-induced intestinal oxidative stress, gut leakiness, and liver injury in a rat model of alcoholic steatohepatitis. *Alcohol,* **43**, 163–172.

Geier, M.S., Butler, R.N. and Howarth, G.S. (2007) Inflammatory bowel disease: current insights into pathogenesis and new therapeutic options; probiotics, prebiotics and synbiotics. *Int. J. Food Microbiol.,* **115**, 1–11.

Glass, M.D., Courtneyb, P.D., LeJeunea, J.T., and Warda, L.A. (2004) Effects of *Lactobacillus acidophilus* and *Lactobacillus reuteri* cell-free supernatants on *Cryptosporidium* viability and infectivity *in vitro. Food Microbiol.,* **21**, 423–429.

Gotteland, M., Andrews, M., Toledo, M., Muñoz, L., Speisky,H. and Salazar, G. (2008) Modulation of Helicobacter pylori colonization with cranberry juice and *Lactobacillus johnsonii* La1 in children. *Nutrition,* **24**, 421–426.

Gratz, S.W., Mykkanen, H. and El-ezami, H.S. (2010) Probiotics and gut health: a special focus on liver diseases. *World J. Gastroenterol.,* **16**, 403–410.

Guo, Z., Liu, X.M., Zhang, Q.X., Shen Z., Tian, F.W., Zhang, H., Sun, Z.H., Zhang H.P. and Chen, W. (2011) Influence of consumption of probiotics on the plasma lipid profile: a meta-analysis of randomized controlled trials. *Nutrition Metab. Cardiovasc. Dis.*, **21**, 844–850.

Hamilton-Miller, J.M.T. (2003) The role of probiotics in the treatment and prevention of Helicobacter pylori infection. *Int. J. Antimic. Agents*, **22**, 360–366.

Hatakka, K., Holma, R., El-Nezami, H., Suomalainen, T., Kuisma, M., Saxelin, M., Poussa, T., Mykkänen, H. and Korpela, R. (2008a) The influence of *Lactobacillus rhamnosus* LC705 together with *Propionibacterium freudenreichii* ssp. shermanii JS on potentially carcinogenic bacterial activity in human colon. *Int. J. Food Microbiol.*, **128**, 406–410.

Hatakka, K., Mutanen, M., Holma, R., Saxelin, M. and Korpela, R. (2008b) *Lactobacillus rhamnosus* LC705 together with *Propionibacterium freudenreichii* ssp shermanii JS administered in capsules is ineffective in lowering serum lipids. *J. Am. Coll. Nutrition*, **27**, 441–447.

Hemsworth, J., Hekmat, S. and Reid, G. (2011) The development of micronutrient supplemented probiotic yogurt for people living with HIV: laboratory testing and sensory evaluation. *Innovative Food Sci. Emerg. Technol.* **12**, 79–84.

Hoesl, C.E. and Altwein, J.E. (2005) The probiotic approach: an alternative treatment option in urology. *Eur. Urol.*, **47**, 288–296.

Isolauri, E. (2004) The role of probiotics in paediatrics. *Curr. Paediatrics*, **14**, 104–109.

Jeun, J., Kim, S., Cho, S., Jun, H., Park, H., Seo J., Chung, M. and Lee, S. (2010) Hypocholesterolemic effects of *Lactobacillus plantarum* KCT3928 by increased bile acid excretion in C57BL/6 mice. *Nutrition*, **26**, 321–330.

Jonkers, D. and Stockbrügger, R. (2007). Review article: probiotics in gastrointestinal and liver diseases. *Alimentary Pharmacol. Therap.*, **26**, 133–148.

Kirpich, I.A., Solovieva, N.V., Leikhter, S.N., Shidakova, N.A., Lebedeva, O.V., Sidorov, P.I., Bazhukova, T.A., Soloviev, A.G., Barve, S.S., McClain, C.J. and Cave, M. (2008) Probiotics restore bowel flora and improve liver enzymes in human alcohol-induced liver injury: a pilot study. *Alcohol*, **42**, 675–682.

Kumar, M., Verma, V., Nagpal, R., Kumar, A., Gautam, S.K., Behare, P.V., Grover, C.R. and Aggarwal, P.K. (2011) Effect of probiotic fermented milk and chlorophyllin on gene expressions and genotoxicity during AFB1-induced hepatocellular carcinoma. *Gene*, **490**, 54–59.

Lam, E.K.Y, Yu, L., Wong, H.P.S., Wu, W.K.K, Shin, V.Y., Tai, E.K.K, So, W.H.L., Woo, P. C.Y, and Cho, P.C.Y. (2007) Probiotic *Lactobacillus rhamnosus* GG enhances gastric ulcer healing in rats. *Europ. J. Pharmacol.*, **565**, 171–179.

LeBlanc, A.M., Matar, C., Thériault, C. and Perdigón, G. (2005) Effects of milk fermented by *Lactobacillus helveticus* R389 on immune cells associated to mammary glands in normal and a breast cancer model. *Immunobiology*, **210**, 349–358.

Lewis, S.J. and Burmeister, S.A. (2005) A double-blind placebo-controlled study of the effects of Lactobacillus acidophilus on plasma lipids. *Eur. J. Clin. Nutrition*, **59**, 776–780.

Linsalata, M. and Russo, F. (2008) Nutritional factors and polyamine metabolism in colorectal cancer. *Nutrition*, **24**, 382–389.

Lorca, G.L., Wadstrom, T., Valdez, G.F. and Ljungh, A. (2001) *Lactobacillus acidophilus* autolysins inhibit *Helicobacter pylori in vitro. Curr. Microbiol.*, **4**2, 39–44.

Ly, N.P, Litonjua, A., Gold, D.R. and Celed. J.C. (2011) Gut microbiota, probiotics, and vitamin D: interrelated exposures influencing allergy, asthma, and obesity? *J. Allergy Clin. Immunol.*, **127**, 1087–1094.

Lye, H., Rusul, G. and Liong M. (2010) Removal of cholesterol by lactobacilli via incorporation and conversion to coprostanol. *J. Dairy Science*, **93**, 1383–1392.

Marco, M.L., Pavan, S. and Kleerebezem, M. (2006) Towards understanding molecular modes of probiotic action. *Curr. Opin. Biotechnol.*, **17**, 204–210.

Marteau, E. (2001) Prebiotics and probiotics for gastrointestinal health. *Clin. Nutrit.*, **20**, 41–45.

Marteau, P., Seksik, P. and Jian, R. (2002) Probiotics and health: new facts and ideas. *Curr. Opin. Biotechnol.*, **13**, 486–489.

Marteau, P. and Shanahan, F. (2003) Basic aspects and pharmacology of probiotics: an overview of pharmacokinetics, mechanisms of action and side-effects *Best Pract. Res. Clin. Gastroenterol.*, **17**, 725–740.

Marteau, P., Sokol, H., Dray, X. and Seksik, P. (2009) Bacteriotherapy for inflammatory bowel disease: therapeutic tool and/or pharmacological vectors? *Gastroentérologie Clinique Biologique*, **33**, Suppl. 3, S228–S234.

McFarland, L.V. and Elmer, G.W. (1997) Pharmaceutical probiotics for the treatment of anaerobic and other infections. *Anaerobe*, **3**, 73–78.

McFarland, V.L. (2009) Evidence-based review of probiotics for antibiotic-associated diarrhea and *Clostridium difficile* infections. *Anaerobe*, **15**, 274–280.

Mombelli, B. and Gismondo, M.R. (2000) The use of probiotics in medical practice. *Int.J. Antimicr. Agents.*, **16**, 531–536.

Myllyluoma, E., Kajander, K., Mikkola, H., Kyrönpalo, S. Rasmussen,M. Kankuri, E., Sipponen, P., Vapaatalo H. and Korpela, R. (2007) Probiotic intervention decreases serum gastrin-17 in Helicobacter pylori infection. *Digest. Liver Dis.*, **39**, 516–523.

Nackerdien, Z.E. (2008) Perspectives on microbes as oncogenic infectious agents and implications for breast cancer. *Medical Hypotheses*, **71**, 302–306.

Noble, A., Baldassano, R., and Mamula, P. (2008) Novel therapeutic options in the inflammatory bowel disease world. *Dig. Liver Dis.*, **40**, 22–31.

Nomot, K. (2005) Prevention of infections by probiotics. *J. Boiscl. Bioeng.*, **100**, 583–592.

Ockeloen, L.E. and Deckers-Kocken, J.M. (2012) Short- and long-term effects of a lactose-restricted diet and probiotics in children with chronic abdominal pain: a rctrospective study. *Comp. Therap. Clinical Practice*, **18**, 81–84.

Oelschlaeger, T.A. (2010) Mechanisms of probiotic actions—a review. *Int. J. Medical Microbiol.*, **300,** 57–62.

Ooi, L., Ahmad, R., Yuen, K. and Liong, M. (2010) *Lactobacillus acidophilus* CHO-220 and inulin reduced plasma total cholesterol and low-density lipoprotein cholesterol via alteration of lipid transporters. *J. Dairy Sci.*, **93**, 5048–5058.

Ooi, L. and Liong, M. (2010) Cholesterol-lowering effects of probiotics and prebiotics: a review of *in vivo* and *in vitro* findings. *Int. J. Mol. Sci.*, **19**, 2499–2522.

Ouwehand, A.C., Kirjavainen, P.V., Shortt, C. and Salminen, S. (1999) Probiotics: mechanisms and established effects. *Inter. Dairy J.*, **9**, 43–52.

Pagninia, C. and Cominelli, F. (2006) Probiotics in experimental and human inflammatory bowel disease: discussion points. *Digestive Liver Dis.*, **38** Suppl. 2, S270–S273.

Prescott, S.L. and Bjorkstén, B. (2007) Probiotics for the prevention or treatment of allergic diseases. *J. Allergy Clin. Immunol.*, **120**, 255–262.

Rafter, J. (2003) Probiotics and colon cancer. *Best Practice Res. Clin. Gastroenterol.*, **17**, 849–859.

Rautava, S., Kallioma, M. and Isolauri, E. (2005) New therapeutic strategy for combating the increasing burden of allergic disease: probiotics—A

Nutrition, Allergy, Mucosal Immunology and Intestinal Microbiota (NAMI) Research Group Report. *J. Allergy Clin. Immunol.*, **116**, 31–37.

Rautava S, Ruuskanen O, Ouwehand A, Salminen S, and Isolauri E. (2004) The hygiene hypothesis of atopic disease—an extended version. *J. Pediatr. Gastroenterol. Nutr.*, **38**, 378–388.

Reid, G. and Burton, J. (2002) Use of Lactobacillus to prevent infection by pathogenic bacteria. *Microbes Infec.*, **4**, 319–324.

Sabbi, T. and Palumbo, M. (2007) The role of probiotics during the antihelicobacter pylori triple therapy in children. *Digest. Liver Dis.*, **39**, A49–A87.

Salminen, S., Nybom, S., Meriluoto, J., Collado, M.C., Vesterlund, S. and El-Nezami, H. (2010) Interaction of probiotics and pathogens—benefits to human health? *Curr. Opin. Biotechnol.*, **21**, 157–167.

Salvatore, S., Hauser, B., Devreker, T., Vieira, M.C., Luini, C., Arrigo, S.,Nespoli, L. and Vandenplas, Y. (2007) Probiotics and zinc in acute infectious gastroenteritis in children: are they effective? *Nutrition*, **23**, 498–506.

Saxelin, M., Tynkkynen, S., Mattila-Sandholm, T. and de Vos, W.M. (2005) Probiotic and other functional microbes: from markets to mechanisms. *Curr. Opin. Biotechnol.*, **16**, 204–211.

Shin, H. S., Park, S.Y., Lee, D.K., Kim, S.A., An, H.M., Kim, J.R., Kim, M.J., Cha, M.G., Lee, S.W., Kim, K.J., Lee, K.O. and Há, N.J. (2010) Hypocholesterolemic effect of sonication-killed *Bifidobacterium longum* isolated from healthy adult Koreans in high cholesterol fed rats. *Arch. Pharm Res.*, 33, 1425–1431.

Simons, L.A., Amansec, S.G. and Conway, P. (2006) Effect of Lactobacillus fermentum on serum lipids in subjects with elevated serum cholesterol. *Nutrition Metab. Cardiovasc. Dis.*, **16**, 531–535.

Singh, K., Kallali, B., Kumar, A. and Thaker, V. (2011) Probiotics: a review. *Asian Pacific J. Trop. Biomed.*, S287–S290.

So, J-S., Leea, C.G., Kwona, H.K., Yia, H-J., Chaea, C.S. Parka, J.-A. Hwangb K-C. and Ima, S.H. (2008) *Lactobacillus casei* potentiates induction of oral tolerance in experimental arthritis. *Mol. Immunol.*, **46**, 172–180.

Steidler, L. (2001) Microbiological and immunological strategies for treatment of inflammatory bowel disease. *Microbes Infect.*, **3**, 1157–1166.

Stein, K., Borowickia, A., Scharlaua, D., Schettlera, A., Scheub, K., Obstb, U. and Gleia, M. (2012) Effects of synbiotic fermentation products on primary chemoprevention in human colon cells. *J. Nutritional Biochem.*, **23**, 777–784.

Storm, D.W., Koff, S.A., X Horvath, D.J., Li, B. and Justice, S.S. (2011) *In vitro* analysis of the bactericidal activity of *Escherichia coli* Nissle 1917 against pediatric uropathogens. *J. Urol.*, **186**, 1678–1683.

Sullivan, A. and Nord, C.E. (2002) The place of probiotics in human intestinal infections. *Int. J. Antimicrob. Agents,* **20**, 313–319.

Taylor, A. L., Dunstan, J.A. and Prescott, S.L. (2007) Probiotic supplementation for the first 6 months of life fails to reduce the risk of atopic dermatitis and increases the risk of allergen sensitization in high-risk children: a randomized controlled trial. *J. Allergy Clin. Immunol.*, **119**, 184–191.

Tuohy, K.M. Probert, H.M. Smejkal, C.W. and Gibson, G R. (2003) Using probiotics and prebiotics to improve gut health. *Drug Discovery Today,* **8**, 692–700.

Tuomola, E.M., Ouwehand, A.C. and Salminen, S.J. (1999) The effect of probiotic bacteria on adhesion of pathogens to human intestinal mucus. *FEMS Immunol Med Microbiol,* **26**, 137–142.

Uehara, S., Monden, K., Nomoto, K., Seno, Y., Kariyama, R., and Kumona, H. (2006) A pilot study evaluating the safety and effectiveness of *Lactobacillus* vaginal suppositories in patients with recurrent urinary tract infection. *Int. J. Antimicrob. Agents,* **28**, S30–S34.

Vasiljevic, T. and Shah, N.P. (2008) Probiotics—from Metchnikoff to bioactives. *Int. Dairy J.,* **18**, 714–728.

Viljanen, M., Pohjavuori, E., Haahtela, T., Korpela, R., Kuitunen, M., Sarnesto, A. Vaarala, O. and Savilahti, E. (2005) Induction of inflammation as a possible mechanism of probiotic effect in atopic eczema–dermatitis syndrome. *J. Allergy Clin. Immunol.*, **115**, 1254–1259.

Van Overtvelta, L. Moussua, H., Horiota, S., Samsonb, S., Lombardia,V., Mascarella, L., van de Moerb, A., Bourdet-Sicard, R. and Moingeona, P. (2010) Lactic acid bacteria as adjuvants for sublingual allergy vaccines. *Vaccine,* **28,** 2986–2992.

Zhang, M., Cheng J., Lu, Y., Yi, Z., Yang, P. and Wu, X. (2010) Use of pre-, pro- and synbiotics in patients with acute pancreatitis: A meta-analysis. *World J. Gastroenterol.*, **16**, 3970–3978.

Zhao, H.Y., Wang, H.J., Lu, Z. and Xu, S.Z. (2004) Intestinal microflora in patients with liver cirrhosis. *Chin J Dig Dis.*, **5**, 64–67.

Wade, W.G. (2010) New aspects and new concepts of maintaining "microbiological" health. *J. Dentistry*, **38**, S21–S25.

Wilson, N.L., Moneyham, L.D. and Alexandrov, A.N. (2008) A systematic review of probiotics as a potential intervention to restore gut health in HIV infection. *Mol. Immunol.*, **46**, 172–180.

Wullt M., Hagslatt M.J. and Odenholt I. (2003) *Lactobacillus plantarum* 299v for the treatment of recurrent *Clostridium difficile*-associated diarrhoea: a double-blind, placebo-controlled trial. *Scand. J. Infect. Dis.*, **35**, 365–367.

Chapter 4

Food as Vehicles of Probiotics

Ana C. Freitas,[a,b] **Dina Rodrigues,**[b] **Sérgio Sousa,**[c] **Ana M. Gomes,**[c] **and Manuela M. Pintado**[c]

[a]*ISEIT/Viseu-Instituto Piaget, Estrada do Alto do Gaio, Galifonge, 3515-776 Lordosa, Viseu, Portugal*

[b]*CESAM & Department of Chemistry, University of Aveiro, 3810-193 Aveiro, Portugal*

[c]*CBQF, Biotechnology School of Portuguese Catholic University, Rua Dr. António Bernardino Almeida, 4200-072 Porto, Portugal*

ana.freitas@viseu.ipiaget.pt, acfreitas@ua.pt

4.1 Introduction

The demand for functional foods has, over recent years, increased markedly (Siro *et al.*, 2008). These foods, when include probiotics and prebiotics as biologically active components, produce metabolic and physiological health benefits in addition to their nutritional properties or at least enhance the normal homeostatic mechanisms in the intestine. Considering that scientific evidences indicate that ingestion of some microbial strains provokes health benefits, which are extensively discussed in previous chapters, no clear indications exist about the effective dose for these strains; however, it has been consensual that high numbers of viable bacteria are recommended to assure probiotic foods efficiency. The viability and metabolic activity of probiotic microorganisms are important factors that should be controlled throughout processing operations, maturation

Probiotic Bacteria: Fundamentals, Therapy, and Technological Aspects
Edited by J. Paulo Sousa e Silva and Ana C. Freitas

ISBN 978-981-4411-62-2 (Hardcover), 978-981-4411-63-9 (eBook)
www.panstanford.com

period and storage of the food. Furthermore, the amount of intake and form of the probiotic food should be adequate for dietary purposes. The most popular functional food products on the market are those designed for improvement of gut health, particularly those that contain probiotics (Siró *et al.*, 2008). Probiotic bacteria are currently used to be incorporated in food products; however, some technological challenges must be faced when included in food matrices with more aggressive environments, namely high salt, acid or oxygen concentrations, or low temperatures. Nonetheless, in general, the beneficial effect of probiotic bacteria depends on its viability, requiring that food matrices as carriers assure their viability at high levels for entire shelf-life, to guarantee their passage throughout the gastrointestinal tract (GIT) and colonization of gut mucosa in order to exert beneficial effects.

The aim of this chapter is to provide a comprehensive overview on the advances in probiotic food, covering the technological issues, functionality aspects, and limitations of some foods as carriers of probiotics.

4.2 Dairy Products

Dairy products constitute the major group of products able to carry and deliver probiotic bacteria, and among them, fermented milks and cheeses are the most consumed around the world. Milk and dairy products possess nutritional characteristics that allow the growth and the survival of probiotic bacteria, namely the high content of lactose. In addition, some dairy products, especially fermented milks and cheeses, due to some of their characteristics such as pH and buffer capacity, their dense matrix, and their fat content offer additional protection to these microorganisms in their passage through the GIT, in particular against the acidic environment of the stomach (Grattepanche *et al.*, 2008; Cruz *et al.*, 2009a; Kiliç *et al.*, 2009; Souza and Saad, 2009).

4.2.1 Fermented Milks

Fermented milks are a traditional food, produced by mankind for thousands of years, which was created as a means to extend the shelf-life of different milks (e.g., cow, goat, sheep, mare, buffalo, camel, or yak). Historical evidence indicates the Middle East and the Balkans as the likely origin of these products, also responsible for the evolution of fermented milks through time as a consequence of their inhabitants culinary skills (Tamime, 2002). Nowadays, fermented milks are produced and widely consumed in many countries worldwide combining the traditional craftsmanship of the past with science development of the present where microbiology, enzymology, physics engineering, chemistry, and biochemistry all play an important role.

4.2.1.1 Definition, classification, market, and physiological role

There are many types of fermented milks. In the late past century, Kurmann (1984) attempted a classification scheme on the basis of starter culture growth requirements building a family tree for such purpose; in order to further account for the different metabolites produced by the prevailing microorganisms, Robinson and Tamime (1990) proposed an additional classification strategy (Fig. 4.1). Such specific cultures are responsible for the properties of fermented milks, such as consistency, texture, taste, aroma as well as the health benefits they may confer. Currently, existing legal standards have been set by the Codex Alimentarius (2003) in which fermented milks are described as belonging to one of four different groups (Fig. 4.1). According to the Codex Alimentarius (2003), standard fermented milks are those that are prepared from pasteurised or raw—whole, partially, or fully skimmed—milk or milk products (concentrated or powdered milk, whey, buttermilk powder, edible casein, or caseinates) by the specific action of detailed bacteria (Table 4.1) and/or yeasts, which proceed to multiply and convert lactose into organic acids, resulting in pH reduction with or without coagulation (isoelectric precipitation). The removal of whey after fermentation is not allowed in their manufacture, except for concentrated fermented milk. An important requirement is that the starter microorganisms added shall be abundant as well as viable and active in the product throughout the shelf-life; nevertheless, if the product is treated by heat after fermentation, naturally the requirement for viable microorganisms does not apply (Codex Alimentarius, 2003). Such specifications of live microorganisms are transversal to the probiotic concept and in many aspects may constitute real opportunities despite the major challenges for the food industry—the development of functional fermented milks. Apart from the standard fermented milks the Codex Alimentarius Standard (2003) also includes (i) concentrated fermented milks, which correspond to fermented milks in which the protein has been increased to a minimum of 5.6% before to or after fermentation (labneh is a common example); (ii) flavored fermented milks, which contain a maximum of 50% (w/w) of nondairy ingredients (sweeteners, fruits, or vegetables such as juices, purees, pulps, preparations, and preserves derived therefrom, cereals, honey, chocolate, nuts, coffee, spices, and natural flavoring compounds); and (iii) drinks based on fermented milks, which are also composite milk products, obtained by mixing standard fermented milk [minimum of 40% (w/w)] with water with or without the addition of other ingredients such as whey, other nondairy ingredients as well as flavorings.

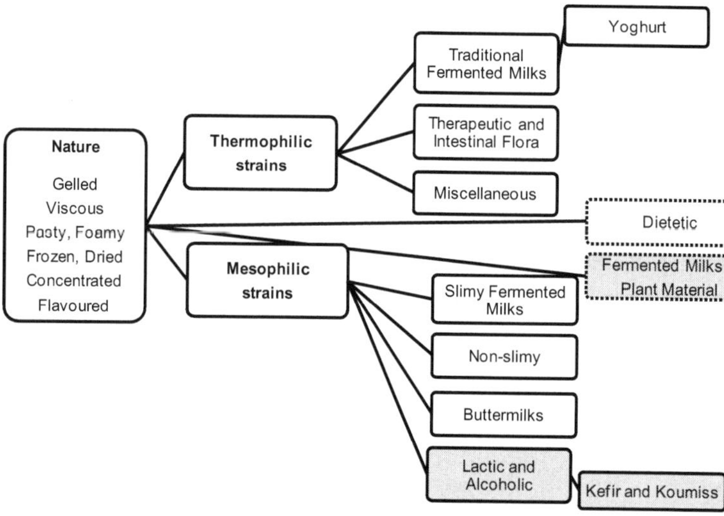

Figure 4.1 The family tree of fermented milks. Adapted from Kurmann (1984) and Robinson and Tamime (1990). All fermented milks are lactic fermentations (largest group worldwide) with exception of shaded boxes that may include lactic-yeast fermentations.

Table 4.1 Commercial products containing *Bifidobacterium* spp. and *Lactobacillus acidophilus* spp.

Product	Country	Microorganisms
Arla A-38	Denmark	*Lactobacillus acidophilus, Bifidobacterium bifidum, Leuconostoc mesenteroides* ssp. *cremoris,* mesophilic lactococci

Product	Country	Microorganisms
Acidophilus buttermilk	USA	*L. acidophilus, Lc. mesenteroides* ssp. *cremoris,* mesophilic lactococci
Progurt		*B. bifidum, L. acidophilus,* mesophilic lactococci
Acidophilus milk	Several countries	*L. acidophilus*
A-B Yoghurt	France, Serbia	*B. bifidum, L. acidophilus*
Cultura	Denmark	Ibidem
Milky	Italy	Ibidem
Nu-Trish A/B Milk	USA	Ibidem
Biomild	Several countries	*Bifidobacterium* spp., *L. acidophilus*
Acidophilus yoghurt	Several countries	*L. acidophilus, L. delbrueckii* subsp. *bulgaricus, Streptococcus thermophilus*
B-Active	France	*L. acidophilus, B. bifidum, L. delbrueckii* subsp. *bulgaricus, S. thermophilus*
Fresh BA	UK	Ibidem
Kyr	Italy	Ibidem
Yoplus	Australia	Ibidem
Biogarde	Germany	*L. acidophilus, B. bifidum, S.thermophilus*
Ofilus	France	Ibidem
Philus	Norway	Ibidem
Bifidus milk	Several countries	*B. bifidum, B. longum*
Bifighurt	Germany	*B. bifidum, S. thermophilus*
Biogurt	Germany	*L. acidophilus, S. thermophilus*
Biokys	Czech Republic	*B. bifidum, L. acidophilus, Pediococcus acidilactici*
Mil-Mil	Japan	*L. acidophilus, B. bifidum, B. breve*
Yakult	Japan	*L. acidophilus, B. bifidum, B. breve, L. casei* subsp. *casei*

(*Continued*)

Table 4.1 (*Continued*)

Product	Country	Microorganisms
Bifidus Milk/ Bifidus yogurt	Japan	*B. longum* BB536, *L. delbrueckii* subsp. *bulgaricus, S. thermophilus*
DanActive, Actimel	USA, Several countries	*L casei* DN114001, *L. delbrueckii* subsp. *bulgaricus, S. thermophilus*
BioK+	USA, Canada	*L. acidophilus* CL1285®, *L. casei* LBC80R
Activia	Several countries	*B. animalis* DN173 010, *L. delbrueckii* subsp. *bulgaricus, S. thermophilus*
Gefilus	Finland	*L. rhamnosus* GG

Source: Adapted from Gomes and Malcata (1999) and Douglas and Sanders (2008).

From a nutritional/functional perspective, functional fermented milks provide positive health benefits to the host either directly, via the interactions of ingested live microorganisms therewith (probiotic effect), or indirectly via the ingestion of a wide range of important nutrients and microbial metabolites generated as a consequence of fermentation (biogenic effect). Microbial metabolites may include bioactive peptides with antihypertensive activity, for example (Papadimitriou *et al.*, 2007; Gonzalez-Gonzalez *et al.*, 2011) or conjugated linoleic acid (Rodríguez-Alcalá *et al.*, 2011). Moreover, the production of several antimicrobial compounds (organic acids, bacteriocins, hydrogen peroxide) during fermentation contributes to increased protection against food contaminants or pathogens, thus playing an important biopreservation role. Increasing scientific evidence confirms that the risk for many chronic diseases such as cancer, osteoporosis, coronary heart disease, and hypertension can be diminished by the regular consumption of fermented milks and fermented milk supplemented with probiotics and/or prebiotics (Sanchez *et al.*, 2009; Panesar, 2011). The ingestion of probiotic fermented milks, in particular, has been shown to cure antibiotic-associated diarrhea, prevent intestinal tract infections, prevent ulcers related to *Helicobacter pylori,* prevent colon cancer, control rotavirus, promote alleviation of lactose intolerance symptoms, reduce irritable bowel syndrome inflammatory effects, improve immune system response, and lower cholesterol (Özer and Kirmaci,

2010). The health benefits of probiotics were reviewed in detail in Chapter 3.

Several probiotic fermented milks are available on the worldwide market, mainly incorporating members of the *Lactobacillus* and *Bifidobacterium* genera, and their existing positive image is well positioned to capitalize the growth of healthy foods consumed for their benefits as well as refreshing organoleptic quality. Some of these are listed in Table 4.1. The probiotic product segment of the functional foods market is continuously on the rise as specified by recent statistical data. Market research by Euromonitor (2008) revealed that the North-American market of probiotic spoonable yogurt market went from US$ 112 million in 2001 to US$ 294 million in 2006. For example, the sales growth rate of fresh probiotic dairy products in the USA in 2004 was much higher than cheese (9–10% vs. 2%) (Granato *et al.*, 2010; Özer and Kirmaci, 2010). Similarly in Europe, Euromonitor (2008) reported that the consumption grew 13% and nearly 18% per annum in Western Europe and in Eastern Europe between 2002 and 2007, respectively. The probiotic yogurt market in Latin America expanded 32% per annum between 2005 and 2007, and accounted for 30% of total yogurt market value in 2007 (Euromonitor, 2009). The European probiotic food and beverage market is estimated to reach $163 million by 2013 (Champagne, 2009; Özer and Kirmaci, 2010).

4.2.1.2 Technological challenges for probiotic fermented milks

Growth of the functional fermented milk sector is an opportunity to enhance the development of probiotic fermented milks into products with nutritional and sensory properties without resorting to costly and complex technology (Seleet *et al.*, 2011). Criterious management of technological and sensory aspects of the probiotic foods are very important aspects because only the satisfaction of consumers demand can lead food industry to success and promote the consumption of functional products (Mattila-Sandholm *et al.*, 2002). Apart from the sensory aspects, viability of probiotic bacteria in fermented milks and the associated probiotic effect also need to be accounted for by manufacturers. These factors have been the objective of many studies and are well documented in the scientific literature (Lacroix and Yidirim 2007; Özer and Kirmaci, 2010; Sanders and Marco, 2010).

4.2.1.2.1 *Milk selection*

The delivery vehicle in itself is an important starting point to consider, as its composition (inherently present compounds, eventual presence of other bioactive ingredients, fermentation end-products) influences probiotic viability and functionality, inducing changes in the cell composition and physiological status of the strain during production and throughout product shelf-life (Sanders and Marco, 2010). As mentioned in this chapter's introductory note, milk and derived products have a distinct role in delivery of probiotic bacteria to the human gut, as these products provide probiotic bacteria with a suitable environment in which not only their growth, viability, and stability are favored, but also their enzyme portfolio and consequent metabolic potential for the production of bioactive metabolites and flavor compounds is intensified (Gomes and Malcata, 1999; Saarela 2009; Özer and Kirmaci, 2010). Undoubtedly, bovine milk has been the most used carrier for fermented milk production worldwide; nonetheless, caprine and ovine milks have gained interest, especially in smaller traditional markets in different countries in the Middle East and Southern Europe where small ruminants milk is commonly produced (Gomes and Malcata, 1998; Gomes *et al.*, 1998a; Minervini *et al.*, 2009; Tamime *et al.*, 2011). From a fermented milk point of view, ovine milk is quite adequate for its manufacture, given its high protein and fat contents; on the contrary, caprine milk quite often requires undergoing protein fortification as well as adaptation of processing conditions in order to obtain sensory attractive products for the consumer (Hilali *et al.*, 2011; Tamime *et al.*, 2011). Albeit this technological handicap as far as good consistency is concerned, goat's milk has been successfully employed for the production of probiotic fermented milks with adequately selected strains. The mixed starter including *L. acidophilus* La5, *Bifidobacterium lactis* Bb12, and *Streptococcus thermophilus* has been reported to manufacture good fermented goat's milk with an inhibitory activity against *Escherichia coli* strains (Cutic *et al.*, 2004) and the same *Lactobacillus* and *Bifidobacterium* species attained high viable cell numbers in goat's milk fermented in a bioreactor and maintained good viability throughout 10 days of storage at 4°C (Kongo *et al.*, 2006). More recently, a selected multiple starter (*S. thermophilus* CR12, *L. casei* LC01, *L. helveticus* PR4, *L. plantarum* 1288) was shown to be adequate for the manufacture of a potentially functional fermented goat's milk, which maintained adequate viable cell numbers after 45 days of storage at 4°C and contained additional functional properties, that is, γ-aminobutyric acid and a significant Angiotensin-converting-enzyme (ACE)-inhibitory activity (Minervini *et al.*, 2009). In addition to milk type, agro-system production mode also seems to influence growth behavior of *B. lactis* in fermented milks. Although many defend that organic and conventional milks are similar in nutritional quality and wholesomeness, Florence *et al.* (2012) were able to show that organic milk was more suitable for production of fermented milks by *B. animalis* subsp. *lactis* strains Bb12 and BL04, thanks to its technological characteristics evidenced by the improvement in probiotic counts and superior levels of conjugated linoleic acid (CLA) isomers and α-linolenic acid (ALA) in the fermented products.

4.2.1.2.2 *Strain selection*

Despite milk qualities, production of high-quality fermented milk products containing *Bifidobacterium* spp. and *L. acidophilus* remains a major challenge to dairy industries owing to the vulnerability of the microorganisms in these products. In particular, bifidobacteria tend to exhibit weaker growth and acid production in milk, which implies longer fermentation periods and anaerobiosis conditions (Gomes and Malcata, 1999), low redox potential at least in the early phase of growth (Dave and Shah, 1997) and often the addition of bifidogenic and growth-promoting factors to the milk (Gomes *et al.*, 1998a; Özer and Kirmaci, 2010). Bifidobacteria produce acetic and lactic acids at the ratio 3:2 during fermentation, so excessive growth may yield unacceptable to consumers, yet such organoleptic hurdles have been duly overcome by tailor-made technological strategies.

As previously demonstrated in the case of caprine milk, strains need to be carefully selected and monitored throughout manufacture in order to guarantee desirable pH values and end-product metabolites. The use of combined cultures of bifidobacteria and other lactic acid bacteria, viz. *L. delbrueckii* subsp. *bulgaricus* and *S. thermophilus*, *S. thermophilus* alone, or mesophilic aromatic cultures, has been indicated as a way to overcome many of these problems (Tamime, 2002), reduction of fermentation time, control of sensory and texture defects, and nutritional improvement of probiotic fermented milks are some of the advantages that can be achieved by the use of combined cultures. In their recent study,

Xantophoulos *et al.* (2012) have been able to demonstrate the success of such binomial: nutritive value of carrier with potential functional properties of mixed strains. Yogurt was successfully produced from caprine milk by using two beneficial (cholesterol removal, resistance to bile salts, low pH, and lysozyme) lactobacilli isolates from newborn infant feces (*L. paracasei* subsp. *paracasei* DC412 and *L. acidophilus* DC602) as costarters with two strains of *S. thermophilus* and two *L. delbrueckii* subsp. *bulgaricus* isolates from traditional goat's milk yogurt. Growth of both *S. thermophilus* [$>10^9$ colony-forming units (cfu) per ml] and total lactobacilli ($>10^8$ cfu/mL) was enhanced along with improved acidification ability in milk, increased production of acetaldehyde, and a desirable consistency and organoleptic evaluation (4.4/5). However, in the case of mixed cultures, one must bear in mind the need to assess strain interactions in order to accurately select compatible strains and that the traceability of the probiotic strains becomes more difficult. Nonetheless, enumeration of culturable and nonculturable methods have evolved greatly and many validated solutions are available in literature (Gomes *et al.*, 2009; Rodrigues *et al.*, 2012a)

The probiotic species most frequently employed in the production of fermented milks are tentatively of human intestinal origin because it is generally accepted that they are better suited to the physiological needs of the host and can more easily colonize its intestine than wild strains or strains from the colon of other animals; however, it is important to note that human origin is not a requirement for probiotic functionality (Douglas and Sanders, 2008). Common strains include *Bifidobacterium adolescentis, B. bifidum, B. breve, B. infantis, B. longum, L. acidophilus, L. casei*, and *L. rhamnosus* (Gomes and Malcata, 1999; Sanders and Marco, 2010). A more comprehensive list is provided in Table 4.2.

General accounts of the physicochemical and technological aspects of commercial fermented milk products containing *Bifidobacterium* spp. and *L. acidophilus* have been provided by Tamime (2002), Sanchez *et al.* (2009), Ranadheera *et al.* (2010), and Panesar (2011).

A number of studies have been published related to characteristics of good probiotics and criteria for selection thereof (Sanders and Marco, 2010) as far as milk culturing capacity is concerned, simultaneous with the inherently required probiotic effect; these are summarized in Fig. 4.2.

Table 4.2 Species currently employed in the manufacture of probiotic products and respective sources

Species	Strain	Source
***Bifidobacterium* spp.**		
B. infantis	35264	Procter & Gamble
B. lactis	Bb12	Christian Hansen
	Ceska®-star B100	CSK Food Enrichment
	HN019 (DR10)	Danisco
B. animalis	LAFTI B94	DSM Food Specialities
	DN173 010 (*Bifidis regularis*™)	Danone
B. longum	BB536	Morinaga Milk Industry Co. Ltd.
B. breve	Yakult	Yakult Japan
***Lactobacillus* spp.**		
L. acidophilus	Ceska®-star A900	CSK Food Enrichment
	LA-1	Chr. Hansen
	LAFTI L-10	DSM Food Specialities
	LB	Lacteol Laboratory
	NCFM®	Danisco
	R0052	Institute Rosell-Lallemand
L. casei	DN114001 (*L. casei defensis*™)	Danone
	LAFTI L26	DSM Food Specialities
	Shirota	Yakult
L. fermentum	VRI003 (PCC)	Probiomics, Australia
L. johnsonii	Lj-1	Nestle
L. paracasei	CRL 431	Chr. Hansen
	F 19	Medipharm
L. plantarum	299V	Probi AB
L. reuteri	RC-14™	Chr. Hansen
	SD2112	Biogaia
	ATTC 55730	Arla-Ingman
L. rhamnosus	GG (LGG)	Valio Dairy Ltd.
	GR-1™	Urex Biotech
	HN001 (DR20)	Danisco
	LB21	Essum AB

(*Continued*)

Table 4.2 (*Continued*)

Species	Strain	Source
	271	Probi AB
	R0011	Institute Rosell-Lallemand
L. salivarius	UCC118	University College Cork
Others		
Lactococcus lactis	L1A	University College Cork
Propionibacterium freudenreichii ssp. shermanii	JS (DSM 7076)	Valio Dairy Ltd.

Source: Data compiled from Gomes and Malcata (1999), Douglas and Sanders (2008) and Ozer and Kirmaci (2010).

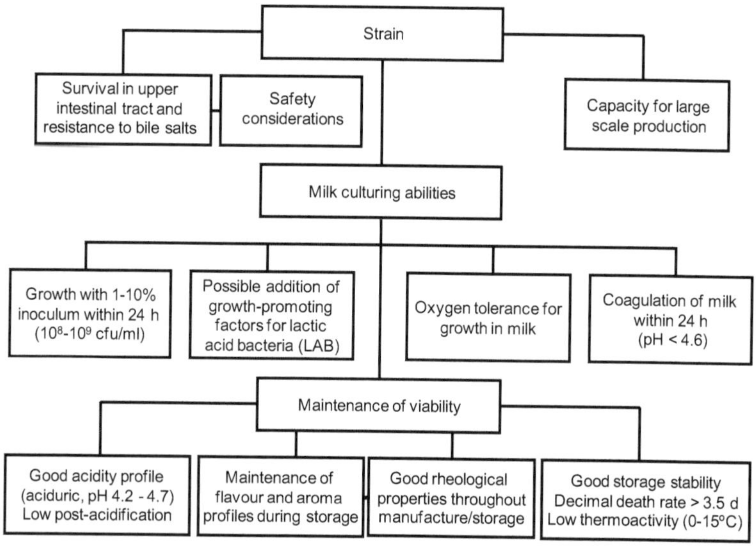

Figure 4.2 Criteria for selection of probiotic strains, in particular *Bifidobacterium* spp., for application as dietary adjuncts.

Important properties include tolerance to acid and bile, fundamental to maintain high numbers of viable cell throughout storage and passage in the digestive tract upon consumption (Gomes and Malcata, 1999; Douglas and Sanders, 2008), and production of antimicrobial substances and concomitant inhibition of pathogens. The strains selected also need to produce a final product with good sensory properties concerning flavor and texture; the delivery vehicle also plays an important role in this case, as it may enable improved product palatability, thus promoting regular consumption by the consumer. In order to improve the texture of fermented milks and yoghurts, several approaches have been proposed. For example, the application of hydrostatic or dynamic high pressure and the use of probiotic strains able to produce exopolysaccharides have been suggested as alternatives to the use of additives, which although allowed by the Codex Alimentarius standard (2003), may negatively affect the fermented milk taste, flavor, aroma, and mouth-feel (Patrignani *et al.*, 2006).

Not less important is that the strains selected are able to be produced in large scale (Sanders and Marco, 2010) and starter manufacturing technologies have largely evolved in such direction; strains selected for Direct-Vat-Set (DVS) starters must undergo concentration of up to 10^{10}–10^{11} cfu/g in order to permit the desired performance in commercial manufacture of fermented milk products. In addition, the starter must also have good stability (usually guaranteed for 3–12 months during processing, storage, and distribution). Direct inoculation of a dairy product with a frozen concentrated culture (ca. 5–10 x 10^{10} cfu/g) is recommended at a rate of 1 kg per 10,000 l of milk (Sanders and Marco, 2010). Finally, safety assessment of the probiotic strains is also a mandatory requirement; a tentative strain must be nonpathogenic for technological uses. There is a large consensus that lactic acid bacteria are benign microorganisms with a well-established record of safety and no record of food poisoning outbreaks. Updated reviews on safety of probiotic bacteria have been made available by Saarela *et al.* (2000), Borriello *et al.* (2003), Donohue (2006), and Bernardeau *et al.* (2008).

From a technological perspective, it is essential that designing of probiotic fermented milks considers five basic factors as a foundation for optimizing probiotic stability, namely (i) probiotic activity, (ii) manner of addition, (iii) composition of the finished food, (iv) processing condition and procedures, and (v) storage and other conditions prior to consumption. A more detailed description of each of these factors and its implications on probiotic fermented milk manufacture is addressed in Table 4.3. The selection of probiotic strains as well as manufacturing optimization (both formulation and storage conditions) are of utmost importance for growth and viability of probiotic bacteria in fermented milks (Martinez-Villaluenga *et al.*, 2006; Saarela *et al.*, 2006; Özer and Kirmaci, 2010).

Table 4.3 Main factors affecting probiotic viability and functionality from production to storage supported by recent studies.

Factor	Description	Case studies	References
		Improvement of stability in powders can be achieved by use of cryoprotectants, use of encapsulation technology where cysteine may be added to encapsulating material, or by application of mild sublethal stresses either during or after fermentation.	Corcoran *et al.*, 2004; Sousa *et al.*, 2012; Borges *et al.*, 2012.
		Selection of naturally occurring strains that lack post-acidification capacity enables development of fermented milks with acceptable sensory and rheological properties.	Damin *et al.*, 2008
Probiotic strain metabolic activity	- Besides added value to food, probiotics need to be cost effectively produced, maximizing substrate-to-biomass yield and stability during processing and shelf life.	Aerotolerance is a desired trait in probiotic strains intended for fermented milk production: Li *et al.* have isolated and selected an aerotolerant strain (high relative bacterial growth ratio), *B. animalis* subsp *lactis* Qq08, with high tolerance to low pH (84% survival at pH 2) and to bile (90% survival after 4.5 h incubation at 0.01 g mL^{-1} bile.	Li *et al.*, 2010
	- Probiotics need to maintain their functionality during storage as frozen or freeze-dried cultures.		

	- Different strains will behave differently under different manufacturing and storage conditions— tolerance to harsh conditions can be due to an intrinsic resistance or to an adaptive response.	Study of the technological and probiotic potential of the bile-adapted strain *B. animalis* subsp. *lactis* 4549dOx with respect to its parental strain IPLA4549 revealed its better ability to survive the simulated GIT conditions, and slightly higher adhesion capability to the model epithelial intestinal line HT29-MTX. Both parental and bile-resistant derivative strains maintained viability throughout fermented milk shelf-life.	Sanchez *et al.*, 2010
	- Different growth conditions may affect physiological activity and alter bacterial components with claimed probiotic activity or flavour-producing capacity. - Certain strains are capable of intense post-acidification contributing to loss of quality, off-flavours or texture deficiencies.	*In vitro* antimicrobial activity of probiotic strains depended on both growth temperature and growth stage for cell harvesting.	Fayol-Messaoudi *et al.*, 2005

(*Continued*)

Table 4.3 (*Continued*)

Factor	Description	Case studies	References
		L. plantarum harvested at different growth phases or when heat treated promoted different modulation profiles of NF-kB-dependent pathways in human mucosa (duodenal biopsies).	Van Baarlen *et al.*, 2009
		L. johnsonii grown in fatty acid–enriched minimal medium (oleic, linoleic or linolenic acids) revealed different membrane composition which impacted acid and heat tolerance, adhesion properties and caused a 2-fold decrease in *Salmonella enterica* serovar *typhimurium* UK1-lux invasion of HT-29 epithelial cells compared with bacteria grown in minimal medium alone.	Muller *et al.*, 2011
Manner of addition	- Reconstitution conditions may affect probiotic viability and stability in food matrix.	Reconstitution conditions such as buffer, pH, duration, sugar type and content and temperature may lead to variations in final viable cell numbers as large as 1 log cycle difference.	Mille *et al.*, 2004; Muller *et al.*, 2010
	- Addition of probiotic strains in a controlled delivery system may help regulate acidification capacity.	Incorporation of free and encapsulated probiotic bacteria did not significantly affect the overall sensory characteristics of yogurts yet microencapsulation promoted better survival of probiotic bacteria in yogurts during storage.	Kailasapathy, 2006

Composition of fermented milk	- Matrix properties inevitably affect probiotic functionality: oxygen content, high temperature, low pH, high water activity, elevated solute concentration and the presence of antimicrobial compunds and certain food additives may all affect probiotic strain viability.	Tailored (addition of carbon and nitrogen sources) fermented milk was able to maintain viability and *in vitro* stress-tolerance of potential probiotic *Propionibacterium freudenreichii* strain during minimum 15 days at 4 °C. *In vivo* efficiency was demonstrated by viability and short-chain fatty acids content in the colon of piglets. When given in the form of lyophilizate the *Propionibacterium* strain was not able to exert any positive effect.	Cousin *et al.*, 2012
	- Delivery vehicle is also essential for potential probiotic activity—metabolic activity and probiotic properties are, in some cases, only stimulated if fermented milk is the delivery vector.	A meta-analysis has shown that delivering probiotic strains via fermented milk products may be more efficient in eradication of intestinal *H. pylori* than delivering them via capsules or sachets.	Sachdeva and Nagpal, 2009
		Presence of available carbon sources such as glucose significantly increase survival of *L. rhamnosus* GG in simulated acidic stomach conditions.	Corcoran *et al.*, 2005

(*Continued*)

Table 4.3 (*Continued*)

Factor	Description	Case studies	References
Processing conditions and procedures		Compared to control fermentations without lactulose, the addition of such a prebiotic in skim milk increased counts of probiotics: *L. acidophilus, L. rhamnosus, L. bulgaricus and B. lactis* in co-culture with S. *thermophilus,* the acidification rate and the lactic acid acidity, and concurrently reduced the time to complete fermentation (tpH4.5) and the pH at the end of cold storage upon 35 days.	Oliveira *et al.*, 2011
	- Milk supplementation, culture composition and processing conditions may affect acidification, textural properties, and microbiological stability of fermented milks.	Fermented milk quality was influenced by both the co-culture composition (probiotic added to *S. thermophilus)* and the selected prebiotic: maltodextrin, polydextrose or oligofructose.	Oliveira *et al.*, 2009a
	- Manufacturing processes and matrix may affect the functionality of the strains and impact outcomes of clinical intervention studies.	Among 15 different *L. rhamnosus* isolates, 14 of which labelled and confirmed as *L. rhamnosus* GG, all revealed similar acid tolerance and binding capacity to human colonic mucus; yet, pathogen exclusion by inhibition and competition varied significantly among the different *L. rhamnosus* isolates and pathogens tested.	Grze kowiak *et al.*, 2011

Storage and other conditions prior to consumption	- Harsh environmental conditions or abuse in storage temperature or time may affect probiotic functionality.	Encapsulated probiotic bacteria were able to survive up to 1 log cycle better in stirred yoghurt than as free cells.	Krasaekoopt *et al.*, 2006
	- Microencapsulation is a protective technology that may increase stress tolerance and improve viability and stability during storage of fermented milks.	Viability of commercial *B. lactis* Bb12 and *L. acidophilus* La-5 in fermented milk was improved by 12% upon 21 d of refrigerated storage when raffinose was added.	Martinez-Villaluenga *et al.*, 2006;
		Viability of commercial *Bifidobacterium* spp. was improved by 55% upon 4 weeks of storage at 4°C when FOS was added.	Shin *et al.*, 2000

4.2.1.3 Survival characteristics

Strain viability in fermented milks by the time of consumption is mainly related to the aforementioned technological requirements. Suggested ranges for the minimum level for probiotic bacteria in probiotic fermented milks may vary according to the strain employed; nevertheless, a minimum value of 10^7 cfu/ml or 10^7 cfu/g of product is recommended (FAO/WHO, 2001; Codex Alimentarius 2003). Maintenance of this level is a challenging objective and industry normally applies significant overages during initial formulation in order to compensate drop in viability throughout storage. There are, however, many internal and external variables to the environment of fermented milks that may influence probiotic integrity, efficacy, and shelf-life. Acidity, pH, dissolved oxygen content, redox potential, sugar concentrations, solids content, presence of competitive microorganisms, storage temperature, and presence of microbial inhibitors (e.g., NaCl and H_2O_2) have been identified as having an effect on probiotic viability during the manufacture and storage of fermented milks (Siró *et al.*, 2008; Ranadheera *et al.*, 2010).

Examples with loss of viability have been reported for both *Bifidobacterium* and *L. acidophilus*, which are more often during refrigerated storage at low pH and high levels of dissolved oxygen (Dave and Shah, 1997; Donkor *et al.*, 2006), and reflect the need for careful strain selection. The use of microencapsulated cells to diminish dissolved oxygen and the addition of prebiotics are some of the most effective strategies of keeping the numbers of probiotic bacteria high enough for therapeutic effects (Özer *et al.*, 2005). Electrochemical reduction of milk, deaeration, or the addition of reducing agents such as cysteine enhanced the survival of oxygen-sensitive bifidobacteria in fermented milks (Gomes and Malcata, 1998; Gomes *et al.*, 1998a; Bolduc *et al.*, 2006). Probiotic bacteria, in particular *Bifidobacterium* strains, also need bifidogenic compounds or growth factors to be able to grow and survive in milk (Gomes and Malcata, 1999; Østlie *et al.*, 2003; Roy, 2005). Various substances have been added to milk for such purpose and favorable results have been achieved with fructooligosaccharides (Shin *et al.*, 2000; Varga *et al.*, 2006; Oliveira *et al.*, 2009b, 2011), raffinose family oligosaccharides (Martínez-Villaluenga *et al.*, 2006), maltodextrin and polydextrose (Oliveira *et al.*, 2009a), caseinomacropeptides and whey protein concentrate (Janer *et al.*, 2004), soy protein concentrate, soy flour and lentil flour (Zare *et al.*, 2012), lactulose (Oliveira *et al.*, 2011), tryptone, yeast extracts, certain amino acids, nucleotide precursors (Gomes *et al.*, 1998a), and a mineral source such as iron or zinc (Seleet *et al.*, 2011).

Other options currently pursued for improving viability include enhancement of bacterial stress response (Corcoran *et al.*, 2008) and quorum-sensing interference. The release of quorum-sensing signal molecules by probiotics may interact with human intestinal epithelial cells and contribute to the modulation of the different physiological functions mentioned previously in Chapter 2.

Although survival in fermented milks has been discussed herein as a challenge for probiotic strain stability, the relevance of the protective effect of fermented milk on passage through the GIT (Ranadheera *et al.*, 2010) should not be overlooked. Indeed, buffering capacity and pH have been indicated as the major reasons for such protection, yet how these properties regulate the metabolism and cellular processes of the probiotics at the molecular level is still unknown. Recent findings by Wang *et al.* (2012) unravel some of these phenomena for *L. casei* Zhang, a strain isolated from koumiss in Inner Mongolia, China. The authors used microarray technology to detect the gene expression profile of the *L. casei* strain with and without fermented milk (strain suspension) used as a carrier during transit in simulated gastrointestinal juice. Interestingly, a large proportion of genes involved in translation and cell division were downregulated in the bacteria that were in strain suspension during transit in simulated intestinal juice. This may hamper protein biosynthesis and cell division and may partially explain the lower viability of *L. casei* Zhang during transit in the GIT without the fermented milk (Wang *et al.*, 2012).

4.2.2 Cheeses

In the last decade, research efforts on the development of probiotic cheeses containing viable cells of *Lactobacillus* and *Bifidobacterium* sp. with potential health benefits have been made to lead this type of product into the functional foods category (Ross *et al.*, 2002). Cheese has been claimed as a good carrier of probiotic bacteria because it enables their passage as viable cells throughout the GIT (Gomes *et al.*, 1995; Mäkeläinen *et al.*, 2009). In addition, the organoleptic characteristics, nutritional values, and the suitability of cheeses to be consumed by several age groups (Gomes and Malcata, 1999) increase the importance of this kind of functional dairy product.

4.2.2.1 Strains, cell probiotic concentration, and viability

Nowadays, it is well known that probiotics are microorganisms, which, when present in adequate amount in food, should be able to resist to the passage through the GIT as well as to adhere to intestinal cells, in order to provide beneficial effects (Gomes and Malcata, 1999; Oliveira *et al.*, 2009c) and therefore viability of probiotics is a key parameter in a probiotic cheese. Due to the fact that cultures can vary significantly in their performance in cheese manufacture and ripening as well as in the intestinal environment, the selection of strains is crucial to the development of probiotic cheeses (Ross *et al.*, 2002). Apart from the clinical evidence that should support the health-promoting activity of probiotic cultures, the technological suitability of the probiotic strains is also a crucial parameter to their use in functional foods (Ross *et al.*, 2005). The main probiotic strains that have been used in different types of cheeses with more or less success are displayed in Table 4.4. The success of using these strains into cheeses is dependent on several factors, namely strain resistance to aggressive factors associated with the composition of cheese, the conditions of processing and ripening, as well as tolerance and competiveness to the lactic acid starters that must assure their viability in the cheese matrix.

Research studies on cheeses with bifidobacteria demonstrate that not all bifidobacteria species exhibit the same survivability or have equal role on the cheese characteristics. Some of the main constraints for the bifidobacteria are related with their susceptibility to oxygen, as they are generally anaerobic in nature (Boylston *et al.*, 2004). In addition, these strains differ in their ability to grow in milk, curdled milk, and in acidified matrices in the presence of starter cultures. However, studies especially with Cheddar, semi-hard, and white-brined cheeses demonstrate that some of the bifidobacteria such as *B. lactis*, *B. longum*, and *B. bifidum* are able to survive through relatively long periods of ripening such as 60 days at 12°C to 6 months at 4°C (Table 4.4). According to a review of Boylston *et al.* (2004) about the challenges of using bifidobacteria in cheeses, an evaluation of bifidobacteria strains viability in several cheeses such as cottage, Crescenza (Italian cheese), Canestrato Pugliese (Italian hard cheese), Fesco cheese, white-brined Tallaga (Egyptian

Table 4.4 Diversity of potential probiotic strains that have been tested in different types of cheese.

Strain	Type of cheese/ Ripening period	References
Bifidobacteria		
B. adolescentis	White brined cheese/60 days	Ghoddusi and Robinson, 1996
B. breve	Fresh cheese/57 days—4 or 12°C	Roy *et al.*, 1997
B. lactis B94	Semi-hard cheese/60 days—12°C Gouda semi-hard	Rodrigues *et al.*, 2011b
B. lactis BO	cheese/9 weeks—13°C	Gomes *et al.*, 1995
B. longum 1941	Cheddar cheese/6 mo—4°C	Ong *et al.*, 2006, 2007
B. bifidum Bb-02	White-brined cheese/90 days—4°C Cottage	Yilmaztekin *et al.*, 2004
B. infantis	cheese/30 days	Blanchette *et al.*, 1996
Lactobacilli		
L. acidophilus 4962	Cheddar cheese/6 mo—4°C	Ong *et al.*, 2006, 2007
L. acidophilus La-5	Curdled milk matrices/60 days—12°C Semi-soft	Rodrigues *et al.*, 2011a
L. acidophilus NCFM	Goudda cheese	Makelainen *et al.*, 2009
L. acidophilus ki	Goat cheese/70 days—5 and 10°C	Gomes *et al.*, 1998b
L. casei 279	Cheddar cheese/6 mo—4°C	Ong *et al.*, 2006, 2007
L. casei-01	Semi-hard cheese/60 days—12°C	Rodrigues *et al.*, 2011b
L. fermentum AB5-18	Turkish Beyaz cheese/120 days—4°C	Kiliç *et al.*, 2009
L. helveticus H100	Cheddar cheese/6 mo—4–12°C	Ong and Shah, 2008
L. paracasei L26	Cheddar cheese/6 mo—4°C	Ong *et al.*, 2006, 2007
L. plantarum AB16-65	Turkish Beyaz cheese/120 days—4°C	Kiliç *et al.*, 2009
L. rhamnosus	Cheddar cheese/32 weeks—9–10°C	Philips *et al.*, 2006
Enterobacteria		
Enterococcus faecium PR88	Cheddar cheese/9 or 15 mo—8°C	Gardiner *et al.*, 1999a,b
Propionibacteria		
P. freudenreichii ssp. *sherrmanii*	Cheese-based dips	Tharmaraj and Shah, 2004
P.freudenreichii	Suisse type cheese	Jan *et al.*, 2000
Lactococci		
Lact. lactis ssp. *lactis*	Fresh cheese/57 days—4 or 12°C	Roy *et al.*, 1997

cheese), Kariesh (Egyptian cheese) indicates that *B. bifidum* and *B. longum* were among the strains with higher levels of viability during the processing and storage, whereas *B. infantis* and *B. adolescentis* revealed lower survivability. According to Rodrigues *et al.* (2011 b, c), good levels of survivability of *B. lactis* B94 (10^9–10^{10} cfu/g cheese) were observed after 45–60 days of ripening, in a potential probiotic semi-hard cheese despite the harsh conditions of low pH values (4.1–5.1) and low moisture content (<30%, w/w).

The diversity of different strains of potential probiotic lactobacilli that have been incorporated in the cheese matrix is higher than those of bifidobacteria (Table 4.4). The use of facultative heterofermentative lactobacilli as mesophilic starters has a long tradition in cheese manufacture. More recently, the concept of using the lactobacilli strains as probiotic adjunct cultures has emerged (Johnson and Lucey, 2006; Cogan *et al.*, 2007). Potential probiotic lactobacilli strains isolated from traditional foods such as cheese have been proposed and studied in order to develop new functional foods (Bertazzoni-Minelli *et al.*, 2004). Lactobacilli strains possess a long history of safe use (Maragkoudakis *et al.*, 2006), and according to Bernardeau *et al.* (2008), 32 selected species of lactobacilli possess the Qualified Presumption of Safety (QPS) proposed by European Food Safety Authority (EFSA). These strains possess the added value of being naturally resistant to cheese matrix environment through manufacture and ripening processes being able to reach high levels of viable cells with positive impacts on the cheese sensorial characteristics. The potential probiotic *L. casei*-01 used as a starter, without adjunct cultures, reached values of 10^9–10^{10} cfu/g in a semi-hard cheese after 15 days of ripening, which remained almost constant until 60 days of ripening (Rodrigues *et al.*, 2011b,c). Several studies about the potential probiotic action of lactobacilli of dairy origin in GIT have been performed in the last years. For example, Maragkoudakis *et al.* (2006) evaluated the probiotic potential of 29 *Lactobacillus* strains of dairy origin through *in vitro* tests: *L. acidophilus*, *L. casei* Shirota, *L. casei* Imunitass, several strains of *L. paracasei*, *L. plantarum*, and *L. rhamnosus*. According to the authors, all strains revealed to be unaffected by pH = 3, pancreatin, and bile salts, but they exhibited variable bile salt hydrolase activity; some of the strains, namely *L. casei* Shirota ACA-DC 6002, *L. plantarum* ACA-DC 146, and *L. paracasei* subsp. *tolerans* ACA-DC 4037, were able to adhere to Caco-2 cells and also to inhibit the adhesion of

Escherichia coli and *Salmonella typhimurium* to Caco-2 cells. These results, associated with the fact that these three strains also induced the pro-inflammatory and anti-inflammatory cytokines secretion by human peripheral blood mononuclear cells, become good evidences of their potential probiotic action on human GIT. Probiotic strains such as *L. acidophilus* NCFM and *L. rhamnosus* HN001 incorporated in a semi-soft cheese survived to simulated gastrointestinal digestion in the upper GIT model, and increased their viable cells in the colon simulator in comparison to nonprobiotic cheese (Mäkeläinen *et al.*, 2009).

The use of enterococci in dairy products is controversial, although they have been reported as part of the adventitious flora of many raw or pasteurized milk cheeses and the general idea is that they play an important role in the ripening process. The majority of studies reporting the presence and influence of enterococci in cheese dated from the 1990s. However, some more recent works still point the influence of this group of microorganisms in cheeses such as Bryndza (Jurkovič *et al.*, 2006), Tolminc cheese (Majhenič *et al.*, 2005), Firode Sardo (Cosentino *et al.*, 2004), San Simon (Garcia *et al.*, 2002), and Terrincho (Pimentel *et al.*, 2007). One of the first strains tested and indicated as potential probiotic enterococci strain, *Enterococcus* PR88, was studied as probiotic adjunct cultures in Cheddar cheese (Table 4.4). According to Gardiner *et al.* (1999b), this enterococcal strain revealed being suitable for incorporation in cheese, as it remained viable at high levels (>10^8 cfu/g) after 9 months of ripening. Giraffa and coauthors, who in 1997 reviewed the risks and potential technological use of enterococci isolated from dairy products (Giraffa *et al.*, 1997), published a review about functionality of enterococci in dairy products in 2003 (Giraffa, 2003), exposing evidences that enterococci, furnished as adjunct starters or nonstarters, could have potential application in some fermented dairy products, but some care in terms of safety should be provided, as clinical research on enterococci indicates that the safety in their use must carefully be addressed before their application.

Dairy propionibacteria in food industry as starter cultures also have a long history of safe use. Propionibacteria have been reported as probiotic due to their ability to modulate some enzymatic activities and microbial flora within the gut. Mantere-Alhonen (1995) in a review about the use of propionibacteria as probiotic indicates the evidences that support their use as potential probiotics.

According to Roland *et al.* (1998), *P. freudenreichii* strain, which is normally found in the microflora of Suisse cheese type, is also able to stimulate bifidobacteria *in vitro* and in the human intestine; further studies about bifidogenic properties (enhancement of bifidobacteria strains) of *Propionibacterium* have been performed (Warminska-Radyko *et al.*, 2002; Kouya *et al.*, 2007). According to Vorobjeva *et al.* (2008), propionibacteria possess a set of physiological and biochemical properties that make them promising human probiotics with the added values that some strains are able to produce CLA isomers; these have received increasing interest in the last years because of their potential health effects such as antitumor, antiobese, antiatherogenic, antidiabetic, immunomodulatory activities, and so on.

Some studies were performed about the probiotic potential of *Lactococcus* strains, although they are commonly used as starter bacteria in the manufacture of several types of cheese. Strains of *Lact. lactis* ssp. *lactis* are pointed as potential new probiotics by Kimoto *et al.* (1999), but no intensive research on lactococci strains was published in the last decade.

According to Douglas and Sanders (2008), although it is not possible to accurately generalize about a minimum dose of probiotics needed for a beneficial effect in the gut, studies showing beneficial effects at numbers below 10^8 cfu per day are uncommon. According to trends reported by Health Canada (2009), the probiotic dosage should be referred to a food portion, that is, a serving size of product should contain a minimum level of 1.0×10^9 cfu of one of the eligible microorganism that is the subject of functional claim. Considering these guidelines, probiotic cheeses have been claimed to be adequate food products to deliver probiotic concentrations able to provide potential health benefits throughout the shelf-life of the product, which naturally depends on the strain as well as the technological aspects of cheese production (Fig. 4.3).

A review on developments in cheese cultures with protective and probiotic functionalities by Grattenpache *et al.* (2008) reported the viability of several probiotic cultures in different types of cheese from studies reported between 1994 and 2007; a range between 10^6 and 10^9 cfu/g is reported as cell concentration at the beginning of ripening period, whereas values ranging from 10^4 to 10^9 cfu/g are reported at the end of ripening period; the ripening period ranged between 14 days at 4°C for the Crescenza soft cheese (Gobetti *et al.*, 1998) and 32 weeks at 9–10°C for Cheddar cheese (Philips *et al.*,

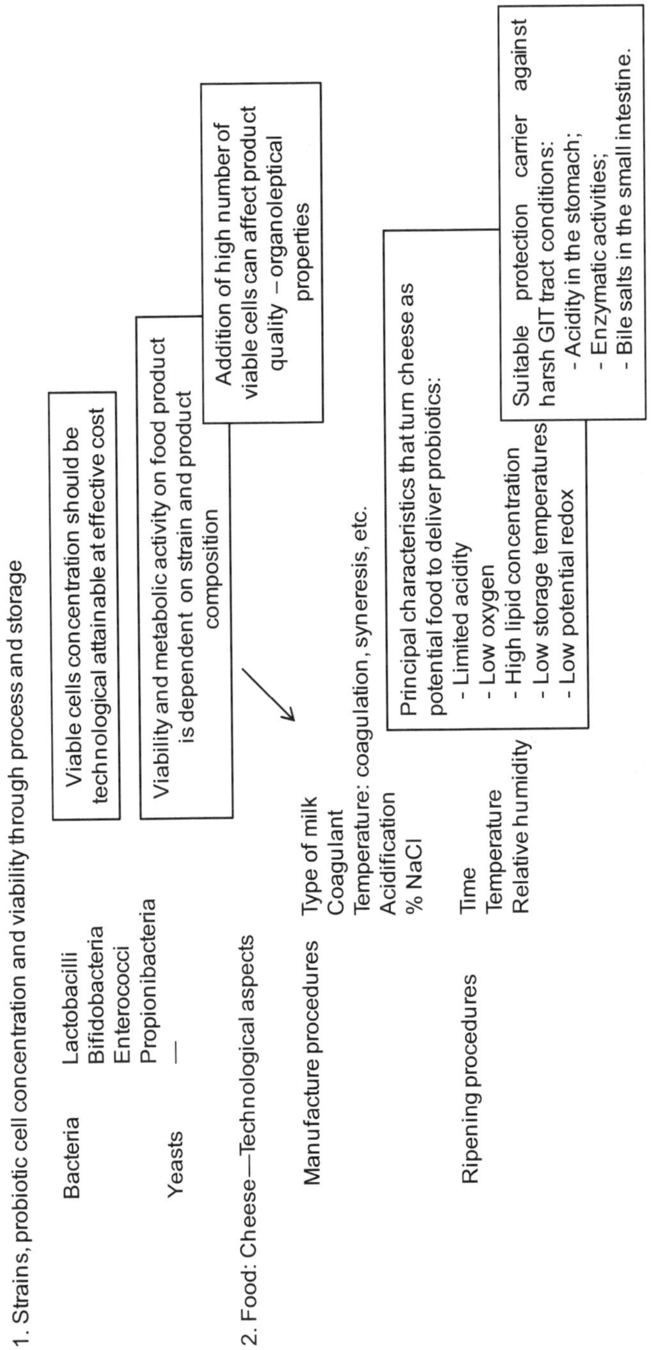

Figure 4.3 Probiotic cheese: parameters, keys, and limitations.

2006). Madureira *et al.* (2008) reported high levels of *L. paracasei* LAFTI L26 (>10^8 cfu/g) in sweet whey cheeses over 21 days at 7°C. The most recent works (2009–2012) concerning the development of probiotic cheeses are reported in Table 4.5. In addition, Karimi *et al.* (2011) in a recent review about viability of probiotic microorganisms in cheese during production and storage described that viability of probiotic bacteria in cheese had been satisfactory in the sense that at the end of ripening/storage, independently of their duration, the numbers of viable cells were above 10^6 cfu/g. According to the data displayed in Table 4.5, the numbers of viable cells varied between 10^7 cfu/g for *L. plantarum* cream cheese for 90 days and 10^{10} cfu/g for *B. lactis* semi-hard cheese for 60 days. These results allow confirming that cheese is a good vehicle of probiotic bacteria for the regular consumer.

Regardless of the high concentration of probiotic bacteria at the moment of consumption, research confirming their survival and resistance through the passage through the GIT is mandatory. Further research should be performed to assess the complex phenomena that probiotic cheese undergoes in each human GIT compartment. Mäkeläinen *et al.* (2009) studied the viability of probiotic lactobacilli in three models that simulated human GIT: upper GIT, human colon, and the colonocytes in cell culture experiments. These findings indicate that the studied lactobacilli strains in cheese matrix were able to survive in GIT.

As the large-scale production of probiotic bacteria at high concentrations of viable cells is sometimes difficult especially for less resistant strains, research efforts have focused its attention in improving the viability of probiotic strains during the production and shelf-life of the product (Ross *et al.*, 2005) such as cheeses. Microencapsulation of probiotic bacteria in suitable and protecting carriers to increase its concentration and improve its viability and functionality is a methodology that has been studied; some of the carriers include milk or whey proteins (Rodrigues *et al.*, 2011d), calcium alginate (Sousa *et al.*, 2012), or complex carbohydrates with prebiotic action (Chen *et al.*, 2005). Different results, however, have been reported; Gobetti *et al.* (1998) reported that immobilization of bifidobacteria strains in calcium alginate did not improved their viability in Crescenza cheese, in comparison to those nonimmobilized. In turn, some benefits of immobilization were reported by Dinakar and Mistry (1994) in Cheddar cheese after 24 weeks. More recent

Table 4.5 Viability of probiotic strains used as starter or as adjunct in different types of cheese reported between 2009 and 2012.

Cheese type	Probiotic strain	Process remarks	Ripening parameters/ Storage conditions	Viable cell counts (log cfu/g)		References
				Fresh cheese	Ripened cheese	
Pategrás cheese (semi-hard cheese)	*L. paracasei* *L. acidophillus* *B. lactis*	Probiotic strain used as adjunct; Starter culture: *Streptococcus thermophilus*	60 days/12°C /80 %HR	6.0–7.8 5.5–7.2 7.0–7.5	9.0 7.5–8.5 7.2–7.8	Bergamini *et al.*, 2009
Cream cheese	*L. plantarum* RL34	Cheese aseptically filled in plastic boxes	90 days/4°C	8.5	7.0	Georgieva *et al.*, 2009
Turkish Beyaz cheese	*L. fermentum* *L. plantarum*	Mixed probiotic culture Cheeses packed in plastic bags with brine	120 days/4°C	9.4	7.9	Kiliç *et al.*, 2009
Cremoso cheese (soft cheese)	*L. casei* I90 *L. plantarum* I91 *L. rhamnosus* I73, I77	Each probiotic strain used as adjunct; Starter culture: *Str. thermophilus.* Vacuum-packed cheeses.	60 days/5°C	–	7.4 8.2 7.3–7.7	Milesi *et al.*, 2009
Pategrás cheese (semi-hard cheese)	*L. casei* I90 *L. plantarum* I91 *L. rhamnosus* I73, I77	Each probiotic strain used as adjunct; Starter culture: *Str. thermophilus.*	60 days/12°C/80 %HR	–	8.7 8.9 8.6–8.7	Milesi *et al.*, 2009

(*Continued*)

Table 4.5 (*Continued*)

Cheese type	Probiotic strain	Process remarks	Ripening parameters/ Storage conditions	Viable cell counts (log cfu/g)		References
				Fresh cheese	Ripened cheese	
Cheddar cheese	*B. longum* 1941 *B. animalis* subsp. *lactis* B94 *L. casei* 279 *L. casei* L26 *L. acidophillus* 4962 *L. acidophilus* L10	Mixed probiotic culture used as adjunct; Starter culture: *Lactococus lactis* subsp. *lactis*, *Lact. lactis* subsp. *Cremoris* Vacuum-packed cheeses in oxygen barrier bags	24 weeks/4–8°C	8.3 8.4 8.0 8.1 8.3 8.2	8.3 8.5 7.9 8.3 8.0 7.9	Ong and Shah, 2009
White-brined Turkish cheese	*B. bifidum* Bb12 *L. acidophilus* La5	Microencapsulated probiotic strains Mixed probiotic culture used as adjunct; Starter culture: *Lact. lactis* subsp. *lactis*, *Lact. lactis* subsp. *cremoris*. Cheese stored in a pasteurized brine solution	90 days/4°C	9.0–10.0 10.0–11.0	8.0–9.0 8.5–9.5	Ozer *et al.*, 2009
Minas fresh cheese	*L. acidophilus* La5	Probiotic added solely or in coculture with starter culture: *Str. Thermophilus* Vacuum-packed cheeses	21 days/5°C	6.0–6.2	6.3–6.6	Sousa and Saad, 2009

Cheese type	Probiotic strain	Process remarks	Ripening parameters/ Storage conditions	Viable cell counts (log cfu/g)		References
				Fresh cheese	Ripened cheese	
Argentinian fresh cheese	*L. paracasei* A13 *B. bifidum* A1 *L. acidophilus* A3	Mixed probiotic culture used as adjunct. Starter culture: *Lact. lactis* A6, *Str. thermophilus* Vacuum-packed cheeses	60 days/12°C	6.6–6.8 7.3 6.5	8.5–8.8 6.7 7.4	Vinderola *et al.*, 2009
Synbiotic cottage cheese	*L. delbrueckii* UFV H2b20	Probiotic strain used as adjunct; Starter: Mesophilic lactic bacteria RA 073. Inulin used as prebiotic. Packed cheese.	20 days/5°C	–	8.2	Araujo *et al.*, 2010
Ras cheese	*L. casei* *L. acidophillus*	Mixed probtioc culture used as adjunct; Starter: *L. delbreukii* subsp. *bulgaricus* and *S. thermophilus*	90 days/12°C	–	8.3–8.4	El-Salam *et al.*, 2011
Curdled milk (similar to fresh cheese)	*L. casei* 01 *L. acidophillus* L10 *B. lactis* B94	Each probiotic bacteria used as starter	60 days/12°C	7.8–8.2 8.2–8.5 8.0–8.5	8.2–8.4 8.4–8.6 7.5–7.8	Rodrigues *et al.*, 2011a

(*Continued*)

Table 4.5 (*Continued*)

Cheese type	Probiotic strain	Process remarks	Ripening parameters/ Storage conditions	Viable cell counts (log cfu/g)		References
				Fresh cheese	Ripened cheese	
Synbiotic curdled milk (similar to fresh cheese)	*L. casei* 01 *L. acidophillus* L10 *B. lactis* B94	Each probiotic bacteria used as starter. 50:50 mix of fructooligosaccharides (FOS)/ Inulin used as prebiotic.	60 days/12°C	7.8–8.2 8.2–8.5 8.0–8.5	8.5–8.7 8.0–8.2 8.2–8.5	Rodrigues *et al.*, 2011a
Semi-hard cheese	*L. casei* 01 *B. lactis* B94	Each probiotic bacteria used as starter	60 days/12°C	8.0 8.0	9.9 10.0	Rodrigues *et al.*, 2011b, c
Synbiotic semi-hard cheese	*L. casei* 01 *B. lactis* B94	Each probiotic bacteria used as starter FOS or 50:50 mix of FOS/ Inulin used as prebiotic	60 days/12°C	8.0 8.0	9.8–10.7 9.9	Rodrigues *et al.*, 2011b, c
White soft cheese	*L. johnsonii* NRRL B-2178 *L. hhlgardi* NRRL B-1843 *L. curvatus* NBIMC 3452	Each probiotic culture used as adjunct; Starter: *L. delbreukii* subsp. *Bulgaricus* and *S. thermophilus.* Dextrin or polydextrose (LitesseTM) used as prebiotics (3%). Packed cheese.	30 days/7±2°C	8.39* 8.71* 8.68*	7.72* 7.75* 7.81*	Effat *et al.*, 2012

Cheese type	Probiotic strain	Process remarks	Ripening parameters/ Storage conditions	Viable cell counts (log cfu/g)		References
				Fresh cheese	Ripened cheese	
Domiati cheese	*L. casei* *E. faecium*	*L. casei* and *E. faecium* (1:1)used as starter Cheese made with reconstituted milk with normal and high content of CLA	60 days/25±5°C	>7.0	>7.0	El-Salam *et al.*, 2012
Caprine coalho cheese	*L. acidophilus* La5	Probiotic culture used as adjunct. Starter culture: *Lact. Lactis* subsp. *lactis, Lact. Lactis* subsp. *cremoris.* Packed cheese.	60 days/10°C	7.12–7.30	7.31–7.39	dos Santos *et al.*, 2012
Brazilian goat semi-hard cheese	*L. acidophilus* *L. paracasei* *B. lactis* *L. acidophilus+ L. paracasei + B. lactis*	Probiotic culture as well as mixed probiotic culture used as adjunct. Starter culture: *Lact. Lactis* subsp. *lactis, Lact. lactis* subsp. *cremoris.*	7 days/10°C	>6.0–7.0	>6.0–7.0	Garcia *et al.*, 2012

Lactobacillus viability obtained in white cheeses made with 3% dextrin studies indicate that cheese factors could affect the integrity of capsules, namely sodium ions, which could exchange with calcium ions responsible for binding alginate and consequently could be responsible for some disintegration of the capsules (Özer *et al.*, 2009). It is not desirable that probiotics changes the organoleptical properties of the final cheese, thus encapsulation could also be regarded as an approach to modulate the effects on cheese matrix. However, no consensual trend has been reported. For example, in Kasar cheese, microencapsulation did not appear to affect the composition, but higher levels of proteolysis were observed in cheeses with encapsulated probiotic bacteria (Özer *et al.*, 2009). In Feta cheese, no significant differences were observed in textural parameters between cheeses containing either free probiotic cells or encapsulated cells (Kailasapathy and Masondole, 2005). According to the facts previously discussed, it is clear that more research is needed to find different strategies to use probiotic strains in cheese, and encapsulation of bacteria in food-grade matrices, which could also protect their viability throughout gastrointestinal transit (Settani and Moschetti, 2010), should be also a subject of further investigation.

4.2.2.2 Cheese: Technological aspects

The viability and metabolic activity of probiotic bacteria are key factors that must be controlled and monitored throughout processing operations, maturation time, and storage of the food. Generally, addition of probiotic bacteria into milk-based food systems, including cheese, becomes a challenge in terms of maintaining probiotic viability and functionality during manufacture and shelf-life. The ripening period of cheeses, except for those consumed as fresh cheeses, is characterized by periods that could range from 20–30 days to months or even years for extremely ripened cheeses. The survival of probiotic strains during this time, at sufficient concentration, is crucial for functionality, namely to exert the probiotic effect in the GIT. What characteristics in cheeses are favorable or represent a limitation for higher levels of viability and metabolic activity of probiotic bacteria as well as a list of constraints that probiotic bacteria need to resist from both technological and intestinal perspectives are summarized in Table 4.6 in order to give the reader a global and simple perspective of the main constraints. The influence of the main factors that could affect the viability of

Table 4.6 List of constraints that probiotic bacteria need to resist, from both technological and intestinal perspectives, and cheese characteristics that could be favourable or unfavourable to overcome.

Physiological constraint	Description	Favourable/U nfavourable cheese characteristic	Examples of studied cases
Oxygen tolerance	Probiotic bifidobacteria and lactobacilli of gut origin are in general anaerobic or microaerophilic-strain dependent.	Cheese core can be considered as anaerobic environment with low redox potential.	Reported values of potential redox for Camembert core cheese through ripening were of –330 ± –30 mV (Abraham *et al.*, 2007).
Acid tolerance	Poor resistance under prolonged acidic conditions; In general bifidobacteria is more susceptible than lactobacilli.	In general, cheese presents higher and favourable pH values than fermented milks or yoghurts. The pH of hard and semi-hard cheeses, generally above 5.0 after production, remains relatively constant through ripening.	In 35-day ripened Camembert cheese pH values are 6.8 and 7.5 (Abraham *et al.*, 2007).
Ability to grow in milk	Probiotic bifidobacteria and lactobacilli of gut origin need to be able to grow in milk and raise the number of viable cells through cheese manufacture.	Milk is a very nutritive product and the majority of probiotic strains are able to ferment lactose.	10^9–10^{10} cfu g of *B. lactis* B94 and of *L.* casei-01 were reported in curdled matrices throughout 30 d of storage at 12 °C (Rodrigues *et al.*, 2011a).

(*Continued*)

Table 4.6 (*Continued*)

Physiological constraint	Description	Favourable/U nfavourable cheese characteristic	Examples of studied cases
Heat tolerance	Manufacturing process of some types of cheese involve steps of heating to temperatures above 40 °C.	Temperatures above 40 °C affect especially bifidobacteria survival in cheese. Modification on manufacture procedures should be accomplished to improve probiotic strains survival.	Higher viability of bifidobacteria due to lower heating temperature was achieved in Canestrato Pugliese cheese (Corbo *et al.*, 2001) .
NaCl	NaCl content in cheese influences directly water activity, which in turn affects the microbial growth and various enzyme activities. Additionally it contributes to the flavour of cheese.	Viability of probiotic strains is limited for NaCl concentrations above 4%.	Salt has been reported as the major limiting factor for the growth of probiotics in white-brined cheeses (Özer *et al.*, 2009).
Ripening	Days to weeks at 4 to 12 °C under high relative humidities (75–85 %RH) characterize the ripening process of the majority of cheeses.	The refrigeration temperatures associated with high levels of humidity help to limited water diffusion from cheese matrix.	High levels of probiotic lactobacilli or bifidobacteria (>10^8 cfu g^{-1}) have been reported in several types of cheese (Table 4.5).

Physiological constraint	Description	Favourable/U nfavourable cheese characteristic	Examples of studied cases
Non starter LAB (NSLAB) with antagonistic activity	The role of NSLAB is still not totally clarified. In ripened cheese, non-pathogenic adventitious bacteria (lactobacilli, etc.) can proliferate and become the dominant microflora of cheese.	The NSLAB presence in cheese could be minimized through incorporation of high levels of probiotic as adjuncts, starters or both.	The addition of *L. casei*-01 or *B. lactis* as starter, without adjunct cultures, reached values of 10^9–10^{10} cfu g^{-1} in 15 to 60 days semi-hard cheese and were the microflora present in the cheese throughout ripening (Rodrigues *et al.*, 2011b,c).
Passage through gastrointestinal tract	Lactobacilli are mainly acid tolerant or aciduric; Isolates of lactobacilli and bifidobacteria from harsh environment of the GIT are normally more resistant to both acid and bile.	Dairy products enhance microbial survival in gastric juice due to a buffering or protecting effect that could be related to milk proteins. Cheese matrix seems to protect probiotic bacteria in simulated GIT.	High survival for *B. bifidum*, *L. acidophilus* and *L. casei* in Argentinian Fresco cheese when subjected to a pH of 3.0 for 3 h at 37°C (Vinderola *et al.*, 2000). Probiotic strains in cheese survived in the simulated upper GIT and resulted in higher numbers of lactobacilli in the simulated human colon (Makelainen *et al.*, 2009).

probiotic bacteria in cheese has been the target of several published reviews. Karimi *et al.* (2011) discussed the main factors affecting viability of probiotic bacteria in cheese and categorized them into three areas, which include formulation, processing, and packaging. Technological aspects of probiotics were also recently reviewed by Bhadoria and Mahapatra (2011) updating some information reported by Cruz *et al.* (2009a) and Saarela *et al.* (2000).

It is well known that microorganisms in cheese play essential roles in their manufacture and ripening processes leading to the development of sensorial characteristics through their metabolism and enzymatic activities; they also have an impact in the microbiological safety of the product because they produce several low-molecular weight compounds with antimicrobial activity (Grattepanche *et al.*, 2008). Phenomena such as glycolysis, proteolysis, and lipolysis are the main biochemical reactions that take place during cheese ripening and are responsible for the degradation of carbohydrates, proteins, and lipids present in the curdled milk matrix. These reactions occur in a controlled environment as a result of the action of different enzymes that leads to the production of a wide range of metabolic compounds that are responsible for the organoleptic characteristics of cheese during maturation (Azarnia *et al.*, 2006) as well as to the generation of hurdle factors (organic acids, pH, and so on) that guarantee the safety of the cheeses.

In terms of gross chemical composition of cheese such as total protein and fat, salt content, and moisture, these are normally not influenced by the added probiotic strains. Variation of pH as well as the extension of glycolysis. In general cheeses with probiotic lactobacilli and bifidobacteria possess higher acetic acid content due to heterofermentation (Gomes *et al.*, 1998). According to Desai *et al.* (2004), acetic and lactic acid are produced by bifidobacteria in a molar ratio of 2:3; in terms of lactobacilli, they also produce acetic acid, but not so much as bifidobacteria.

Lactose maldigestion can be alleviated by β-galactosidase activities of probiotic bacteria, and according to Rodrigues *et al.* (2011a), lactic acid was significantly produced in both *L. acidophilus* and *B. lactis* B94 probiotic matrices and correlated well with lactose degradation.

According to several authors, the use of probiotic cultures in cheese does not affect necessarily the primary proteolysis, which is mainly derived from activity of the coagulant agent and plasmin and to a lesser extent from residual coagulant and starter microflora enzymes through ripening time. Reported results from Rodrigues *et al.* (2011a,b) pointed that enzymes from probiotic cultures could also have an important role in both primary and secondary proteolysis. Higher increases of water-soluble and nonprotein nitrogen fractions were observed throughout ripening time than with control matrices, which were coagulated with animal rennet but noninoculated (Rodrigues *et al.*, 2011a). In semi-hard probiotic cheeses, there was a significant increase of nonprotein nitrogen fraction in the first 30 days that was more pronounced for the probiotic cheeses (Rodrigues *et al.*, 2011b).

Influences on the secondary proteolysis with increases in free amino acid content are facts that have been reported in cheeses containing probiotics-viable cells (Ong *et al.*, 2006, 2007); higher levels for total amino acids were recorded in probiotic cheese inoculated with *L. casei*-01 than those inoculated with *B. lactis* B94 (Rodrigues *et al.*, 2011b). According to Requena *et al.* (1993), high activity of aminopeptidases is a characteristic of *L. casei* that is probably responsible for the higher contents of free amino acids in cheeses inoculated with this bacterium. Peptides and amino acids influence cheese flavor and they are potential precursors of flavor and aroma compounds.

Lipolysis during ripening is a phenomenon that also influences the development of the cheese organoleptic characteristics. Several authors agree in the fact that the addition of probiotic cultures does not appear to affect the free fatty acid (FFA) profile of cheese, probably due to a higher lipolytic activity of starters and some nonstarter lactic acid bacteria (NSLAB) than probiotic cultures (Gomes *et al.*, 1998b). Interesting results about FFA are reported by Rodrigues *et al.* (2011c) in their study about lipolysis in probiotic cheese and in particular about CLA production. The role of bacterial lipolytic esterases (lipases) was confirmed, as lipolytic agents in cheese, as no increase of FFA was observed in noninoculated curdled matrices over 60 days of ripening at 12°C (Rodrigues *et al.*, 2011a). According to Rodrigues *et al.* (2011c), increases in total FFA, three different CLA, ALA, and γ-linolenic acids were observed during the ripening period, especially in synbiotic cheeses containing fructooligosaccharides (FOS) and inulin. Synbiotic food products result from the combination of prebiotics and probiotics; their combination promotes health in a synergistic manner, offering more beneficial effects over either probiotics or prebiotics alone. Prebiotics are known as nondigestible dietary components that can reach the colon essentially intact; in the colon, they stimulate proliferation and activity of desirable bacteria *in situ* such as probiotic bacteria (Mattila-Sandholm *et al.*, 2002). FOS and inulin are among the most used prebiotic compounds to formulate synbiotic foods.

The production of new functional cheeses such as synbiotic cheese with an improved performance (with higher content of CLA) or with selected mixed cultures of probiotic bacteria providing several beneficial effects should be the base of the future research; this process will require the adaptation and reformulation of manufacturing protocols involving food technologists for the revision of the traditional manufacture of cheese (Settani and Moschetii, 2010).

4.3 Nondairy Products

4.3.1 Beverages

Alternative functional foods with probiotics and dairy products aside such as juices are of potential interest (Rodrigues *et al.*, 2012b). The growing interest in the development of nondairy beverages is associated with the potential alternative ways to deliver probiotic strains to lactose-intolerant people with reduced cholesterol content, which is of interest to many regular consumers. According to the review by Espírito Santo *et al.* (2011), the probiotic food with fruits as ingredients has been indicated as consumers' predilection. However, fermented milks are still the preferred product to develop probiotic beverages. Calcium and vitamin-fortified juices as functional drinks are consumed regularly (Bhadoria and Mahapatra, 2011), and therefore, probiotic beverages based on fruit juices are of utmost interest, as full benefits of probiotics are increasingly recognized by the regular consumer. Apart from allergy to dairy products, other factors such as tradition and economic reasons limiting the consumption of dairy products in countries such as China or Japan reinforce the need of alternative nondairy products to deliver probiotic agents (Granato *et al.*, 2010).

In several reports, fruit drinks have been indicated as good probiotic carriers if some care is taken relating to organoleptic characteristics and pH (Tuorila and Cardello, 2002; Luckow and Delahunty, 2004; Champagne and Gardner, 2008). Fruits and vegetables are in general considered as potential matrices because they are rich in nutrients such as vitamins, dietary fibers, sugars, minerals, and polyphenols known by its antioxidant properties (Parkar *et al.*, 2008; Soccol *et al.*, 2010).

Champagne and Gardner (2008) studied the survival of different lactobacilli in a commercial fruit drink based on a blend of different fruits concentrates and yoghurt powder with a pH of 4.2, through 80 days at 4°C; strains of *L. rhamnosus*, *L. fermentum*, *L. reuteri*, and *L. plantarum* were most resistant through the 80 days of storage, whereas strains of *L. acidophilus* showed lower resistance to the juice matrix. This fact demonstrates that acidic environment of some fruit juices represents a technological challenge to overcome (Sheehan *et al.*, 2007), as probiotics should be delivered to the consumers in adequate concentrations to provide a potential health benefit. A strategy to increase pH in a fruit juice is blending it with milk ingredients, as observed in the commercial juice studied by Champagne and Gardner (2008), which alter the sensory characteristics of the juice (Suomalainen *et al.*, 2006) and do not overcome the constraint of lactose and allergy to milk proteins.

The main results from studies of potential probiotic beverages based on fermented or nonfermented juices that have been reported between 2006 and 2011 are displayed in Table 4.7. *L. paracasei* is the most pointed with potential as a functional supplement in fruit juices, especially not only in orange, peach, or apple juices, but also in pineapple juice. Interesting results are reported with fermented carrot juice with *L. rhamnosus* and *B. lactis*. High values of viable cells in fruit juices, namely between 10^9 and 10^{10} cfu/ml, are reported after 28–50 days of storage at 4°C of carrot, peach, or orange juices. These results are in fact good evidences that fruit juices have a potential to deliver adequate concentration of probiotic bacteria to consumer without the use of dairy additives.

The trends displayed in Table 4.7 agree with those reported by a review by Espírito Santo *et al.* (2011) in which it is summarized that—strains of lactobacilli such as *L. casei*, *L. acidophilus*, and *L. rhamnosus* and of bifiobacteria such as *B. lactis* are among the

Table 4.7 Potential probiotic beverages based on fermented/non-fermented juices, reported between 2006 and 2011.

Juice composition	Probiotic strains	Other relevant information	Storage conditions	Viable cell counts (log cfu/mL)/pH		Remarks	References
				Start	End		
Pomegranate	*L. plantarum* *L. delbrueckii* *L. paracasei* *L. acidophilus*	Fermented through 72 h at 30 °C	4°C 4 weeks	8.6 8.6 8.5 8.5	NA NA NA NA	Increments of all probiotic strains between 24 and 48 h, followed by a general decrease until 72 h of fermentation; *L. plantarum* and *L. delbruecki* survived until two weeks of storage with 10^5 cfu/mL.	Mousavi *et al.*, 2011
Cashew apple	*L. casei*	Fermented through 24 h at 30 °C	4°C 42 days	8.4/6.4	8.6/3.6–3.8	Significant increment of *L. casei* through 24 h of fermentation; Cashew apple juice as potential probiotic juice.	Pereira *et al.*, 2011

Juice composition	Probiotic strains	Other relevant information	Storage conditions	Viable cell counts (log cfu/mL)/pH		Remarks	References
				Start	End		
Orange Peach	*L. paracasei* L26	Free cells and alginate microcapsules in juices.	5°C 50 days	9.2–9.5/±3.6 9.5–9.6/2.9–3.4	9.2–9.5/3.7–3.8 9.5–10.5/2.9–3.4	*L. paracasei* 26 with potential as functional supplement in fruit juices as free or encapsulated.	Rodrigues *et al.*, 2011e
Model juice	*L. rhamnosus* HN001 *B. lactis* HN001 *L. paracasei* LPC37	A model juice was prepared with sucrose, sodium citrate and citric acid. It was studies model juice with and without vitamins and antioxidants.	4°C 6 weeks	8.2/3.8 8.3/3.8 8.4/3.8	NA/3.6 NA/3.4 NA/3.3	Higher survivability of all strains in model juice containing grape extract, tea extract or vitamin C; after 6 weeks 10^6 to 10^7 cfu/mL was observed for the three strains in model juice with vitamin C.	Shah *et al.*, 2010

(*Continued*)

Table 4.7 (*Continued*)

Juice composition	Probiotic strains	Other relevant information	Storage conditions	Viable cell counts (log cfu/mL)/pH		Remarks	References
				Start	End		
Noni	*L. casei* *L. plantarum* *B. longum*	Fermented through 48 h.	4°C 4 weeks	NA	NA	*L. casei* did not exhibited cell viability after 3 weeks of storage; *L.plantarum* and *B. longum* survived the 4 weeks.	Wang *et al.*, 2009
Orange Apple	*L. rhamnosus* *B. longun* *L. salivarius* *L. plantarum* *L. acidophilus* *L. paracasei* *B. lactis* Bi-04/Bi-07	Free cells and alginate microcapsules in juices.	4°C 6 weeks	±8.0 /2.8	Orange: 5.0–5.5/2.5–2.8 Apple: 5.0–5.5/2.2–2.9	Encapsulated probiotic bacteria survived in fruit juices throughout six weeks whereas free cells lost their viability within five weeks.	Ding and Shah, 2008

Juice composition	Probiotic strains	Other relevant information	Storage conditions	Viable cell counts (log cfu/mL)/pH		Remarks	References
				Start	End		
Carrot	*B. lactis* Bb12 *B. bifidum* B7.1 *B. bifidum* B3.2	Fermented through 48 h at 37°C without juice supplementation.	No storage	NA	NA	0.7 to 1.7 log increments after 24 h of fermentation reaching values of 10^8–10^9 cfu/mL.	Kun *et al.*, 2008
Carrot	*L. rhamnosus* *L. bulgaricus*	Fermented through 48 h at 37°C; Study of influence of FOS and inulin.	4°C 4 weeks	9.7/3.4–3.6/ 9.7/3.5–3.7	9.2–9.5/3.2–3.3 9.5/3.3–3.4	The presence of FOS or inulin altered neither the viable cells of both lactobacilli nor the biochemical characteristics of fermented juices.	Nazzaro *et al.*, 2008

(*Continued*)

Table 4.7 (*Continued*)

Juice composition	Probiotic strains	Other relevant information	Storage conditions	Viable cell counts (log cfu/mL)/pH		Remarks	References
				Start	End		
Orange Pineaple Cranberry	*L. salivarius* UCC118	Non-fermented juices.	4°C 12 weeks	7.9/±3.5	NA/±3.5	Strains of *L. salivarus* were detected only after 1 week (10^3–10^7 cfu/mL) whereas *B. lactis* were detected after 6 weeks (10^3–10^7 cfu/mL) in both juices. *L. rhamnosus*, *L. casei* and *L. paracasei* demonstrated good potential as functional supplements in fruit juices.	Sheenan *et al.*, 2007
	L. sallvarus UCC500			8.2–8.3/±3.5	NA/±3.5		
	B. lactis Bb-12			7.6/±3.5	NA/±3.5		
	L. casei DN-114001			8.0–8.2/±3.5	6.3–7.8/±3.5		
	L. rhamnosus GG			7.9/±3.5	6.3–7.9/±3.5		
	L. paracasei NBFC43338			8.4±3.5	7.4/±3.5		

Juice composition	Probiotic strains	Other relevant information	Storage conditions	Viable cell counts (log cfu/mL)/pH		Remarks	References
				Start	End		
Carrot and beetroot	*L. acidophilus* NCDO 1748	Vegetables juices enriched with brewers yeast isolate and fermented though 8 h ate 37°C	No storage.	**NA**	**NA**	One to two log increments after 8 h of fermentation.	Rakin *et al.*, 2007
Orange Grape Passion fruit	B. animalis ssp. lactis VTT E-012010	Different forms to prepare *B. animalis* ssp. *lactis* were tested.	4 and 20°C 6 weeks	7.5–8.4/3.7	20 °C—NA 4 °C—NA to ±5.0	In juices sucrose-protected cells survived better than skim milk protected cells.	Saarela *et al.*, 2006
Cabbage	*L. plantarum* C3 *L. casei* A4 *L. delbrueckii* D7	Cabbage juice was fermented through 48 h at 30°C.	4°C 4 weeks	±8.0 ±8.0 ±8.0	7.6 NA 5.6	Fermented cabbage juice with some potential as healthy juice.	Young *et al.*, 2006

Note: NA - Not available

most used in the formulation of new fruity probiotic products—the viability of *L. acidophilus* is variable and dependent on fruit juice, whereas *L. rhamnosus* has been pointed as a potential probiotic with adequate viable counts in the most tested fruit juices.

Other attempts have been reported to increase storage stability of *Bifidobacterium* strains in low pH fruit juice such as the use of ultraviolet (UV) mutagenesis combined with a stress step in low pH to generate acid-resistant strains (Saarela *et al.*, 2011, 2010). Such recent attempts reveal that other strategies could be interesting to improve probiotic viability and stability in low pH juice matrices. The use of microencapsulation to encapsulate probiotic strains as a way to improve viability and survivability in juices is another approach studied. It is known that microencapsulation could provide a favorable micro-environment for the bacteria enabling their survival throughout processing and storage, and their release in the appropriate location(s) in the GIT (Weinbreck *et al.*, 2010). According to Ding and Shah (2008) and Saarela *et al.* (2006), more knowledge is still needed to ascertain the potential of encapsulation as a way to protect probiotic bacteria to organic acids and low pH in fruit juices. According to Rodrigues *et al.* (2012b) and Ding and Shah (2008), encapsulation revealed an efficient way to protect and increase the survival period of probiotic strains in juices over storage time (Table 4.7). Despite the good evidences that fruit juice could be used as a potential food to deliver adequate concentration of probiotic strains to the consumer, according to a review by Prado *et al.* (2008), there are not many examples of probiotic fruit juices in the market, most of them being commercialized in the Northern European countries. Nowadays, an increased demand from consumers for nondairy probiotic products has been observed (Granato *et al.*, 2010).

The incorporation of prebiotics such as inulin and FOS has also been attempted; carrot juice with or without inulin and FOS was demonstrated suitable for *L. rhamnosus* and *L. bulgaricus* (Nazzaro *et al.*, 2008) with preservation of β-carotene content and antioxidant activity through 1 month of cold storage. As in carrot juice with *B. lactis* and *B. bifidum* strains, a significant decrease of carotenoids was observed (Kun *et al.*, 2008) but not with *L. rhamnosus* and *L. bulgaricus*, this suggests that the consumption of carotenoids is genera and/or strain dependent with implications on the antioxidant potential of the fruit juice.

Fermented soy beverages, another suitable alternative as nondairy probiotic product, have been studied and consumed. Probiotic products based on soy extract mixed with fruit juices are some of the new generation of foods on market (Champagne and Gardner, 2008; Granato *et al.*, 2010). Tang *et al.* (2007) studied the fermentation of calcium-fortified soy milk with several strains of lactobacilli (*L. acidophilus*, *L. casei*, *L. plantarum*, and *L. fermentum*); the viability of all strains was high after fermentation and through 14 days of storage at 4°C (>8.5 log cfu/g). According to these authors, the fermentation of soy milk with the selected probiotic strains can potentially enhance the calcium bioavailability and bioactive isoflavones. Champagne *et al.* (2009, 2010) performed studies with probiotic bacteria in combination with *S. thermophilus* on fermented soy beverages. The authors selected *L. helveticus* and *B. longum* to assert the effect of fermentation by pure and mixed cultures on isoflavone and B-vitamin content in the fermented soy beverage (Champagne *et al.*, 2010); fermentation did not significantly improved B1 or B6 vitamins levels, and the addition of *S. thermophilus* to *L. helveticus* culture resulted in lower bioconversion of soy isoflavones. The authors emphasized the need for careful choice of culture for fermentation in order to optimize the quality of the final product.

Functionality of probiotic beverages should also be addressed once some probiotic strains tolerance to the acidic environment in juices is confirmed. In addition, in order to consider the fruit juice a functional food, it will require not only sensory evaluation toward consumer acceptance but will also need to be validated as a suitable carrier for delivery of probiotics to consumers in adequate amounts by performing GIT resistance studies. None of the studies reported in Table 4.7 performed sensory analysis nor analyzed the survival in simulated GIT conditions through storage period. Saarela *et al.* (2006) and Champagne and Gardiner (2008) performed some studies related to GIT resistance. According to these authors, the tested strains in a commercial juice were evaluated for their survival to the exposure to simulated GIT stresses after 35 days of storage at 4°C. Their viability in presence of 0.3% bile salts and pancreatic enzymes was not affected by the storage, but some susceptibility was observed to exposition at simulated gastric stress.

Although fruit juices based functional beverages with probiotics are at first sight appealing to all age groups due to their sensorial characteristics such as freshness, sweetness, and so on and healthy concept associated, unsuitable aromas or flavors could alter sensory profile of the juice. Unpleasant aromas and flavors were reported by Luckow and Delahunty (2004) in juices with *L. plantarum*. According to Luckow *et al.* (2006), who report masking strategies for improving the sensory quality of probiotic juice, the perceptible off-flavors caused by probiotics causing malimpression in the consumers could be masked with addition of tropical fruit juices. Masking some off-flavors and reinforcing the perception in the consumer about associated health benefits could be one strategy to lead consumer preferring the probiotic juice to the conventional juice counterpart.

4.3.2 Other Products

Some lactic acid bacteria with probiotic properties have been used in meat products for a very long time; however, the application of these starter cultures in meat has been performed with the main goal of improving meat safety rather than to produce new functional food (Khan *et al.*, 2011). The environment found in meat products can have positive and negative aspects upon probiotic bacteria: on the one hand, the fermented meat is not usually exposed to high temperatures and it has been reported that matrix components seem to protect the bacteria from passage through GIT (Klingberg and Budde, 2006); on the other hand, the presence of inhibitors such as high levels of salt, some antimicrobials from seasonings, acidic pH, and lower water activity as a consequence of drying and/or smoking can create adverse conditions and limit the survival of these strains (Khan *et al.*, 2011). So, in general, before application of probiotic starter culture, a screening of survival should be performed to assure that bacteria are not inhibited and can be adapted to the specific milieu.

Several probiotic strains have been tentatively introduced in meat products resulting in several positive effects, in particular on the technological and organoleptical characteristics of the final product as well as on the reduction of pathogen growth and related toxin production, providing a probiotic product with additional food safety properties (De Vuyst *et al.*, 2008). Some of these studies are described in Table 4.8, highlighting the probiotic strain used and type of meat product produced.

Table 4.8 Some examples of other food products containing probiotic bacteria.

Probiotic starter culture	Food product type	Reference
L. rhamnosus FERM P-15120 *L. paracasei* ssp. *paracasei* FERMP-15121	Meat sausage of lean pork	Sameshima *et al.*, 1998
L. fermentum HL57 *P. acidilactici*	Traditional Iberian dry-fermented sausages	Ruiz-Moyano *et al.*, 2011
L. reuteri *B. longum*	Dry- fermented sausages	Muthukumarasamy and Holley 2006; 2007
L. rhamnosus E-97800, *L. rhamnosus* LC-705 *L. plantarum* ALC01	Dry sausages	Erkkila *et al.*, 2001; 2003
L. acidophilus LAFTI™L10 *L. paracasei* 5119 *Lactobacillus* ssp. L24 *B. lactis* LAFTI™B94	Hungarian salami	Pidcock *et al.*, 2003
L. helveticus RO52 *B. longum* RO175	Sremska type of fermented sausages	Radulovi *et al.*, 2011
L. casei OCK 0900 *L. casei* CECT 475 + orange fiber	Dry-cured pork loins Spanish non-fermented dry-cured sausage (Longaniza de Pascua)	Stadnik and Dolatowski, 2012 Sayas-Barbera *et al.*, 2012
Bc. subtilis var. Natto	Natto–a fermented soybean	Cutting, 2011
Bc. subtilis CS90 *L. acidophilus* LA-2	Soybean fermented food cheonggukjang Soy bar with improved soy oligosaccharides digestibility	Cho *et al.*, 2011 Chen and Mustapha, 2012

(*Continued*)

Table 4.8 (*Continued*)

Probiotic starter culture	Food product type	Reference
L. acidophilus MJLA1 *B. lactis* *L. rhamnosus* *L. paracasei* ssp. paracasei	Non-fermented frozen vegetarian dessert	Heenan *et al.*, .2004
L. casei ssp. *rhamnosus*	Probiotics dried apple	Betoret *et al.*, 2003
L. acidophilus La-5	Probiotic strawberry	Moayednia *et al.*, 2010
L. rhamnosus GG	Synbiotic fresh-cut apple wedges	Rößle *et al.*, 2010
L. helveticus CNCM I-1722 *B. longum* CNCMI-3470	Dark and milk chocolates	Possemiers *et al.*, 2010
L. paracasei ssp. *paracasei* LBC 82	Probiotic and synbiotic (inulin) chocolate mousse	Aragon-Alegro *et al.*, 2007
L. casei Lc-01 *B. lactis* Bb12	Synbiotic (starch) ice cream	Homayouni *et al.*, 2008

Sameshima *et al.* (1998) incorporated three selected potential probiotics in fermented pork sausage at 10^7 cfu/g, but only two of them showed to be applicable to meat fermentation to assure product safety, namely *L. rhamnosus* FERM P-15120 and *L. paracasei* ssp. *paracasei* FERM P-15121, which satisfactorily inhibited the growth and enterotoxin production of *Staphylococcus aureus.* In addition, these strains also accomplish technological requirements, such as fermentation time and acid production, assuring their use as a starter culture to produce new fermented meat products. Other strains have also been used for pathogen inactivation, namely *L. reuteri* ATCC 55730 and *B. longum* ATCC 15708, which promote the inactivation of *E. coli* O157:H7 throughout sausage manufacturing (Muthukumarasamy and Holley, 2007).

Probiotic or bioprotective *L. rhamnosus* strains GG, LC-705 and E-97800 as well as *Pediococcus pentosaceus* E-90390 and *L. plantarum* E-98098 have been studied in order to know about their ability as main fermenting organisms in the manufacturing process of dry sausages (Erkkilä *et al.*, 2001). The sensorial properties in probiotic sausages were similar to those produced by the commercial meat starter culture, except for the *L. rhamnosus* strains GG LC-705 that reduced final quality; *L. rhamnosus* E-97800, *L. rhamnosus* LC-705 as well as *L. plantarum* ALC01 conveyed additional antilisterial activity at an early stage of the ripening process (Erkkilä *et al.*, 2003). Another study developed by Pidcock *et al.* (2003) reported that *L. paracasei* LAFTI™L26 and *B. lactis* LAFTI™B94 in combination with a traditional meat starter culture did not developed negative effects on the meat sensory properties. The same authors showed that *L. acidophilus* LAFTI™L10, *L. paracasei* 5119, *Lactobacillus* spp. L24, and *B. lactis* LAFTI™B94 could be used as a way to increase Hungarian salami safety because a strong inhibition of both *E. coli* O111 and *Listeria monocytogenes* was observed by these cultures.

Recently, Ruiz-Moyano *et al.* (2011) have studied the use of *L. fermentum* HL57 and *Pediococcus acidilactici* SP979 as potential probiotics to be used in the manufacture of traditional Iberian dry-fermented sausages. Although survival was assured for both strains, Iberian dry-fermented sausages with *P. acidilactici* SP979 guaranteed the production of an equilibrated product from the sensory point of view, though higher amounts of acetic acid and lipid degradation by *L. fermentum* HL 57 were observed, leading to a negative impact on the color and taste, confirming that although several probiotic strains can survive at recommended levels (>10^7 cfu/g), not all can assure the expected quality of product.

Three variants of Sremska type of fermented sausages were produced by Radulović *et al.* (2011) using starter culture Bactoferm T-SPX (Chr. Hansen): (1) control sausage variant; (2) variant with *L. helveticus* RO52 (Lallemand, France); (3) variant with *B. longum* RO175. The probiotic *L. helveticus* RO52 and *B. longum* RO175 were shown to be adequate for the production of dry sausages. During the first ripening stage, the bacterial counts were 10^6 cfu/g, after which they increased to the level of 10^8 cfu/g; afterward, they remained constant until the end of ripening period. The strains did not induce a decrease in sensory quality; nonetheless, slightly better aroma, taste, and texture were detected in sausages produced with *L. helveticus* RO52.

The combination of probiotic strains with fiber as a synbiotic product was also reported. Sayas-Barberá *et al.* (2012) combined the use of *L. casei* CECT 475 and orange fiber to produce Spanish nonfermented dry-cured sausage (Longaniza de Pascua), demonstrating that probiotic strain accelerates the curing process increasing organic acids release, establishing a possible starter culture. The incorporation of 1% orange fiber enhances the growth and survival of lactobacilli and micrococci. This probiotic product may explore several benefits, in particular if proper fibers capable of reducing residual nitrite are added.

The safety of probiotic meat products has also been considered mainly concerning the ability of biogenic amine production by these strains. Stadnik and Dolatowski (2012) compared the contents in 4, 8, and 16-month-old samples of dry-cured pork loins inoculated with *L. casei* ŁOCK 0900 and showed that histamine and spermidine were not detected, and spermine was detected at very low levels, while cadaverine and tryptamin were the most abundant biogenic amines, however below the suggested toxic limits.

Microencapsulation of probiotics for incorporation in meat products as a means of strain protection has also been tested in a study by Muthukumarasamy and Holley (2006, 2007). They reported that microencapsulation increased survival of *L. reuteri* and *B. longum*, maintain sensory properties, but reduced their inhibitory action against *E. coli* O157:H7.

Human studies confirming the eventual functionality of probiotic-fermented sausages are residual up to now. De Vuyst *et al.* (2008) described that the daily consumption of 50 g of probiotic (*L. paracasei* LTH 2579) sausage only resulted moderately successful, indicating a significant increase of *L. paracasei* LTH only in some of the volunteers and exhibiting only modulation of host immunity, but with no significant influence on cholesterol and triacylglycerides serum concentrations. Hence, more research is still required, particularly in terms of human studies, if new probiotics and probiotic fermented sausages are sought.

Other probiotic food products include those with dried probiotics (e.g., breakfast cereals, infant formulas, and dry milk formulations with dried fruit or with high-lipid contents, such as chocolate). In some of these products, microencapsulation has been reported as an approach to improve the viability, namely in products with harsh environment, viz. probiotics in freeze-dried yogurt, in spray-dried milk powder, or in spray-dried kudzu powder, a starch derived from roots of Puerari lobata, which has traditionally been used as a food ingredient in East Asia.

Some dried fruits have been used to incorporate probiotic bacteria. Some years ago, Betoret *et al.* (2003) developed a probiotic dried apple by applying the vacuum impregnation process. They impregnated either orange juice with *Saccharomyces cerevisiae* and with whole milk or apple juice containing 10^7 or 10^8 cfu/ml of *L. casei* ssp. *rhamnosus*. The stability of probiotic fruit was obtained by air drying at 40°C and stored at room temperature for 60 days. The recommended probiotic level was achieved (10^7 cfu/g) throughout storage period.

More recently, Roßle *et al.* (2011) developed potentially synbiotic fresh-cut apple wedges by applying probiotic *L. rhamnosus* GG and prebiotics such as oligofructose and inulin. The wedges were dipped in probiotic solution, and the prebiotic carrier used was alginate assuring a homogeneous layer on fruit surface. Organoleptic properties were almost not changed by applying the functional ingredients, assuring similar quality to apple slices currently available. All samples attained ca. 10^8 cfu/g over the test period, which is sufficient for a probiotic effect. The alginate coating positively affected the stability of polyphenols and was able to preserve apple volatiles slightly better than uncoated apple wedges. Moayednia *et al.* (2010) reported on probiotic fortification of strawberry fruit, combining encapsulated probiotics and fruit-coating techniques, namely dipping the fruit into sodium alginate solution (2%, w/v) containing probiotic and after a short dripping off the residual solution submerging them in a solution of calcium chloride. Other vegetable materials (artichokes, cabbage, table olives, tomato, red beet, carrot juice), mainly in fermented products, have been used as carriers and sources of potentially probiotic lactic acid bacteria and were extensively reviewed by Peres *et al.* (2012). Among plant materials, soybean has been quite explored as matrix for probiotic delivery. As a soybean probiotic product (fermented soybean), Natto is normally consumed either hot or cold. In this example, it is sold as a snack with dried soybeans coated with a fine white powder of *Bacillus subtilis* var. Natto, the active ingredient required for the taste and texture of Natto. However, the health benefits associated with Natto imply the consumption of soybeans and bacteria, rather than just the bacterium. *Bc. subtilis* var. Natto carries as many as 10^8 viable spores per gram of product, and for decades, health benefits have been associated with consumption of Natto including stimulation of the immune system (Cutting, 2011). Another fermented soybean probiotic product was studied by Cho *et al.* (2011), in which they attained the fermentation of soybean fermented food cheonggukjang by a potential probiotic *Bc. subtilis* CS90. They reported that this strain induced changes in 25 phytochemical contents, including isoflavones, flavonols, and phenolic acids during the fermentation, increasing phenolic compounds and consequently antioxidant activity. The final probiotic cheonggukjang extract may be used as a basis for possible commercial production of functional foods in the future.

Chen and Mustapha (2012) introduced a functional probiotic strain (*L. acidophilus* LA-2) into a soy bar product aiming a probiotic bar with *in vivo* enzymatic hydrolysis of soy oligosaccharides (mainly α-galactosides), promoting the digestibility of those oligosaccharides. In order to maintain probiotic strain with high viability in the product, the cells were microencapsulated and freeze-dried using the combination of k-carrageenan and inulin as an optimal formulation at a proportion of 1.9:0.1 (w:w) as capsule wall materials. The probiotic soy bar showed high levels of viable cells throughout a 14-week storage at 4°C with high level of α-galactosidase activity, improving product digestibility.

Another soy-based product, soy low-fat frozen dessert, similar to ice cream, was developed by Heenan *et al.* (2004) and proved to be a suitable product for the delivery of bacterial probiotics with good sensory appeal. They incorporated several probiotic strains (*L. acidophilus* MJLA1, *B. lactis*, *L. rhamnosus*, and *L. paracasei* ssp. *paracasei*), which grow well in this matrix.

Possemiers *et al.* (2010) proposed both dark and milk chocolates as food vectors for oral delivery of a microencapsulated mixture of *L. helveticus* CNCM I-1722 and *B. longum* CNCMI-3470. Both chocolates offered higher protection than plain milk (91% and 80% survival in milk chocolate for *L. helveticus* and *B. longum*, respectively, against 20% and 31%). The coating of the probiotics in chocolate may constitute an excellent strategy to enable protection of these probiotics from environmental stress conditions, opening the opportunity toward new balanced matrices. Furthermore, chocolate mousse, an aerated dairy dessert, has also shown a great market potential, demonstrating high viability of the probiotic under the storage conditions during 21 days with prebiotic ingredients (Aragon-Alegro *et al.*, 2007).

Ice cream and frozen desserts based on dairy or fruit pulp or juice are another group of food products that have demonstrated potential as probiotic culture carrier for the consumers (Ranadheera *et al.*, 2010). Due to the lower storage temperatures, the ice cream is considered favorable for viability of probiotic strains, provided that damage by freezing and thawing, mechanical stresses of mixing and by oxygen incorporation during ice cream manufacture is minimized, as they can lead to decrease of probiotic viable cells at the moment of consumption (Cruz *et al.*, 2009b). As in general ice cream is a well accepted and desirable food product especially for children, it has a great potential for delivering probiotics. A review on ice cream as a probiotic carrier was published by Cruz *et al.* (2009b). More recent studies on probiotic ice cream focus on the use of prebiotic compounds such as inulin and starch and microencapsulated cells (Akin *et al.*, 2007; Homayouni *et al.*, 2008). The addition of inulin improved viscosity and stimulated the growth of *L. acidophilus* and *B. lactis* resulting in higher viability in ice cream with no effect on its sensory properties (Akin *et al.*, 2007). According to Homayouni *et al.* (2008), encapsulation increased significantly the survival rate of probiotic bacteria in the ice cream over storage for 180 days at −20°C.

4.4 Conclusions

The demand for functional foods has been increased over the last years. These foods, including probiotics and prebiotics as biologically active components, produce metabolic and physiological health benefits apart from their nutritional properties. The most common probiotic strains found in functional foods belong to *Lactobacillus* and *Bifidobacterium* genera. Nowadays, a phletora of probiotic food products are available in the market, some of them including prebiotic compounds that demonstrate the interest and potential of these products. The dairy-based products dominate the most consumed probiotic products (mostly fermented milks and cheeses) over the world, but beverages (with or without dairy components) or other products, such as meat products, dry bars, and so on, have been researched and some of them are already found in the market.

The most challenging aspects to overcome by using food as vehicles of probiotics are indeed to assure their viability through the food processing, storage, and resistance to GIT as well as to control their repercussions on organoleptic properties of the final food product. Several approaches have been attempted to increase levels of survival and viability of probiotic strains taking into account minimization of off-flavors. The use of prebiotic compounds, microencapsulation techniques, and so on are some of the ones that were discussed and have the potential to increase the offer of different food products containing viable cells of probiotic in adequate amounts to produce beneficial effects in the host. It is known that viability and metabolic activity of probiotic strains on food product are both dependent on strain itself and on product composition. This interrelationship should be considered under the technological point of view considering the main parameters that influence the final product.

References

Abraham S., Cachon R., Colas B., Feron G. and De Coninck J. (2007) Eh and pH gradients in Camembert cheese during ripening: measurements using microelectrodes and correlations with texture. *Int. Dairy J.*, **17**, 954–960.

Akin M. B., Akin, M. S. and Kirmaci, Z. (2007) Effects of inulin and sugar levels on the viability of yogurt and probiotic bacteria and the physical and sensory characteristics in probiotic ice-cream. *Food Chem.*, **104**, 93–99.

Aragon-Alegro, L. C, Alarcon Alegro, J. H., Cardarelli, H. R., Chiu, M. C. and Isay Saad, S. M. I. (2007) Potentially probiotic and synbiotic chocolate mousse. *LWT-Food Sci. Technol.*, **40**, 669–675.

Araújo E. A., Carvalho A. F., Leandro E. S., Furtado M. M. and Moares C. A. (2010) Development of a symbiotic cottage cheese added with *Lactobacillus delbrueckii* UFV H2b20 and inulin. *J. Functional Foods*, **2**, 85–89.

Azarnia, S., Robert, N. and Lee, B. (2006) Biotechnological methods to accelerate Cheddar cheese ripening. *Crit. Rev. Biotechnol.*, **26**, 121–143.

Bergamini, C.V., Hynes, E. R., Palma, S. B., Sabbag, N. G. and Zalazar, C. A. (2009) Proteolytic activity of three probiotic strains in semi-hard cheese as single and mixed cultures: *Lactobacillus acidophilus*, *Lactobacillus paracasei* and *Bifidobacterium lactis*. *Int. Dairy J.*, **19**, 467–475.

Bernardeau, M., Vernoux, J. P., Henri-Dubernet, S. and Guéguen, M. (2008) Safety assessment of dairy microorganisms: the *Lactobacillus* genus. *Int. J. Food Microb.*, **126**, 278–285.

Bertazzoni-Minelli, E., Benini, A., Marzotto, M., Sbarbati, A., Ruzzenente, O., Ferrario, R., Hendriks, H. and Dellaglio, F. (2004) Assessment of novel probiotic *Lactobacillus casei* strains for the production of functional dairy foods. *Int. Dairy J.*, **14**, 723–736.

Betoret, N., Puente, L. Díaz, M. J, Pagán, M. J, García, M. J, Gras, M. L, Martínez-Monzó, J. and Fito P. (2003) Development of probiotic-enriched dried fruits by vacuum impregnation. *J. Food Eng.*, **56**, 273–277.

Bhadoria, P. B. S. and Mahapatra, S. C. (2011) Prospects, technological aspects and limitations of probiotics: a worldwide review. *Eur. J. Food Res. Rev.*, **1**, 23–42.

Blanchette, D., Roy, D., Belanger, G. and Gauthie, S. F. (1996) Production of cottage cheese using dressing fermented by Bifidobacteria. *J. Dairy Sci.*, **79**, 8–15.

Bolduc, M. P., Raymond, Y., Fustier, P., Chamapgne, C. P. and Vuillemard, J. C. (2006) Sensitivity of bifidobacteria to oxygen and redox potential in non-fermented pasteurized milk. *Int. Dairy J.*, **16**(9), 1038–1048.

Borges, S., Barbosa, J., Camilo, R., Carvalheira, A., Silva, J., Sousa, S., Gomes, A.M., Pintado, M. M., Silva, J. P., Costa, P., Amaral, M. H., Teixeira, P. and Freitas, A. C. (2012) Effects of encapsulation on the viability of probiotic strains exposed to lethal conditions. *Int. J. Food Sci. Technol.*, **47**(2), 416–421.

Borriello, S. P., Hammes, W. P., Holzapfel, W., Marteau, P., Schrezenmeir, J., Vaara, M. And Valtonen, V. (2003) Safety of probiotics that contain Lactobacilli or Bifidobacteria. *Clin. Infect. Dis.*, **36**, 775–780.

Boylston, T. D., Vinderola, C. G., Ghoddusi, H. B. and Reinheimer, J. A. (2004) Incorporation of bifidobacteria into cheese: challenges and rewards. *Int. Dairy J.*, **14**, 375–387.

Capela, P., Hay, T. K. C. and Shah, N.P. (2006) Effect of cryoprotectants, prebiotics and microencapsulation on survival of probiotic organisms in yoghurt and freeze-dried yoghurt. *Food Res. Int.*, **39**, 203–211.

Champagne, C. P., Tompkins, T. A., Buckley, N. D. and Green-Johnson, J. M. (2010) Effect of fermentation by pure and mixed cultures of *Streptococcus thermophilus* and *Lactobacillus helveticus* on isoflavone and B-vitamin content of a fermented soy beverage. *Food Microbiol.*, **27**, 968–972.

Champagne, C. P. (2009) Some technological challenges in the addition of probiotic bacteria to foods, in *Prebiotics and Probiotics Science and Technology,* (ed. Charalampopoulos, D. and Rastall, D.), New York, pp. 761–804.

Champagne, C. P., Green-Johnson, J. M., Raymond, Y., Barrette, J. and Buckley, N. D. (2009) Selection of probiotic bacteria for the fermentation of a soy beverage in combination with *Streptococcus thermophilus. Food Res. Int.*, **42**, 612–621.

Champagne, C. P. and Gardner, N. J. (2008) Effect of storage in a fruit drink on subsequent survival of probiotic lactobacilli to gastro-intestinal stresses. *Food Res. Int.*, **41**, 539–543.

Chen, M. and Mustapha, A. (2012) Survival of freeze-dried microcapsules of α-galactosidase producing probiotics in a soy bar matrix. *Food Microb.*, **30**, 68–73.

Chen, K., Chen, M, Liu, J., Lin, C. and Chiu, H. (2005) Optimization of incorporated prebiotics as coating materials for probiotuc microencapsulation. *J. Food Sci.*, **70**, M260–M266.

Cho, K.M., Lee, J. H., Yun, H. D., Ahn, B. Y., Kim H. and Seo, W. T. (2011) Changes of phytochemical constituents (isoflavones, flavanols, and phenolic acids) during cheonggukjang soybeans fermentation using potential probiotics Bacillus subtilis CS90. *J. Food Comp. Anal.*, **24**, 402–410.

Codex Alimentarius (2003) Codex standard for fermented milks. Codex Stan 243-2003. Revision 2008, 2010.

Cogan, T., Beredsford, T. P., Steele, J., Broadbent, J., Shah, N. P. and Ustunol, Z. (2007) Advanced in starter cultures and cultured foods. *J. Dairy Sci.*, **90**, 4005–4021.

Consentino, S., Pisano, M. B., Corda, A., Fadda, M. E. and Piras, C. (2004) Genotypic and technological characterization of enterococci isolated from artisanal Fiore Sardo cheese. *J. Dairy Res.*, **71**, 444–450.

Corbo, M. R., Albenzio, M., De Angelis, M., Sevi, A. and Gobbetti, M. (2001) Microbiological and biochemical properties of Canestrato Pugliese hard chese supplemented with bifidobacteria. *J. Dairy Sci.*, **84**, 551–561.

Corcoran, B. M., Stanton, C., Fitzgerald, G. and Ross, R.P. (2008) Life under stress: the probiotic stress response and how it may be manipulated. *Curr. Pharm. Des.,* **14**(14), 1382–1399.

Corcoran, B. M., Stanton, C., Fitzgerald, G. F. and Ross, R. P. (2005) Survival of probiotic lactobacilli in acidic environments is enhanced in the presence of metabolizable sugars. *Appl Environ. Microbiol.*, **71**, 3060–3067.

Corcoran, B. M., Ross, R. P., Fitzgerald, G. F. and Stanton, C. (2004) Comparative survival of probiotic lactobacilli spray-dried in the presence of prebiotic substances. *J. Appl. Microbiol.*, **96**, 1024–1039.

Cousin, F. J., Louesdon, S., Maillard, M. B., Parayre, S., Falentin, H., Deutsch, S. M., Boudry, G. and Jan, G. (2012) The first dairy product exclusively fermented by *Propionibacterium freudenreichii*: a new vector to study probiotic potentialities *in vivo*. *Food Microb.*, **32**(1), 135–146.

Cruz, A. G., Buriti, F.C. A., Souza, C. H. B., Faria, J. A. F. and Saad, S. M. I. (2009a) Probiotic cheese: health benefits, technological and stability aspects. *Trends Food Sci. Technol.*, **20**, 344–354.

Cruz, A. G., Antunes, A. E. C., Sousa, A. L. O. P., Faria, J. A. F. and Saad, S. M. I. (2009b) Ice-cream as a probiotic food carrier. *Food Res. Int.*, **42**, 1233–1239.

Cutic, V., Hardi, J., Slacanac, V., Pavlovic, H. and Vukovic, D. (2004) Inhibitory effect of goat and cow milk fermented by ABT-2 culture (*Lactobacillus acidophilus* La-5, *Bifidobacterium lactis* Bb-12 and *Streptococcus thermophilus*) on the growth of some uropathogenic *E. coli* strains. *Ital. J. Food Sci.*, **16**, 209–220.

Cutting, S. M. (2011) Bacillus probiotics. *Food Microb.*, **28**, 214–220.

Dave, R. I. and Shah, N. P. (1997) Characteristics of bacteriocin produced by *Lactobacillus acidophilus* LA-1. *Int. Dairy J.*, **7**, 705–715.

Damin, M. R., Minowa, E., Alcantar, M. R., Oliveira, M. N. (2008) Effect of cold storage on culture viability and some rheological properties of fermented milk prepared with yogurt and probiotic bacteria. *J. Textural Stud.*, **39**, 40–55.

De Vuyst, L., Falony, G. and Leroy, F. (2008) Probiotics in fermented sausages. *Meat Sci.*, **80**, 75–78.

Desai, A. R., Powell, I. B. and Shah, N. P. (2004) Survival and activity of probiotic lactobacilli in skim milk containing prebiotics. *J. Food Sci.*, **69**, 57–60.

Dinakar, P. and Mistry, V.V. (1994) Growth and viability of Bifidobacterium bifidum in Cheddar cheese. *J. Dairy Sci.*, **77**, 2854–2864.

Ding W. K. and Shah N. P. (2008) Survival of free and microencapsulated probiotic bacteria in orange and apple juices. *Int. Food Res. J.*, **15**, 219–232.

Dos Santos, K. M. O., Bomfim, M. A. D., Vieira, A. D. S., Benevides, S. D., Saad, S. M. I., Buriti, F. C. A. and Egito, A. S. (2012) Probiotic caprine coalho cheese naturally enriched in conjugated linoleic acid as a vehicle for *Lactobacillus acidophilus* and beneficial fatty acids. *Int. Dairy J.*, **24**, 107–112.

Donkor, O. N., Henriksson, A., Vasiljevic, T. and Shah, N. P. (2006) Effect of acidification on the activity of probiotics in yoghurt during cold storage. *Int. Dairy J.*, **16**, 1181–1189.

Donohue, D. C. (2006) Safety of probiotics. *Asia Pacific J. Clin. Nutri.*, **15**, 563–569.

Douglas, L. C. and Sanders, M. E. (2008) Perspectives in practice: probiotics and prebiotics in dietetics practice. *J. Am. Diet. Assoc.*, **108**, 510–521.

Effat, B. A. M, Mabrouk, A. M. M., Sadek, Z. I., Hussein, G. A. M. and Magdoub, M. N. I. (2012) Production of novel functional white soft cheese. *J. Microb. Biotechnol. Food Sci.*, **1**, 1259–1278.

El-Salam, M. H. Abd, Hippen, A. R., Salem, M. M., Assem, F. M. and El-Aassar, M. (2012) Survival of probiotic *Lactobacillus casei* and *Enterococcus faecium* in Domiati cheese of high conjugated linoleic acis content. *Emirates J. Food Agr.*, **24**, 98–104.

El-Salam, M. H. Abd, Hippen, A. R., Assem, F. M., El-Shafei, K., Tawfik N. F. and El-Aassar M. (2011) Preparation and properties of probiotic cheese high in conjugated linoleic acid content. *Int. J. Dairy Technol.*, **64**, 64–74.

Erkkilä, S., Markkula, A., Petäjä, E., Suihko, M. L., and Mattila-Sandholm, T. (2003) Survival of *Listeria monocytogenes* in North European type dry sausages fermented by bioprotective meat starter cultures. *Food Control*, **14**, 181–185.

Erkkilä, S., Markkula, A., Petäjä, E., Mattila-Sandholm, T. and Suihko, M. L. (2001) Flavour profiles of dry sausages fermented by selected novel meat starter cultures. *Meat Sci.*, **58**, 111–116.

Euromonitor (2008) Soy yoghurts as carrier of probiotic bacteria. Euromonitor International, London. Functional Times, Food Business.

Euromonitor (2009) Functional foods: a world survey. Euromonitor International, London.Functional Times, Food Business, February, 35. 6 p.

Espírito Santo, A. P., Perego, P., Converti, A. and Oliveira, M. N. (2011) Influence of food matrices on probiotic viability: a review focusing on the fruity bases. *Trends Food Sci. Technol.*, **22**, 377–385.

FAO/WHO (2001) Report on joint FAO/WHO expert consultation on evaluation of health and nutritional properties of probiotics in food including powder milk with live acid bacteria, Cordoba, Argentina.

Fayol-Messaoudi, D., Berger, C. N., Coconnier-Polter, M. H., Lievin-Le, M. V. and Servin, A. L. (2005) pH-, lactic acid-, and non-lactic acid dependent activities of probiotic lactobacilli against *Salmonella enterica* Serovar *Typhimurium*. *Appl. Environ. Microbiol.*, **71**, 6008–6013.

Florence, A. C. R., Oliveira, R. P. S., Silva, R. C., Soares, F. A. S. M., Gioielli, L. A. and Oliveira, M. N. (2012) Organic milk improves *Bifidobacterium lactis* counts and bioactive fatty acids contents in fermented milk. *LWT-Food Sci.Technol.*, **49**, 89–95.

Garcia, E. F., Gomes de Oliveira, M. E., Queiroga, R. C. R. E., Machado, T. A. D. and Leite de Souza, E. (2012) Development and quality of a Brazilian semi-hard goat cheese (coalho) with added probiotic lactic acid bacteria. *Int. J. Food Sci. Nutr.*, **63**(8), 947–956.

Garcia, M. C., Rodríguez, M. J., Bernardo, A., Tornadijo, M. E. and Carballo, J. (2002) Study of enterococci and micrococci isolated throughout manufacture and ripening of San Simón cheese. *Food Micr.*, **19**, 23–33.

Gardiner, G., Stanton C., Lynch P. B., Collins J. K., Fitzgerald G. and Ross, R. P. (1999a) Evaluation of Cheddar cheese as a food carrier for delivery of a probiotic strain to the gastrointestinal tract. *J. Dairy Sci.*, **82**, 1379–1387.

Gardiner, G. E., Ross, R. P., Wallace J. M., Scanlan F. P., Jagers P. P. J. M., Fitzgerald G. F., Collins J. K. and Stanton C. (1999b) Influence of a probiotic adjunct culture of *Enterococcus faecium* on the quality of Cheddar cheese. *J. Agric. Food Chem.*, **47**, 4907–4916.

Giraffa, G. (2003) Functionality of enterococci in dairy products. *Int. J. Food Microb.*, **88**, 215–222.

Giraffa, G., Carminati, D. and Neviani, E. (1997) Enterococci isolated from dairy products: a review of risks and potencial technological use. *J. Food Protect.*, **6**, 732–738.

Georgieva, R., Iliev, I., Haertlé, T., Chobert, J., Ivanova, I. and Danova, S. (2009) Technological properties of candidate probiotic *Lactobacillus plantarum* strains. *Int. Dairy J.*, **19**, 696–702.

Ghoddusi, H. B. and Robinson, R. K. (1996) The test of time. *Dairy Ind. Int.*, **61**, 25-238

Gomes, A. M. P., Pintado, M. E. and Malcata, F. X. (2009) Probiotics, in *Handbook of dairy food analysis* (ed. Nollet, L.M.L. and Toldra, F.), CRC Press – Taylor & Francis, New York, p. 503.

Gobetti, M., Cosetti, A., Smacchi, E., Zocchetti, A. and De Angelis, M. (1998) Production of crescenza cheese by incorporation of *Bifidobacteria*. *J. Dairy Sci.*, **81**(1), 37–47.

Gomes, A. M. P. and Malcata, F. X. (1999) *Bifidobacterium* spp. and *Lactobacillus acidophilus*: biological, biochemical, technological and therapeutical properties relevant for use as probiotics. *Trends Food Sci. Technol.*, **10**, 139–157.

Gomes, A. M. P. and Malcata, F. X. (1998) Use of small ruminants' milk supplemented with available nitrogen as growth media for *Bifidobacterium lactis* and *Lactobacillus acidophilus*. *J. Applied Microb.*, **85**(5), 839–848.

Gomes, A. M. P., Malcata, F. X. and Klaver, F. A. M. (1998a) Growth enhancement of *Bifidobacterium lactis* Bo and *Lactobacillus acidophilus* Ki by milk hydrolyzates. *J. Dairy Sci.*, **81**(11), 2817–2825.

Gomes, A. M. P., Silva, M. L. P. C. and Malcata, F.X. (1998b) Caprine cheese with probiotic strains: the effects of ripening temperature and relative humidity on proteolysis and lipolysis. *Zeichstrift für Lebensmittel-Untersuchung und -Forschung* A, **207**, 386–394.

Gomes, A. M. P., Malcata, F. X., Klaver, F. A. M., and Grande, H. J. (1995) Incorporation and survival of *Bifidobacterium* sp. strain Bo and *Lactobacillus acidophilus* strain Ki in a cheese product. *Netherlands Milk Dairy J.*, **43**, 71–95.

Gonzalez-Gonzalez, C. R., Tuohy, K. M. and Jauregi, P. (2011) Production of angiotensin-I-converting enzyme (ACE) inhibitory activity in milk fermented with probiotic strains: effects of calcium, pH and peptides on the ACE-inhibitory activity. *Int. Dairy J.*, **21**, 615–622.

Granato D., Branco G. F., Nazzaro F., Cruz A. G. and Faria J. A. F. (2010) Functional Foods and Nondairy probiotic food development: Trends, concepts, and products. *Comprehensive Rev.Food Sci. Food Safety*, **9**, 292–302.

Grattepanche, F., Miescher-Schwenninger, S., Meile, L. and Grattepanche, C. L. (2008) Recent developments in cheese cultures with protective and probiotic functionalities. *Dairy Sci. Technol.*, **88**, 421–444.

Grzeskowiak, L., Isolauri, E., Salminen, S. and Gueimonde, M. (2011) Manufacturing process influences properties of probiotic bacteria. *Brit J Nutr.*, **105**, 887–994.

Health Canada (2009) The use of probiotic microorganisms in food. Section 8.7. http://www.inspection.gc.ca/english/fssa/labeti/guide/ch8ae.shtml#a8_7 (last accession 10.07.12)

Heenana, C. N., Adams, M. C., Hoskena, R. W. and Fleet, G. H. (2004) Survival and sensory acceptability of probiotic microorganisms in a non fermented frozen vegetarian dessert. *Lebensm.-Wiss. u.-Technol.*, **37**, 461–466.

Hilali, M., El-Mayda, E. and Rischkowsky, B. (2011) Characteristics and utilization of sheep and goat milk in the Middle East. *Small Rum. Res.*, 101, 92–101.

Homayouni, A., Azizi A., Ehsai M. R., Yarmand M. S. and Razavi S. H. (2008) Effect of microencapsulation and resistant starch on the probiotic survival and sensory properties of synbiotic ice cream. *Food Chem.*, **111**, 50–55.

Jan G., Rouault A. and Maubois J. L. (2000) Acid stress susceptibility and acid adaptation of *Propionibacterium freudenreichii* subsp. *sherrmanii*. *Lait*, **80**, 325–336.

Janer, C., Pelaez, C. and Requena, T. (2004) Caseinomacropeptide and whey protein concentrate enhance *Bifidobacterium lactis* growth in milk. *Food Chem.*, **86** 263–267.

Johnson, M. E. and Lucey, J. A. (2006) Major technological advances and trends in cheese. *J. Dairy Sci.*, **89**, 1174–1178.

Jurkovič, D., Križkova, L., Dušinský, R., Belicová, A., Sojka, M., Krajčovič, J. and Ebringe,r L. (2006) Identification and characterization of enterococci from Bryndza cheese. *Letter Appl. Microbiol.*, **42**, 553–559.

Kailasapathy, K. (2006) Survival of free and encapsulated probiotic bacteria and their effect on the sensory properties of yoghurt. 2005. *LWT-Food Sci. Technol.*, **39**(10), 1221–1227.

Kailasapathy, K. and Masandole, L. (2005) Survival of free and microencapsulated *Lactobacillus acidophilus* and *Bifidobacteria lactis* and their effect on texture of Feta cheese. *Australian J. Dairy Technol.*, **60**, 252–258.

Karimi R., Mortazavian A. M. and Cruz A. G. (2011) Viability o probiotic microorganisms in cheese during production and storage: a review. *Dairy Sci. Technol.*, **91**, 283–308.

Khan, M. I., Arshad, M.S., Anjum, F.M., Sameen, A., Aneeq-ur-Rehman and Gill, W. T. (2011) Meat as a functional food with special reference to probiotic sausages. *Food Res. Int.*, **44**, 3125–3133.

Kiliç, G. B.; kuleaşan, H.; Eralp, I. and Kaharan, A. G. (2009) Manufacture of Turkish Beyaz cheese added with probiotic strains. *LWT- Food Sci. Technol.*, **42**, 1003–1008.

Kimoto, H., Kurisaki, J., Tsuji, N. M., Ohmoto, S. and Okamoto, T. (1999) Lactococci as probiotic strains: adhesion to human enterocyte-like Caco-2 cells and tolerance to low pH and bile. *Letter Appl. Microbiol.*, **29**, 313–316.

Klingberg T. D. and Budde B. B. (2006) The survival and persistence in the human gastrointestinal tract of five potential probiotic lactobacilli consumed as freeze dried cultures or as probiotic sausage. *Int. J. Food Microb.*, **109**, 157–159.

Kongo, J. M., Gomes, A. M. and Malcata, F. X. (2006) Manufacturing of fermented goat milk with a mixed starter culture of *Bifidobacterium animalis* and Lactobacillus acidophilus in a controlled bioreactor. *Letter Appl. Microbiol.*, **42**, 595–599.

Kouya, T., Misawa, K., Horiuchi, M., Nakayama, E., Deguchi, H., Tanaka T. and Taniguchi M. (2007) Production of extracellular bifidogenic growth stimulator by anaerobic and aerobic cultivations of several *Proponibacteria* strains. *J. Biosci. Bioengineering*, **103**, 46–471.

Krasaekoopt, W., Bhandari, B. and Deeth, H. (2006) Survival of probiotics encapsulated in chitosan-coated alginate beads in yoghurt from UHT and conventionally treated milk during storage. *LWT-Food Sci. Technol.*, **39**, 177–183.

Kun S., Rezessy-Szabó J. M., Nguyen Q. D. and Hoschkle A. (2008) Changes of microbial population and some components in carrot juice during fermentation with selected *Bifidobacterium* strains. *Process Bioch.*, **43**, 816–821.

Kurmann, J. A. (1984) Aspects of the production of fermented milks, in *Fermented Milks*, pp. 16–26, Bulletin no. 179. Brussels: International Dairy Federation.

Lacroix, C. and Yidirim, S. (2007) Fermentation technologies for the production of probiotics with high viability and functionality. *Curr. Opin. Biotechnol.*, **18**(2), 176–183.

Li, Q. Q., Chen, Q. H., Hui, R., Zhu, D. S. and He, G. Q. (2010) Isolation and characterization of an oxygen, acid and bile resistant *Bifidobacterium animalis* subsp *lactis* Qq08. *J. Sci. Food Agric.*, **90**, 1340–1346.

Luckow, T., Sheehan, V., Fitzgerald, G. and Delahunty, C. (2004) Exposure, health information and flavour-masking strategies for improving the sensory quality of probiotic juice. *Appetite*, **47**(3), 315–323.

Luckow, T. and Delahunty, C. (2004) Which juice is healthier? A consumer study of probiotic non-dairy juice drinks. *Food Qual. Preference*, **15**, 751–759.

Madureira, A. R., Soares, J. C., Pintado, M. E., Gomes, A. M. P., Freitas, A. C. and Malcata, F. X. (2008) Sweet whey cheese matrices inoculated with the probiotic strain *Lactobacillus paracasei* LAFTI L26. *Dairy Sci. Technol.*, **88**, 649–665.

Majhenic, A. C., Rogelj, I. and Perko, B. (2005) Enterococci from Tolmic cheese: population structure, antibiotic susceptibility and incidence of virulence determinants. *Int. J. Food Microb.*, **102**, 239–244.

Mantere-Alhonen, S. (1995) *Propionibacteria* used as probiotics: a review. *Lait*, **75**, 447–452.

Maragkoudakis, P. A., Zoumpopoulou, G., Miaris, C., Kalantzopoulos, G., Pot, B. and Tsakalidou, E. (2006) Probiotic potential of *Lactobacillus* strains isolated from dairy products. *Int. Dairy J.*, **16**, 189–199.

Martinez-Villaluenga, C., Frias, J., Gomez, R. and Vidal-Valverde, C. (2006) Influence of addition of raffinose family oligosaccharides on probiotics survival in fermented milk during refrigerated storage. *Int. Dairy J.*, **16**, 768–774.

Mattila-Sandholm, T., Myllarinen, P., Crittenden, R., Mogensen, G., Fondén, R. Saarela, M. (2002) Technological challenges for future probiotic foods. *Int. Dairy J.*, **12**, 173–182.

Mäkeläinen, H., Forssten, S., Olli, K., Granlund, L., Rautonen, N. and Ouwehand, A. C. (2009) Probiotic lactobacilli in a semi-soft cheese survive in the simulated human gastrointestinal tract. *Int. Dairy J.*, **19**, 675–683.

Milesi, M. M., Vinderola, G., Sbbag, N., Meinardi, C. A. and Hynes, E. (2009) Influence of cheese proteolysis and sensory characteristics of non-starter lactobacilli strains with probiotic potencial. *Food Res. Int.*, **42**, 1186–1196.

Mille, Y., Obert, J. P., Beney, L., Gervais, P. (2004) New drying process for lactic bacteria based on their dehydration behaviour in liquid medium. *Biotechnol Bioeng.*, **88**, 71–76.

Minervini, F., Bilancia, M.T., Siragusa, S., Gobbetti, M. and Caponio, F. (2009) Fermented goats' milk produced with selected multiple starters as a potentially functional food. *Food Microb.*, **26**, 559–564.

Moayednia, N., Ehsani, M. R., Emamdjomeh, Z., Asadi, M. M., Mizani, M., Mazaheri, A. F. (2010) Effect of refrigeration on viability of immobilized probiotic bacteria in alginate coat of strawberry. *World Appl. Sci. J.*, **10**, 472–476.

Mousavi, Z. E., Mousavi, S. M., Razavi, S. H., Emam-Djomeh, Z. and Kiani, H. (2011) Fermentation of pomegranate juice by probiotic lactic acid bacteria. *World J. Microb. Biotechnol.*, **27**, 123–128.

Muller, J. A., Ross, R. P., Sybesma, W. F. H., Fitzgerald, G. F. and Stanton, C. (2011) Modification of the technical properties of *Lactobacillus johnsonii* NCC 533 by supplementing the growth medium with unsaturated fatty acids. *Applied Env. Microb.*, **77**, 6889–6898.

Muller, J. A., Stanton, C., Sybesma, W., Fitzerald, G. F. and Ross, R. P. (2010) Reconstitution conditions for dried probiotic powders represent a critical step in determining cell viability. *J. Appl. Microb.*, **108**, 1369–1379.

Muthukumarasamy, P. and Holley, R. A. (2007) Survival of *Escherichia coli* O157:H7 in dry fermented sausages containing micro-encapsulated probiotic lactic acid bacteria. *Food Microb.*, **24**, 82–88.

Muthukumarasamy, P. and Holley, R. A. (2006) Microbiological and sensory quality of dry fermented sausages containing alginate-microencapsulated *Lactobacillus reuteri*. *Int. J. Food Microb.*, **111**, 164–169.

Nazzaro, F., Fratianni, F., Sada, A. and Orlando, P. (2008) Synbiotic potential of carrot juice supplemented with *Lactobacillus* spp. and inulin or fructooligosaccharides. *J. Sci. Food Agric.*, **88**, 2271–276.

Oliveira, R. P. S., Florence, A. C. R., Perego, P., Oliveira, M. N. and Converti, A. (2011) Use of lactulose as prebiotic and its influence on the growth, acidification profile and viable counts of different probiotics in fermented skim milk. *Int. J. Food Microb.*, **145**, 22–27.

Oliveira, R. P. S., Florence, A. C. R., Silva, R. C., Perego, P., Converti, A., Gioielli, L .A. an Oliveira, M.N. (2009a) Effect of different prebiotics on the fermentation kinetics, probiotic survival and fatty acids profiles in nonfat symbiotic fermented milk. *Int. J. Food Microb.*, **128**, 467–472.

Oliveira, R. P. S., Perego, P., Converti, A. and Oliveira, M. N. (2009b) Effect of inulin on growth and acidification performance of different probiotic bacteria in co-cultures and mixed culture with *Streptococcus thermophilus*. *J. Food Eng.*, **91**, 133–139.

Oliveira, R. P. S., Perego, P., Converti, A. and Oliveira, M. N. (2009c) Growth and acidification performance of probiotics in pure culture and co-culture with *Streptococcus thermophilus*: the effect of inulin. *LWT-Food Sci. Technol.*, **42**, 1015–1021.

Ong, L. and Shah, N. P. (2009) Probiotic Cheddar cheese: Influence of ripening temperatures on survival of probiotic microorganisms, cheese composition and organic acid profiles. *LWT-Food Sci. Technol.*, **42**, 1260–1268.

Ong, L. and Shah, N. P. (2008) Influence of Probiotic *Lactobacillus acidophilus* and *L. helveticus* on proteolysis, organic acid profiles, and ACE-iInhibitory activity of Cheddar cheeses ripened at 4, 8, and 12°C. *J. Food Sci.*, **73**, M111–M120.

Ong, L., Henriksson, A. and Shah, N. P. (2007) Proteolytic pattern and organic acid profiles of probiotic cheese as influenced by probiotic strains of

Lactobacillus acidophilus, Lb. casei, Lb. paracasei or *Bifidobacterium* spp. *Int. Dairy J.*, **17**, 67–78.

Ong, L., Henriksson, A. and Shah, N. P. (2006) Development of probiotic Cheddar cheese containing *Lactobacillus acidophilus, Lb. casei, Lb. paracasei* and *Bifidobacterium* spp. and the influence of these bacteria on proteolytic patterns and production of organic acid. *Int. Dairy J.*, **16**, 446–456.

Østlie, H. M., Helland, M. H. and Narvhus, J. A. (2003) Growth and metabolism of selected strains of probiotic bacteria in milk. *Int. J. Food Microb.*, **87**, 17–27.

Özer, B. and Kirmaci, H. A. (2010) Functional milks and Dairy beverages. *Int. J. Dairy Technol.*, **63**(1), 1-15.

Özer, B., Kirmaci, H. A., Şenel, E., Atamer, M., Hayaloğlu Özer, B., Kirmaci, H. A., Şenel, E., Atamer, M. and Hayaloğlu, A. (2009) Improving the viability of *Bifidobacterium bifidum* BB-12 and *Lactobacillus acidophilus* LA-5 in white-brined cheese by microencapsulation. *Int. Dairy J.*, **19**, 22–29.

Özer, D., Akin, M. S. and Özer, B. (2005) Effects of inulin and lactulose on survival of *Lactobacillus acidophilus* LA-5 and *Bifidobacterium bifidum* BB-02 in acidophilus-bifidus yoghurt. *Food Sci. Technol. Int.*, **11**, 19–24.

Panesar, P. (2011) Fermented dairy products: starter cultures and potential nutritional benefits. *Food Nutr. Sci.*, **2**(1), 47–51.

Papadimitriou, C. G., Vafopoulou-Mastrojiannaki, A., Silva, S. V., Gomes, A. M., Malcata, F. X. And Alichanidis, E. (2007) Identification of peptides in traditional and probiotic sheep milk yoghurt with angiotensin I-converting enzyme (ACE)-inhibitory activity. *Food Chem.*, **105**(2), 647–656.

Parkar, S. G., Stevenson, D. E., and Skinner M. A. (2008) The potential influence of fruit polyphenols on colonic microflora and human gut health. *Int. J. Food Microb.*, **124**, 295–298.

Patrignani, F., Lanciotti, R., Mathara, J. M., Guerzoni, M. E. and Holzapfel, W.H. (2006) Potential of functional strains, isolated from traditional Maasai milk, as starters for the production of fermented milks. *Int. J. Food Microb.*, **107**, 1–11.

Pereira, A. L. F., Maciel, T. C. and Rodrigues, S. (2011) Probiotic beverage from cashew apple juice fermented with *Lactobaciilus casei*. *Food Res. Int.*, **44**, 1276–1283.

Peres, C. M., Peres, C., Hernández-Mendoza, A. and Malcata F. X. (2012) Review on fermented plant materials as carriers and sources of potentially probiotic lactic acid bacteria: with an emphasis on table olives. *Trends Food Sci. Technol.*, **26**, 31–42.

Pidcock, K., Heard, G. M. and Henriksson, A. (2003) Application of nontraditional meat starter cultures in production of Hungarian salami. *Int. J. Food Microb.*, **76**, 75–81.

Pimentel, L. L., Semedo, T., Tenreiro, R., Crespo, M. T. B, Pintado, M. M. E and Malcata, F. X. (2007) Assessment of safety of *Enterococci* isolated throughout traditional Terrincho cheesemaking: virulence factors and antibiotic susceptibility. *J. Food Prot.*, **70**, 2161–2167.

Philips, M., Kailasapathy, K. and Tran, L. (2006) Viability of commercial probiotic cheese cultures (*L. acidophilus, Bifidobacterium sp., L. casei, L. paracasei* and *L. rhamnosus* in cheddar cheese. *Int. J. Food Microb.*, **108**, 276–280.

Possemiers, S., Marzorati, M., Verstraete, W. and Van de Wiele, T. (2010) Bacteria and chocolate: a successful combination for probiotic delivery. *Int. J. Food Microb.*, **141**, 97–103.

Prado F. C., Parada J. L., Pandey A. and Soccol C. R. (2008) Trends in non-dairy probiotic beverages. *Food Res. Int.*, **41**, 111–123.

Radulović, Z., Živković, D., Mirković, N. Petrušić, M., Stajić, S. Perunović,M. and Paunović, D. (2011) Effect of probiotic bacteria on chemical composition and sensory quality of fermented sausages. *Procedia Food Sci.*, **1**, 1516–1522.

Rakin, M., Vukasinovic, M., Siler-Marinkovic, S. and Maksimovic, M. (2007) Contribution of lactic acid fermentation to improve nutritive quality vegetable juices enriched with brewer's yeast autolysate. *Food Chem.*, **100**, 599–602.

Ranadheera, R. D. C. S, Baines, S. K. and Adams, M. C. (2010) Importance of food in probiotic efficacy. *Food Res. Int.*, **43**, 1–7.

Requena, T., Pelaez, C. and Fox, P.F. (1993) Peptidase and proteinase activity of *Lactococcus lactis, Lactobacillus casei* and *Lactobacillus plantarum. Z. Lebensm.-Unters. Forsch.*, **196**, 351–355.

Robinson, R. K. and Tamime, A. Y. (1990) Microbiology of fermented milks, in *Dairy Microbiology*, (ed. Robinson, R. K.) 2nd ed., Elsevier Applied Science, London, Vol. 2, pp 291–343.

Roy, D. (2005) Technological aspects of related to the use of bifidobacteria in dairy products. *Lait*, **85**, 39–56.

Roy D., Mainville I. and Mondou F. (1997) Selective enumeration and survival of *Bifidobacteria* in fresh cheese. *Int. Dairy J.*, **7**, 785–793.

Rößle, C., Brunton, N. Ronan, Gormley, T., Ross, P. R. and Butler, F. (2010) Development of potentially synbiotic fresh-cut apple slices. *J. Functional Foods*, **2**, 245–254.

Rodrigues, D., Rocha-Santos, T. A. P., Freitas, A. C., Gomes, A. M. P., Duarte, A. C. (2012a). Analytical strategies for characterization and validation of functional dairy foods. *Trends in Anal. Chem.*, **41**, 27–45.

Rodrigues, D., Sousa, S., Gomes, A. M., Pintado, M. M., Silva, J. P., Costa, P., Amaral, M. H., Rocha-Santos, T. A. P. and Freitas, A. C. (2012b) Storage stability of *L. paracasei* as free cells or encapsulated in alginate based microcapsules in low pH fruit juices. *Food Bioprocess Technol.*, **5**, 2478–2757.

Rodrigues, D., Rocha-Santos, T. A. P., Pereira, C. I., Gomes, A. M., Malcata, F. X. and Freitas, A.C. (2011a) The potential effect of FOS and inulin upon probiotic bacterium performance in curdled milk matrices. *LWT–Food Sci. Technol.*, **44**, 100–108.

Rodrigues, D., Santos, C. H., Rocha-Santos, T. A. P., Gomes, A. M., Goodfellow, B. J. and Freitas A. C. (2011b) Metabolic profiling of potential probiotic or synbiotic cheeses by nuclear magnetic resonance (NMR) spectroscopy. *J. Agric. Food Chem.*, **59**, 4955–4961.

Rodrigues, D., Rocha-Santos, T. A. P., Gomes, A. M., Goodfellow, B. J. and Freitas, A. C. (2011c) Lipolysis in probiotic and synbiotic cheese: The influence of probiotic bacteria, prebiotic compounds and ripening time on free fatty acid profiles. *Food Chem.*, **131**, 1414–1421.

Rodrigues, D., Sousa, S., Rocha-Santos, T., Silva, J., Sousa Lobo, J., Costa, P., Amaral, M. H., Gomes, A., Pintado, M. M., Malcata, F. X. and Freitas, A. C. (2011d) Influence of L-cysteine, oxygen and relative humidity upon survival throughout storage of probiotic bacteria in whey protein-based microcapsules. *Int. Dairy J.*, **21**, 869–876.

Rodríguez-Alcalá, L. M., Braga, T., Malcata, F. X., Gomes, A. and Fontecha, J. (2011) Quantitative and qualitative determination of CLA produced by *Bifidobacterium* and lactic acid bacteria by combining spectrophotometric and Ag^+-HPLC techniques. *Food Chem.*, **125**(4), 1373–1378.

Roland, N., Bougle, D., Lebeurrier, F., Arhan, P., Maubois, J. L. (1998) *Propionibacterium freudenreichii* stimulates the growth of *Bifidobacterium bifidum in vitro* and increases fecal bifidobacteria in healthy human volunteers. *Int. Dairy J.*, **8**, 587–588.

Ross, R. P., Fitzgerald, G. F., Collins, K. and Stanton, C. (2002) Cheese delivering biocultures: probiotic cheese. *Austr. J. Dairy Technol.*, **57**, 71–78.

Ross, R. P., Desmond, C., Fitzgerald, G. F. and Stanton, C. (2005) Overcoming the technological hurdles in the development of probiotic foods. *J. Applied Microb.*, **98**, 1410–1417.

Ruiz-Moyano, S., Martín, A., Benito, M. J., Hernández, A., Casquete, R. and Córdoba, M.G. (2011) Application of *Lactobacillus fermentum* HL57 and *Pediococcus acidilactici* SP979 as potential probiotics in the manufacture of traditional Iberian dry-fermented sausages. *Food Microb.*, **28**, 839–847.

Saarela, M. (2009) Probiotics as ingredients in functional beverages, in *Functional and speciality beverage technology* (ed. Paquin P.) CRC Press, New York, pp. 55–70.

Saarela, M., Alakomi, H. L., Mättö, J., Ahonen, A. M., Puhakka, A. and Tynkkynen, S. (2011) Improving the storage stability of *Bifidobacterium breve* in low pH fruit juice. *Int. J. Food Microb.*, **149**, 106–110.

Saarela, M., Alakomi, H. L., Mättö, J., Ahonen, A. M., Puhakka, A. and Tynkkynen, S. (2010) Acid tolerant mutants of *Bifidobacterium animalis* subsp. lactis with improved stability in fruit juice. *LWT-Food Sci. Technol.*, **44**, 1012–1018.

Saarela, M., Virkajärvi, I., Alakomi, H., Sigvart-Matilla, P., Mätto, J. (2006) Stability and functionality of freeze-dried probiotic *Bifidobacterium* cells during storage in juice and milk. *Int. Dairy J.*, **16**, 1477–1482.

Saarela, M., Mogensen, G., Rangne, F., Mättö, J. and Mattila-Sandholm T. (2000) Probiotic bacteria: safety, functional and technological properties. *J. Biotechnol.*, **84**, 197–215.

Sachdeva, A. and Nagpal, J. (2009) Effect of fermented milk-based probiotic preparations on *Helicobacter pylori* eradication: a systematic review and meta-analysis of randomized-controlled trials. *Eur. J. Gastroenterol. Hepatol.*, **21**(1), 45–53.

Sameshima, T., Magome, C., Takeshita, K., Arihara, K., Itoh, M. and Kondo Y. (1998) Effect of intestinal *Lactobacillus* starter cultures on the behaviour of *Staphylococcus aureus* in fermented sausage. *Int. J. Food Microb.*, **41**, 1–7.

Sánchez, B., Fernández-García, M., Margolles, A., De los Reyes-Gavilán, C. G. and Ruas-Madiedo, P. (2010) Technological and probiotic selection criteria of a bile-adapted Bifidobacterium animalis subsp. Lactis strain. *Int. Dairy J.*, **20**, 800–805.

Sánchez, B., de Los Reyes-Gavilán, C. G., Margolles, A. and Gueimonde, M. (2009) Probiotic fermented milks: present and future. *Int. J. Dairy Technol.* **62**(4), 472–483.

Sanders, M. E. and Marco, M. L. (2010) Food formats for effective delivery of probiotics. *Annual Rev. Food Sci. Technol.*, **1**, 65–85.

Sayas-Barberá, E. Viuda-Martos, M., Fernández-López, F., Pérez-Alvarez, J. A. and Sendra, E. (2012) Combined use of a probiotic culture and citrus fiber in a traditional sausage 'Longaniza de Pascua'. *Food Control*, **27**, 343–350.

Settani, L. and Moschetti, G. (2010) Non-starter acid bacteria used to improve cheese quality and provide health benefits. *Food Microb.*, **27**, 691–695.

Seleet, F. L., El-Kholy, W. I. and Abd-Rabou, N. S. (2011) Evaluation of milk drinks fermented by probiotic bacteria and fortified with zinc Salts. *Polish J. Food Nutr. Sci.*, **61**(1), 55–60.

Shah, N. P., Ding, W. K., Fallourd, M. J. and Leyer, G. (2010) Improving the stability of probiotic bacteria in model fruit juices using vitamins and antioxidants. *J. Food Sci.*, **75**(5), M278–M282

Sheehan, V. M., Ross, P. and Fitzgerald, G. F. (2007) Assessing the acid tolerance and the technological robustness of probiotic cultures for fortification in fruit juices. *Innovative Food Sci. Emerging Technol.*, **8**, 279-284.

Shin, H.S., Lee J.H., Petska J.J. and Ustunol Z. (2000) Growth and viability of commercial *Bifidobacterium* spp. in skim milk containing oligosaccharides and inulin. *J. Food Sci.*, **65**(5), 884–887.

Siró, I., Kápolna, E., Kápolna, B., and Lgasi, A. (2008) Functional food. Product development, marketing and consumer acceptance – A Review. *Appetite*, **51**, 456–467.

Soccol C. R., Vandenberghe L. P. S., Spier M. R., Medeiros A. B. P., Yamaguishi C. T., Lindner J. D., Pandey A. and Thomaz-Soccol V. (2010) The potential of probiotics: A review. *Food Technol. Biotechnol.*, **48**, 413-434.

Sousa, C. H. B. and Saad, S. M. I. (2009) Viability of *Lactobacillus acidophilus* La-5 added solely or in co-culture with a yoghurt starter and implications on physic-chemical and related properties on Minas fresh cheese during storage. *LWT-Food Sci. Technol.*, **42**, 633–640.

Sousa, S., Gomes, A. M., Pintado, M. M., Malcata, F. X., Silva, J. P., Sousa Lobo, J. M., Costa, P., Amaral, M. H., Rodrigues, D., Rocha-Santos, T. A. P. and Freitas, A. C. (2012) Encapsulation of probiotic strains into in plain or cysteine-supplemented alginate improve viability at storage below freezing temperatures. *Eng. Life Sci.*, **12**(4), 1–9.

Stadnik, J. and Dolatowski, Z. J. (2012) Biogenic amines content during extended ageing of dry cured pork loins inoculated with probiotics. *Meat Sci.*, **91**, 374–377.

Suomalainen, T., Lagström, H., Mättö, J., Saarela, M., Laitinen, L, Ouwehands, A.C. and Salminen, A. (2006) Influence of whey-based fruit juice containing *Lactobacillus rhamnosus* on intestinal well-being and humoral immune response in healthy adults. *LWT-Food Sci. Technol.*, **39**(7), 788–795.

Tamime, A.Y. (2002) Fermented milks: a historical food with modern applications: a review. *Eur. J. Clinical Nutr.*, **56**(4), S2–S15.

Tamime, A. Y., Wszolek, M., Bo¡zani, C, R. and Özer, B. (2011) Popular ovine and caprine fermented milks. *Small Rumin. Res.*, **101**, 2–16.

Tang, A. L., Shah, N. P., Wilcox, G., Walker, K.Z. and Stojanovska, L. (2007) Fermentation of calcium-fortified soymilk with *Lactobacillus*: Effects on calcium solubility, isoflavone conversion, and production of organic acids. *J. Food Sci.*, **72**, M431–M436.

Tharmaraj, N. and Shah, P. N. (2004) Survival of *Lactobacillus acidophilus, Lactobacillus paracasei* ssp. *paracasei, Lactobacillus rhamnosus, Bifidobacterium animalis* and *Propionibacterium* in cheese-based dips and the suitability of dips as effective carriers of probiotic bactéria. *Int. Dairy J.*, **14**, 1055–1066.

Tuorila, H. and Cardello, A. V. (2002) Consumer responses to an off-flavor in juice in the presence of specific healh claims. *Food Qual. Preference*, **13**, 561–569.

Van Baarlen, P., Troost, F., Van Hemert, S., Van der Meer, C., De Vos, W. M., Hooiveld, G. J. E. J., Brummer, R. J. M and Kleerebezem, M. (2009) Differential NF-κB pathways induction by *Lactobacillus plantarum* in the duodenum of healthy humans correlating with immune tolerance. *Proc. Natl. Acad. Sci. USA*, **106**, 2371–2376.

Varga, L., Szigeti, J. and Gyenis, B. (2006) Influence of chicory inulin on the survival of microbiota of a probiotic fermented milk during refrigerated storage. *Ann. Microbiol.*, **56**(2), 139–141.

Vinderola, G., Prosello, W., Molinari, F., Ghiberto, D. and Reinheimer, J. (2009) Growth of *Lactobacillus paracasei* A13 in Argentinian probiotic cheese and its impact on the characteristics of the product. *Int. J. Food Microb.*, **135**, 171–174.

Vinderola, C. G., Prosello, W., Ghilberto, D. and Reinheimer, J. A. (2000) Viability of probiotic *Bifidobacterium, Lactobacillus acidophilus* and *Lactobacillus casei* and nonprobiotic microflora in Argentinean Fresco cheese. *J. Dairy Sci.*, **83**, 1905–1911.

Vorobjeva, L. I., Khodjaev, E. Y. and Vorobjeva, N. V. (2008) Propionic acid bacteria as probiotics. *Microbial Ecol. Health Dis.*, **20**, 190–112.

Wang, J., Zhong, Z., Zhang, W., Bao, Q., Wei, A., Meng, H. and Zhang, H. (2012) Comparative analysis of the gene expression profile of probiotic *Lactobacillus casei* Zhang with and without fermented milk as a vehicle during transit in a simulated gastrointestinal tract. *Res. Microbiol.*, **163**, 357-365.

Wang, C., Ng, C., Su, H., Tzeng, W. and Shyu, Y. (2009) Probiotic potential of noni juice fermented with lactic acid bacteria and bifidobacteria. *Int. J. Food Sci. Nut.*, **60**, 98–109.

Warmiska-Radyko I., Laniewska-Moroz L. and Babuchowski A. (2002) Possibilities for stimulation of *Bifidobacterium* growth by propionibacteria. *Lait*, **82**, 113–121.

Weinbreck, F., Bodnár, I. and Marco, M. L. (2010) Can encapsulation lengthen the shelf-life of probiotic bacteria in dry products? *Int. J. Food Microb.*, **136**, 364–367.

Xanthopoulos, V., Ipsilandis, C. G. and Tzanetakis, N. (2012) Use of a selected multi-strain potential probiotic culture for the manufacture of set-type yogurt from caprine milk. *Small Ruminant Res.*, **106**(2–3), 145–153.

Yilmaztekin, M., Özer, B.H. and Atasoy, F. (2004) Survival of *Lactobacillus acidophilus* LA-5 and *Bifidobacterium bifidum* BB-02 in white-brined cheese. *Int. J. Food Sci. Nutr.*, **55**, 53–60.

Yoon, K. Y., Woodams, E. E. and Hang, Y. D. (2006) Production of probiotic cabbage juice by lactic acid bacteria. *Biores. Technol.*, **97**, 1427–1430.

Zare, F., Champagne, C. P., Simpson, B. K., Orsat, V. and Boye, J. I. (2012) Effect of the addition of pulse ingredients to milk on acid production by probiotic and yoghurt starter cultures. LWT-*Food Sci.Technol.*, **45**, 155–160.

Chapter 5

Immobilization and Microencapsulation of Probiotics

Paulo J. C. Costa,[a] **Teresa Rocha-Santos,**[b,c] **Ana M. Gomes,**[d] **Manuela M. Pintado,**[d] **Sérgio Sousa,**[d] **Maria H. Amaral,**[a] **J. Paulo Sousa e Silva,**[a] **and Ana C. Freitas**[b,c]

[a]*Faculty of Pharmacy, University of Porto, Rua de Jorge Viterbo Ferreira, 228, 4050-313 Porto, Portugal*

[b]*ISEIT/Viseu-Instituto Piaget, Estrada do Alto do Gaio, Galifonge, 3515-776 Lordosa, Viseu, Portugal*

[c]*CESAM & Department of Chemistry, University of Aveiro, 3810-193 Aveiro, Portugal*

[d]*CBQF, Biotechnology School of Portuguese Catholic University, Rua Dr. António Bernardino Almeida, 4200-072 Porto, Portugal*

pccosta@ff.up.pt

5.1 Introduction

The preparation of microparticles is in great development in several industrial areas, especially in the pharmaceutical and food industries. In recent years, the food industry has been incorporating probiotics in microparticles in order to develop new and more diversified functional foods that could cause an enhancement in health state of consumer. Probiotics have also been encapsulated for incorporation on pharmaceutical dosage forms.

Probiotic Bacteria: Fundamentals, Therapy, and Technological Aspects
Edited by J. Paulo Sousa e Silva and Ana C. Freitas

ISBN 978-981-4411-62-2 (Hardcover), 978-981-4411-63-9 (eBook)
www.panstanford.com

The terms immobilization and encapsulation are used as synonyms in most of the scientific literature. Although encapsulation is the process of forming a continuous coating around an internal matrix that is fully contained within the wall of the capsule, immobilization refers to the capture of material within or along a matrix (Kailasapathy 2002, Vidhyalakshmi *et al.* 2009). Therefore, a small percentage of the material fixed can be exposed at the surface, which is not the case for encapsulated material (King Alan 1995, Kailasapathy 2002). For the sake of systematization, we will use the term encapsulation in a more comprehensive way, also including the concept of immobilization.

The substance that is encapsulated may be called the core material, fill, internal phase, or payload phase and the substance that is encapsulating may be called the coating, membrane, shell, carrier material, wall material, or external phase (Barbosa-Cánovas *et al.* 2005, Augustin and Sanguansri 2008, Zuidam and Shimoni 2010). All the raw material used for encapsulation intended for food products or processes should be natural food components or other ingredients that have GRAS (Generally Regarded As Safe) status (Barbosa-Cánovas *et al.* 2005, Augustin and Sanguansri 2008) or be food-grade materials (Zuidam and Shimoni 2010).

The different current techniques of encapsulation make it possible to obtain particles with diameters from a few nanometres to a few millimetres. Generally, it is considered that the process of microencapsulation produces solid particles with a size varying between 1 μm and 1000 μm (Heinzen *et al.* 2002, Burgess and Hickey 2006, Kinam and Yoon 2006). Other authors consider a different range of sizes (Arshady 1989, Gibbs *et al.* 1999, Desai and Park 2005, Chen and Chen 2007, Vidhyalakshmi *et al.* 2009).

The technology associated with the encapsulation of drugs, colorings, flavoring and aromatic substances, bacteria, and so on is vast. Among these technologies, the polymeric matrix systems are widely applied in the form of microparticles. The microparticles are subdivided according to their structure, in reservoir type (microcapsules) and in matrix type (microspheres) and other combinations of these main types (Arshady 1989, Gibbs *et al.* 1999, Barbosa-Cánovas *et al.* 2005). They are called microspheres if they are compact particles consisting of a network in which the substance is homogeneously distributed in its solid or molecular state. They are called microcapsules if they are particles composed of an inner core containing the bioactive agent covered with a layer of varying thickness (Fig. 5.1).

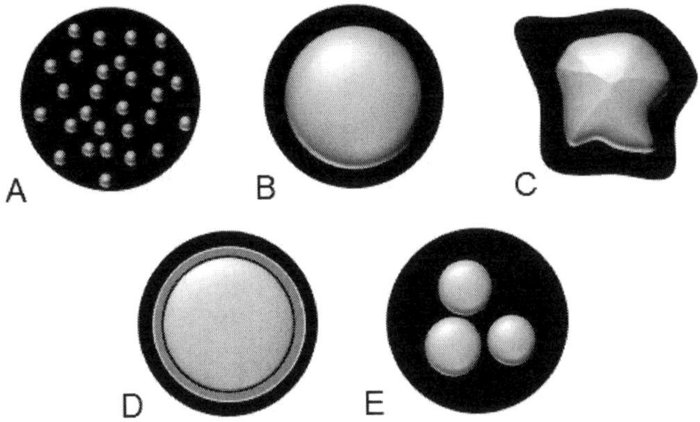

Figure 5.1 Some forms of microparticles. (A) Matrix type (microsphere); (B) Regular reservoir type (plain microcapsule); (C) Regular reservoir type (irregular microcapsule); (D) Multi-wall reservoir type (microcapsule); (E) Multi-core reservoir type (microcapsule). Adapted from Arshady (1989) and Gibbs *et al.* (1999).

Microencapsulation can be defined as a technology of packaging solids, liquids, or gaseous materials in miniature sealed capsules that can release their contents at controlled rates under the influence of specific conditions (Nixon 1985, Anal and Singh 2007, Champagne and Fustier 2007, Rokka and Rantamäki 2010).

In a general way, we can classify the objectives of encapsulation into five categories: immobilization, protection, controlled release, structuration and functionalization of active ingredients (Poncelet 2006).

The first records of attempts of application of this technique dates from the years 1930s, but the first product with microencapsulated material only came in 1954 (Dziezak 1988, Burgess and Hickey 2006, Kinam and Yoon 2006). The American company National Cash Register (NCR) pioneered when it developed a carbonless copy paper (Green 1953). This paper received a thin layer of microcapsules of a suitable pigment. The pressure from the tip of the pencil on the paper surface broke the microcapsules, releasing the pigment, which, by direct contact with the acid coating applied to the front surface of the second sheet, changed color depending on the pH, allowing to obtain a copy (Green 1955). In the food industry, the first researches took place from the late 1950s (Gouin 2004). Lactic acid bacteria (LAB) was first immobilized on Berl saddles in 1975 and later *Lactobacillus lactis* was encapsulated in calcium alginate beads (Gibbs *et al.* 1999, Desai and Park 2005). In the pharmaceutical industry, the early research also occurred in the same period. In this field, there was an important contribution because microencapsulation permitted the development of controlled-release formulas, that is, those with the capacity to release active agents in the organs where they shall act only or where they will be absorbed (Suave *et al.* 2006).

The microparticles continue to be employed in different sectors of industry in the present day, performing a variety of functions. The protection afforded by the wall of polymeric microparticles increases the lifespan of a volatile compound, extending the shelf time of many food products and cosmetics (Leimann 2008). In the pharmaceutical industry, the applications are very varied: concealment of flavors or odors, converting liquids into solids, protection in relation to atmospheric agents (light, heat and humidity, and/or oxidation), reduction or elimination of gastric irritation or secondary effects caused by certain drugs, reducing volatility, production of modified-release dosage forms, and so on (Kas and Oner 2000, Yoshizawa 2004, Burgess and Hickey 2006, Jyothi *et al.* 2010).

The use of microparticles in the food industry is also of great importance, because it increases the stability of oils, flavorings, vitamins, and so on (Leimann 2008). In this area, they have the ability to reduce the reactivity of the core material with the environment; decrease the rate of evaporation or the transfer of the core material toward the outer space; facilitate the encapsulated material handling; promote the controlled release of some substances; mask unpleasant odor and flavor; and promote homogeneous dilution of the material encapsulated in a food matrix (Favaro-Trindade *et al.* 2008).

Probiotic encapsulation was developed from the technology involved in cell culture (immobilized cell culture technology, ICT) (Heidebach *et al.* 2012). Probiotics have two limitations regarding encapsulation, namely the size of the microorganisms (with diameters typically between 1 and 5 μm), which prevents the use of nanotechnology, and the fact that the cells must be kept viable (Burgain *et al.* 2011). This aspect has been crucial to the choice of encapsulation technology (Champagne and Fustier 2007). The main purpose of the encapsulation of probiotics is to increase viability of these products during its shelf life, protect cells against an unfavorable environment that occurs in food matrices and in the gastrointestinal tract, and to enable their release in a viable and metabolically active state in the gut (Sun and Griffiths 2000, Picot and Lacroix 2004, Burgain *et al.* 2011, Nazzaro *et al.* 2012).

Different approaches have been proposed to increase the resistance of these sensitive microorganisms against adverse conditions (Anal and Singh 2007) such as an appropriate selection of acid and bile-resistant strains, the use of oxygen-impermeable containers, a two-step fermentation, a stress adaptation, an incorporation of micronutrients such as peptides and amino acids, protectors such as sugars and oligosaccharides, and, as previously referred, the usage of microencapsulation.

After a successful encapsulation, the inner bioactive material should be released to the outside, where it might implement its beneficial action. There are four typical mechanisms by which the core material can be released from a microparticle: mechanical rupture of the capsule wall, dissolution of the wall, melting of the wall, and diffusion through the wall. Less common release mechanisms include ablation (slow erosion of the shell) and biodegradation (Franjione and Vasishtha 1995, Barbosa-Cánovas *et al.* 2005).

5.2 Microencapsulation

Several procedures from many fields of application with different goals led to a great number of encapsulation methods (Dziezak 1988, Arshady 1989, Dulieu *et al.* 1999, Gibbs *et al.* 1999, Heinzen *et al.* 2002, Gouin 2004, Anal and Singh 2007). The terminology employed varies between the different scientific domains. Therefore, the same technology may have different names in different fields.

The selection of the microencapsulation method depends on the properties of the core and the coating materials, the size and morphology of the particle, and the release mechanism desired. Many of these processes have been adapted from the pharmaceutical and chemical industries. The use of low-cost materials and manufacturing processes is very important because food products generally have lower profit margins than pharmaceutical products (Augustin and Sanguansri 2008). Generally, microencapsulation can be divided into three main stages (Poncelet 2006, Burgain *et al.* 2011) as shown in Fig. 5.2.

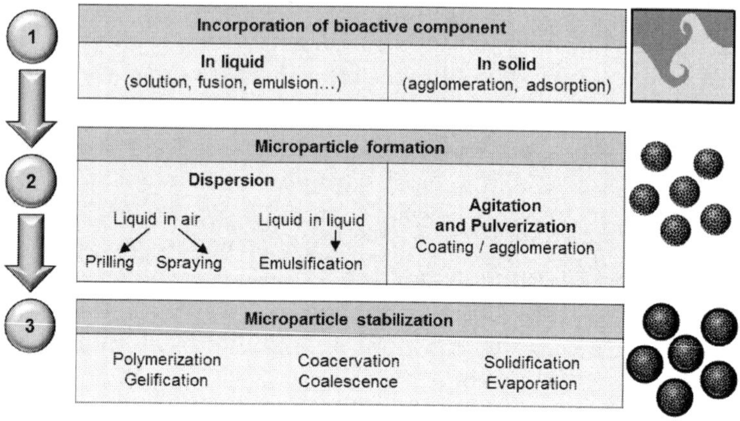

Figure 5.2 General plan describing the three main phases of microparticles production. Adapted from Poncelet (2006) and Burgain *et al.* (2011).

The incorporation of the bioactive compound in a solid or liquid phase is a prior step to microencapsulation itself, but is always necessary. If this phase is liquid, this step may involve processes of mixing or dispersion. If this phase is solid, this step may involve processes of agglomeration, adsorption, drying, and so on.

The second step, division into smaller particles, consists of mechanical operations: for a liquid system, it is dispersed in air (dropping or spraying) or in another immiscible liquid (emulsification); for a solid system, the division can be done by grinding and/or sieving; after that, a solution is sprayed on the microparticles in agitation (fluid bed or pan coating) until a good and uniform coating is obtained.

The third step consists in the stabilization of the microparticles formed in the previous phase, by chemical, physicochemical, or physical process (Heinzen *et al.* 2002, Poncelet 2006).

5.2.1 Encapsulating Materials

Several materials have been used for the encapsulation of probiotic bacteria, including alginate, gums (gellan gum and xanthan gum), k-carrageenan, cellulose acetate phthalate, chitosan, starch, gelatine, milk proteins, whey proteins, and many others (Table 5.1) (de Vos *et al.* 2010, Rokka and Rantamäki 2010, Ain Riaz and Masud 2011,

Burgain *et al.* 2011, Rodrigues *et al.* 2011, Huq *et al.* 2012, Sousa *et al.* 2012).

The choice of the encapsulate agent depends on a number of factors, among them, the nonreactivity with the material to be encapsulated, the process used for the microparticle formation, and release mechanism are the most relevant. The ideal encapsulant must present low viscosity at high concentrations and be easy to handle during the process; have low hygroscopicity, for ease of handling and preventing agglomeration; have the ability to seal and hold the active material within the structure of the capsule; provide maximum protection to the active material against adverse conditions, such as light, pH, oxygen, and reactive ingredients; be soluble in solvents commonly used; have the desired release properties of the active material; not have an unpleasant flavor in the case of oral consumption; and be costeffective (Shahidi and Han 1993, Barbosa-Cánovas *et al.* 2005, Desai and Park 2005). Biodegradable polymers and blends of biodegradable polymers natural or synthetic are often used in controlled release of drugs (Cerini 2001).

Table 5.1 Commonly used coating materials for food applications

Material class	Example
Carbohydrates	Starch and starch products, (dextrins, natural starches, modified starches) Sugars (fructose, glucose, maltose sucrose, corn syrup) Celluloses (carboximethyl cellulose, hydroxymethylpropyl cellulose, cellulose acetate phthalate) Chitosan Gums (gellan gum, xanthan gum arabic gum, alginates, carrageenan, agar, pectin) Cyclodextrins
Lipids	Waxes (beeswax, carnauba wax) Monoglycerides and diglycerides Natural fats and oils Phospholipids Hydrogenated fats
Proteins	Peptides, gluten, casein, gelatine, albumin, and other proteins

Source: Adapted from Augustin and Sanguansri (2008)

5.3 Methods of Microencapsulation

The objective of this section is to provide a short review of commonly used methods of microencapsulation and is certainly not a complete list. More details about these processes can be found in the references.

Microencapsulation itself can be divided into two main stages, including the stage of division into smaller particles and the stage of stabilization of the particles formed.

5.3.1 Microparticle Formation

The first stage of microencapsulation is the division of probiotic-containing phase into small particles with diameters in the micrometres order. The formation of the microparticles depends on the liquid or solid state of the dispersing system containing the active substance. So, we can have liquid matrix dispersion (extrusion, spraying, emulsification) or several solid matrix techniques (air suspension coating, pan coating).

5.3.1.1 Liquid matrix dispersion

The dispersion of the liquid matrix can be done in air or in another liquid. If done in air, it can be made simply by the action of gravity, by dripping, giving rise to a prill, or by atomization (or spraying). Dripping is the simplest technology for production of microparticles. Usually by dripping, the particles formed are very large (2–5 mm diameter) and consequently nonsuitable for many biotechnological or medical applications, and it is therefore necessary to reduce the size of the particles using auxiliary techniques (Heinzen *et al.* 2002, Burgess and Hickey 2006).

A prill is a small aggregate of a material, most often a solid sphere, formed from a melted substance. The material to be prilled must be a low-viscosity liquid when melted and a solid at room temperature. It is formed by allowing the drops of the melted substance to solidify (congeal, freeze, or coagulate).

The atomization usually forms an aerosol that is a dynamic set of very small liquid droplets or solid particles dispersed in a gas. If the dispersion of the liquid matrix is made in another liquid, the technique used is the emulsification.

5.3.1.1.1 *Extrusion*

The extrusion can be defined as a forced passage through an opening (or openings) giving the substance a defined format. One of the most important features in this procedure is the size of the hole that will require a higher or lower division of the material to extrude. The smaller is the inner diameter of the opening (nozzle), the smaller are the particles.

This technique has been used for many years in the food industry. The work that originally led to the extrusion/encapsulation process was done by Schultz *et al.* of the United States Department of Agriculture Albany Laboratory (Schultz *et al.* 1956). Encapsulation of flavors via extrusion was first patented in 1957 (Swisher 1957). The main referred advantage of the extrusion method referred is the increased stability of flavors or other heat-labile food components, because in this method, it is not necessary to use high temperatures (Dziezak 1988, Gibbs *et al.* 1999, Madene *et al.* 2006). The extrusion method is one of the most used techniques for probiotic encapsulation for food applications (Heidebach *et al.* 2012). This category of extrusion technologies presents generally no risks but sometimes is a very complex technique for microencapsulation (de Vos *et al.* 2010).

The probiotic encapsulation by extrusion thus consists in forcing the liquid dispersion containing the cells through a nozzle using high pressure at a low temperature. If the extrusion occurs slowly, droplets that will be formed will fall when the action of gravity exceeds the surface tension. If the extrusion occurs faster, a jet of liquid will be formed. If the extrusion (droplet formation) occurs in a controlled mode (as opposed to atomization—spraying), the technique is known as prilling (Heinzen 2002, Kailasapathy 2002, Burgain *et al.* 2011). Prilling can be a very useful technology if the solidification of the exterior material could occur in an instantaneous way (Meiners 2009). If, as already mentioned, the extrusion is done only by the action of gravity, the particles formed are large and it is therefore necessary to reduce the size of the droplets using auxiliary techniques.

The preparation of microparticles using the extrusion process is well documented (Gibbs *et al.* 1999, Krasaekoopt *et al.* 2003, Gouin 2004, Madene *et al.* 2006, de Vos *et al.* 2010, Kuang *et al.* 2010, Rokka and Rantamäki 2010, Burgain *et al.* 2011, Matalanis *et al.* 2011,

Nazzaro *et al.* 2012), but in general, the microparticles obtained are in a range of few hundred micrometers. In most applications involving immobilization of living cells, the size of microparticles needs to be small (lower than 1 mm) and carefully controlled. The reason for this is mostly because of diffusion limitations of nutrients within the matrix constituting the microparticle. For example, alginate beads made by the extrusion technique generally vary in size from 2 mm to 4 mm (Rokka and Rantamäki 2010). In general, extrusion gives a small range size, but it does not provide particles under 300 μm (Burgain *et al.* 2011). In order to get microparticles by extrusion below the mouth feel detection limit, referred to be 100 μm (Annan *et al.* 2007), some modifications in these techniques are necessary in order to reduce the size of the of the droplets.

Some research groups have often the incorrect assumption that this type of procedure does not allow for the large-scale production and is only suitable for lab-scale processes. However, huge advances have been made in scaling of encapsulation processes using extrusion technologies (de Vos *et al.* 2010) allowing large-scale microparticles production.

One of these modifications is the use of jet-based methods. These approaches have been demonstrated to be most economical and versatile on the basis of the ability to handle a wide range of materials (from micro/nano to living cellular particles) (Jayasinghe and Suter 2006). Among these methods, we can cite some very promising ones such as the electrostatic technique, the coaxial flow jetting, the aerodynamically assisted jetting (AAJ), the nozzle resonances technology, the spinning disk technology, and so on. (Heinzen *et al.* 2002, Poncelet 2006, Prüsse *et al.* 2008, de Vos *et al.* 2010, Sousa *et al.* 2012).

5.3.1.1.1.1 Electrostatic generators

Amsden and Goosen (1997) developed a method on the basis of the extrusion of a liquid through a needle with an electric field applied. By applying an electrostatic potential in the falling drop (Fig. 5.3), electrical charges accumulate on its surface creating a repulsion that opposes the surface tension (Poncelet *et al.* 1999, Poncelet *et al.* 1999, Mattheus *et al.* 2005, Prüsse *et al.* 2008). Generation of microparticles using this equipment is based on the formation of a single droplet at the top of the nozzle.

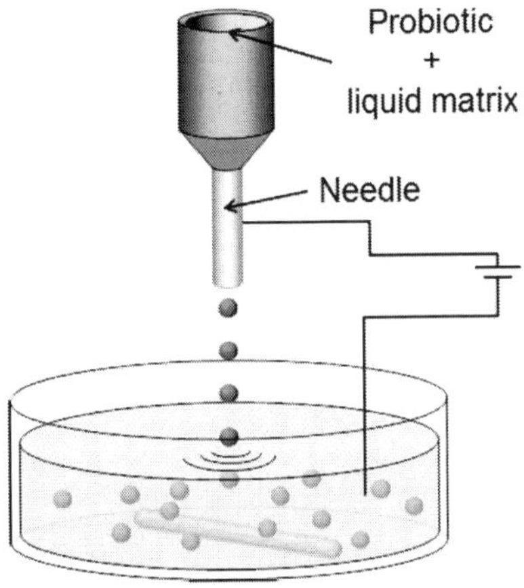

Figure 5.3 Principle of electrostatic generators.

A commercially available equipment is the Nisco Encapsulation Unit—Var V1 (Nisco V1 2009–2011). This equipment mainly consists of a high-voltage power unit 0–10 kV, a switch for tuning of the voltage magnitude, a needle holder, and a safety cage. Other setups have been developed by some research groups using different applied voltage such as 6.5–7.5 kV (Manojlovic *et al.* 2006), 0–25 kV (Prüsse *et al.* 2008), and 0–30 kV (Mattheus *et al.* 2005). The liquid dispersion can be fed via an infusion pump. A shaker keeps the bath, where solidification occurs, in agitation to prevent the union of the microparticles formed.

The diameter of microparticles produced is governed principally by the nozzle diameter, voltage, and distance between needle and solution (Amsden and Goosen 1997, Prüsse *et al.* 2008, Teoh *et al.* 2011). It is possible to obtain small sizes microparticles less than 20 μm for high voltages (10 kV). The potentials used are between 10 and 25 kV (Heinzen *et al.* 2002). The major disadvantage of this technique is the very low flow rate and is, nevertheless, inherently limited to small yield, as drops are only formed one after the other. Therefore, it is only used for the production of small batches (Senuma *et al.* 2000, Heinzen *et al.* 2002, Poncelet 2006, Zuidam and Shimoni 2010).

The Nisco instrument is designed for research uses, that is, for production of smaller quantities of spherical alginate beads ranging in size from around 200 μm to 1000 μm (Nisco V1 2009–2011).

5.3.1.1.1.2 Coaxial flow jetting

The basic principle of this instrument (Fig. 5.4) is to use a coaxial airflow to push the droplets that are formed in the nozzle. With this technology, microparticles with diameters of 200 μm can be produced (Heinzen *et al.* 2002).

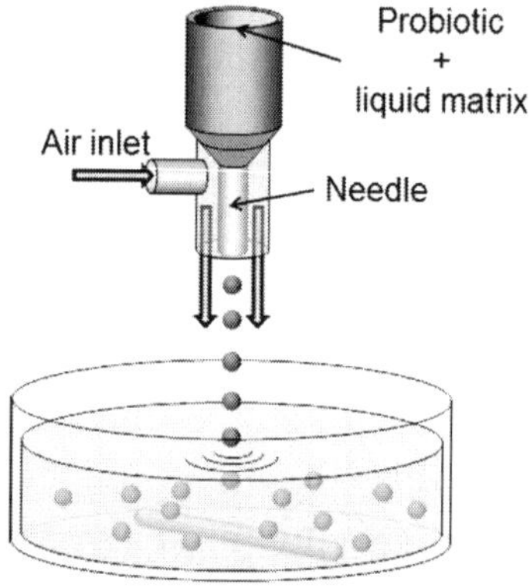

Figure 5.4 Principle of coaxial airflow bead generator.

A commercially available equipment is the Nisco Encapsulation Unit—Var J1 (Nisco J1 2009–2011). This instrument is designed for the production of small quantities of spherical beads (e.g., alginic acid) with diameters smaller than 500 μm (Nisco J1 2009–2011).

The diameter of beads produced is governed principally by the nozzle diameter, the flow rate, and the applied air flow (Prüsse *et al.* 2008). The major disadvantage of this technology is the very low throughput and therefore is only suitable for small-scale production (Heinzen *et al.* 2002, Zuidam and Shimoni 2010).

5.3.1.1.1.3 Aerodynamically assisted jetting

Aerodynamically assisted jetting (AAJ) is one of the main jet-processing approaches (Arumuganathar *et al.* 2009). AAJ is a phenomenon exploring a pressure differential for forming a liquid jet, which subsequently generates a myriad of droplets (Gañán-Calvo and Barrero 1999, Jayasinghe and Suter 2006) (Fig. 5.5).

A commercially available equipment is the Nisco Encapsulation Unit—Var J30 (Nisco J1 2009–2011). The product enters through a central needle, which is enclosed in a pressure chamber with an exit through the orifice. The exit orifice, which is centrally in line with the axis of the needle, has been counter-sunk externally. The counter sunk leads to the aerodynamical effect so that the jet has a smaller diameter when passing the orifice than before at the needle (Fig. 5.5). The size of the drops is determined by the product flow rate and the pressure inside the chamber. The product flow rate is controlled by a syringe pump, which is connected to the product nozzle. With this type of equipment, it is possible to obtain very small and homogeneous particles (up to about 10 μm) with a slight risk of clogging (Nisco J30 2009–2011). This unique technology has the advantage of reaching smaller particles than the needle diameter, depending on the physical properties of the product (Fig. 5.6).

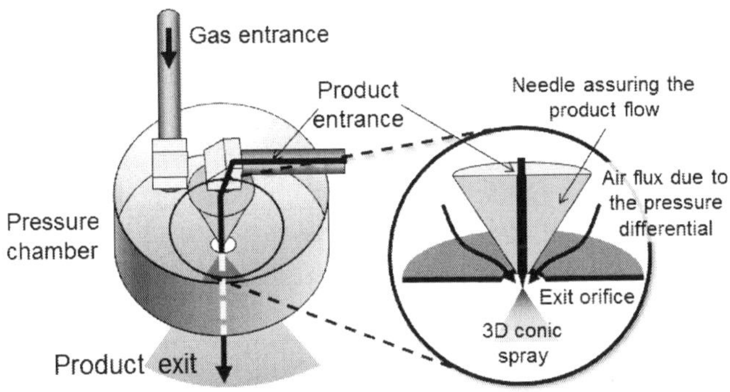

Figure 5.5 Operating principle of AAJ equipment.

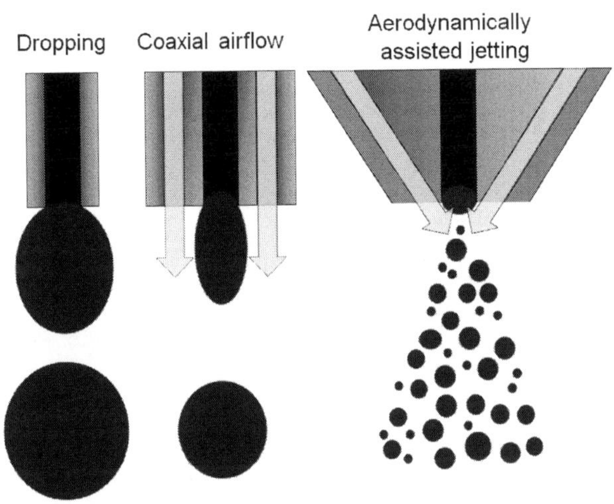

Figure 5.6 Preparation methods and schema size obtained by monoaxial extrusion technologies.

Four probiotic bacteria (*L. paracasei* L26, *L. casei*-01, *L. acidophilus* Ki, and *Bifidobacterium animalis* BB-12) were encapsulated using an AAJ technique in plain alginate or alginate supplemented with L-cysteine·HCl, and stored at different temperatures for a period up to 6 months, and the results showed that the encapsulation was only effective in promoting protection at freezing temperatures, independently of the sensitivity of the strain (Sousa *et al.* 2012).

5.3.1.1.1.4 Nozzle resonances technology

Berkland *et al.* (2001) developed a method on the basis of the extrusion of a liquid through a needle that vibrates at an ultrasonic frequency, in order to obtain microparticles with a narrow size distribution (Fig. 5.7). This technology is based on an old principle described by Joseph Plateau (Plateau 1873), and later confirmed by Lord Rayleigh (Rayleigh 1878) that demonstrates that a laminar liquid jet when subjected to a superimposed vibration breaks into droplets of equal sizes (McCuan 1997). This vibration has to be done in resonance of the Plateau–Rayleigh instability and leads to very uniform droplets size distribution (Berkland *et al.* 2001, Kim and Pack 2006).

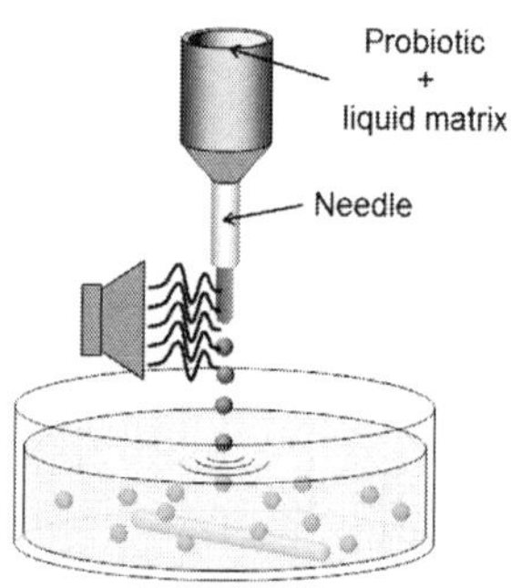

Figure 5.7 Principle of vibration technology.

During the formation of the jet from the nozzle, there is a tendency to split into small droplets. Applying a vibration at a particular frequency, uniform drops with a size of approximately twice the diameter of the jet are formed. The parameters that affect the dimensions of the particles are the frequency, the speed of the liquid jet, and the nozzle diameter (Heinzen *et al.* 2002, Prüsse *et al.* 2008). For large particles of about 1 mm, this method allows a high liquid flow, up to several l/h. For smaller particles, flow decreases proportionally. After defining an optimal vibration, the process becomes highly reproducible. The resonance is damped if the viscosity of the dispersion is too high, preventing or hindering the formation of droplets (Poncelet 2006). The process works very well for generating droplets between 100 and 5000 μm, but applications that can obtain either smaller or larger droplets are known (Vidhyalakshmi *et al.* 2009).

If one needs uniform, monodisperse, and small particles (diameters from 0.1 mm to 2 mm) and an up-scalable technology (from 10 g up to several 100 kg/batch), this technology is the answer (Heinzen *et al.* 2002). This technique is only suitable for lab or small-scale production (Senuma *et al.* 2000, Zuidam and Shimoni 2010).

5.3.1.1.1.5 Jet cutter technology

With this technology, the liquid is pressed at high speed out of the nozzle as a continuous jet. Directly below the nozzle, the jet is mechanically cut in cylindrical segments by a rotating cutting tool made of small wires attached on a stand (Prüsse *et al.* 1998, Prüsse *et al.* 1998, Prüsse *et al.* 2000, Prüsse *et al.* 2008). Driven by surface tension, the cylindrical segments after been cut form spherical droplets (Fig. 5.8). One of the advantages of this method is that the liquid flow rate can be high, but it is especially suitable for high viscosity dispersions (Poncelet 2006). The diameter of microparticles produced is mainly governed by the nozzle diameter, rotation frequency of the cutting tool, and number and diameter of the wires (Prüsse *et al.* 2008). This technique is suitable both for lab-scale production and industrial scale microparticles production (Zuidam and Shimoni 2010).

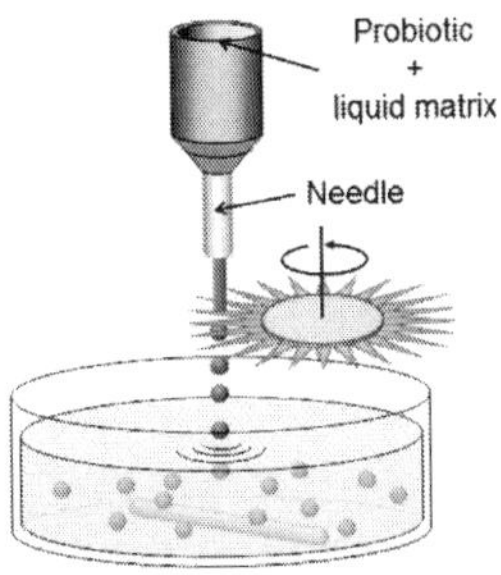

Figure 5.8 Principle of jet cutter technology.

5.3.1.1.1.6 Spinning disk technology

Rotational suspension separation (or centrifugal suspension separation coating or spinning disk method) is a microencapsulation technique that was first developed by Sparks in 1987 (Barbosa-Cánovas *et al.* 2005). This process involves (1) suspending core particles in a liquefied coating material; and (2) pouring the suspension through a rotating disk apparatus under conditions such that excess liquid between the core particles spreads into a film thinner than the core particle diameters. The liquid jet is directed to a rotating disk (Fig. 5.9) that uses centrifugal force to cause the division into droplets (Dziezak 1988, Gouin 2004, Desai and Park 2005, Augustin and Sanguansri 2008, Acosta 2009, Meiners 2009). The microparticles solidify after its departure from the disk. This whole process can take from a few seconds to a few minutes (Barbosa-Cánovas *et al.* 2005).

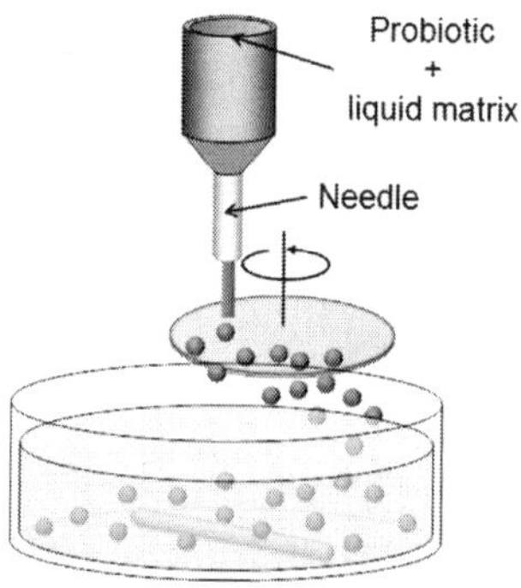

Figure 5.9 Principle of spinning disk technology.

The parameters that affect the size of particles are the speed of rotation, the geometry of the disk, and the liquid jet flow rate (Meiners 2009). This method has the advantage that the liquid flow rate can be high (Poncelet 2006). In addition to the method of jet cutting, this process is the most promising for the food industry because the preparation conditions are mild, there is no problem of plugging, the process is continuous, and power costs are generally low (Teunou and Poncelet 2005).

The main objectives in the disk design are to ensure that the liquid reaches the speed of disk and to obtain a uniform droplet size distribution in atomized liquid. Disk diameters vary from 5 cm in small laboratory models to 40 cm for industrial size dryers. Disk speeds range from 1000 to 50,000 rpm (Teunou and Poncelet 2005). This is a continuous process that makes possible to produce, at a high rate, particles of a given size with a narrow size distribution (Oxley *et al.* 2000, Senuma *et al.* 2000, Anantachoke *et al.* 2006). Particles of 30 μm up to 2 mm can be encapsulated by this process (Barbosa-Cánovas *et al.* 2005, Desai and Park 2005). Bégin *et al.* (1991) studied the use of a rotative flat disk atomizer for the production of biocatalysts immobilized in alginate gel and obtained microparticles with diameters ranging from 1 mm to 3 mm. Spinning disk atomization has been applied to an alginate microsphere preparation with sizes ranging from 300 to 600 μm in which yeast was used as a model system (Senuma *et al.* 2000).

5.3.1.1.1.7 Centrifugal extrusion

The Southwest Research Institute (SwRI), headquartered in San Antonio, Texas, developed the centrifugal extrusion concept in 1960s (Barbosa-Cánovas *et al.* 2005).

This centrifugal extrusion system, which is similar to the spinning disk system, is a liquid coextrusion process that uses rotational forces to create droplets. Spinning disk and centrifugal extrusion are both based in atomization methods (Gouin 2004).

In centrifugal extrusion, liquids are encapsulated using a rotating extrusion head containing a modified double-fluid nozzle in which the active ingredient is pumped through the inner part of the nozzle, whereas the shell material is pumped through the outer part of the nozzle (Dziezak 1988, Kailasapathy 2002, Gouin 2004, Desai and Park 2005, Augustin and Sanguansri 2008, Vidhyalakshmi *et al.* 2009). In this process, a jet of core liquid is surrounded by a layer of shell material (Fig. 5.10). As the jet moves through the air, it breaks, owing to Rayleigh instability, into droplets of core coated with the wall solution. Although the droplets are in flight, a molten wall may be hardened, a solvent may be evaporated from the wall solution, or other mechanism may occur, depending on the encapsulant material, leading to the hardening of the microparticles (Augustin and Sanguansri 2008, Vidhyalakshmi *et al.* 2009). Particles produced by this method have diameters ranging from 150 μm to 2000 μm (Dziezak 1988).

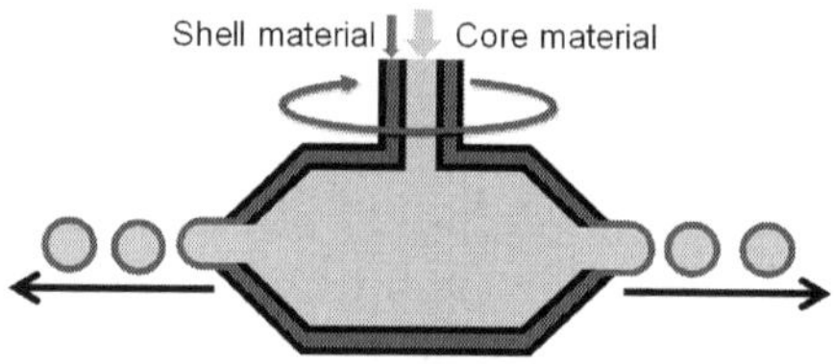

Figure 5.10 Principle of centrifugal extrusion technology.

From an industrial point of view, spinning disk and centrifugal extrusion are alternatives to conventional atomization devices such as double-fluid nozzles, pressure nozzles, and spinning wheels to atomize an emulsion or a suspension in a coating formulation (Gouin 2004). Centrifugal extrusion is an inexpensive process for producing particles with diameter from 400 to 2000 μm with a high production rate, up to 22.5 kg of microparticles per hour per nozzle (Barbosa-Cánovas *et al.* 2005).

5.3.1.1.1.8 Microfluidic techniques

In this kind of technique, uniform droplets are fabricated using precise microchannels through which the encapsulant material was extruded (Seo *et al.* 2005, Hyun-Jik *et al.* 2006, Zhang *et al.* 2007, Oh *et al.* 2008, Matalanis *et al.* 2011). The formation of monodisperse Ca-alginate microparticles using a microfluidic chip and a reaction of internal gelation was reported (Huang *et al.* 2007). The microfluidic chip was capable of generating relatively uniform microparticles and has the advantages of active control of droplet diameter, simple and low-cost process, and a high throughput. It was possible to control the size of microparticles from 80 μm to 800 μm by altering the relative sheath/sample flow rate ratio. The great advantage of microfluidics is the production of highly reproducible droplet sizes (Nie *et al.* 2005, Seo *et al.* 2005, Utada *et al.* 2005, Matalanis *et al.* 2011). Nevertheless, batch process for food industry using this methodology can be difficult to scale up (Matalanis *et al.* 2011).

5.3.1.1.2 *Spraying*

Spraying (also called atomization) is one of the most used methods in the food industry, because in addition to being economical and flexible produces good quality products (Dziezak 1988, Kailasapathy 2002, Gharsallaoui *et al.* 2007, Augustin and Sanguansri 2008, de

Vos *et al.* 2010, Zuidam and Shimoni 2010, Burgain *et al.* 2011, Peighambardoust *et al.* 2011). Atomization followed by hot air drying (spray drying encapsulation) has been used in the food industry since the late 1950s (Gouin 2004, Desai and Park 2005). The spray drying of microorganisms dates back to 1914 to the study of Rogers on dried lactic acid cultures (Peighambardoust *et al.* 2011). In 1932, the first spray-dried flavor powders, in which the flavors were encapsulated in a thin arabic gum film, were produced by an English company A. Boake, Roberts & Co., Ltd (Barbosa-Cánovas *et al.* 2005).

In the spraying process, bacteria are dispersed in a liquid phase and this system is atomized in a stream of air (Sousa e Silva and M. Ferreira 1998, Gharsallaoui *et al.* 2007, de Vos *et al.* 2010). In the case of probiotics, dispersion must be made mandatory in an aqueous phase.

A dispersion or emulsion containing the living cells of the probiotic in a suitable liquid carrier is initially prepared, usually polymeric. This carrier should have good emulsifying properties, have low viscosity at high solids content, and exhibit low hygroscopicity (Barbosa-Cánovas *et al.* 2005). This process is characterized by spraying the liquid dispersion inside a chamber subjected to a controlled stream of warm air (spray drying) or cold air (spray freeze-drying). This dispersion is atomized into millions of small individual droplets by a fast rotating device or a nozzle (Fig. 5.11). Through this process, the contact surface area of the product sprayed is greatly increased, giving rise to microparticles. A rapid vaporization of solvent takes place from the microparticles lying inside the chamber in contact with the stream of air. After evaporation of the solvent, the dried microparticles are retrieved.

Atomization can also occur at low temperatures (spray-congealing or sprayfreezing, (Dziezak 1988, Gouin 2004, Rokka and Rantamäki 2010, Nazzaro *et al.* 2012). In this case, the bacterial cells are in a solution that is atomized in a cold gas phase, which leads to dispersion of frozen droplets. These droplets can then be dried by freeze-drying (Wang *et al.* 2006, Augustin and Hemar 2009, de Vos *et al.* 2010). This technique involves the consumption of large amounts of energy, high processing times, and higher price than that of the spray-drying technique, especially on a large scale (Gölker 1993, Johnson and Etzel 1995, Knorr 1998, Mattila-Sandholm *et al.* 2002, Burgain *et al.* 2011). Despite of this, many LAB cannot tolerate the relatively high temperatures used during spray-drying (Porubcan and Sellars 1979, Ananta *et al.* 2005), and as a consequence, freeze-drying is a very popular method for the production of dried LAB preparations (Mattila-Sandholm *et al.* 2002). However, some more heat-resistant strains of LAB can be spray dried without a drastic loss of viability and activity, which are comparable to that obtained by freeze-drying (Silva *et al.* 2002, Ananta *et al.* 2005). Semyonov *et al.* (2010) developed a new process using spray freeze-drying to produce microparticles of *L. paracasei* with high viability.

Another alternative for atomization is the inclusion of the bacterial cells in materials with a melting point above ambient temperature (spraychilling or and spray-cooling). Initially, these materials are fused and the bacterial dispersion is added. This process is performed in an equipment similar to the one used in spray-drying, except for the fact that the process air is not heated (Augustin and Sanguansri 2008). After spraying, the liquid will split it into droplets that solidify by cooling in contact with the air at room temperature (Pedroso *et al.* 2012).

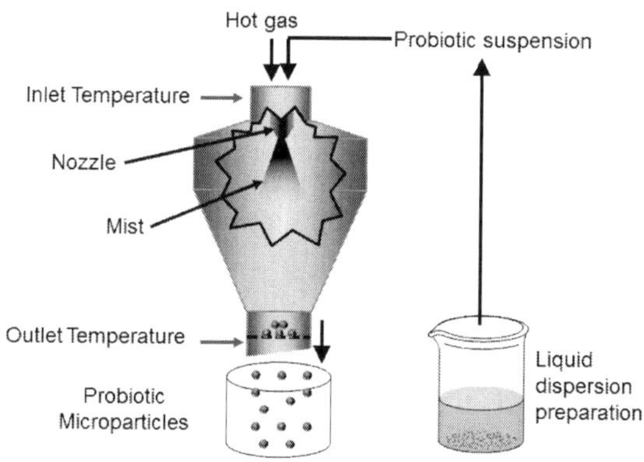

Figure 5.11 Schematic representation of the atomization process (spraying).

Spraying can form microspheres or microcapsules, as the drug is dissolved or dispersed in polymer solution. Formulation factors influencing the characteristics of microparticles are the polymer concentration, surface tension and viscosity of the liquid, temperature, and atomization flow rate (Silva *et al.* 2003, Kinam and Yoon 2006, Kuang *et al.* 2010, Zuidam and Shimoni 2010), which are often optimized by trial and error. In general, spray drying has been found to produce microparticle sizes between 5 and 80 μm (Rokka and Rantamäki 2010).

The advantages of spraying are the speed of preparation and the low cost of the procedure (de Vos *et al.* 2010, Burgain *et al.* 2011). It is a simple technique that allows to obtain the final form without having to resort, to washes, to isolate the microparticles or dispose of waste solvents. This technique is highly reproducible and adaptable to industrial applications. Another advantage of the atomization process is that it can be operated continuously. This process also allows obtaining large amounts, even when operated in a discontinued way. The encapsulation efficiency varies typically between 70 and 85%, regardless of the process parameters (Giunchedi and Conte 1995, Silva *et al.* 2003).

A major disadvantage of this process is that it is an immobilization technology rather than an encapsulation technology, which implies that some bioactive components may be exposed at the surface. This fact is especially problematic when considering the probiotics encapsulation, in which the bacteria may leak when some hydration occurs (de Vos *et al.* 2010). Among the disadvantages of atomization are the cost of the equipment and the difficulty in obtaining spherical particles (Giunchedi and Conte 1995). Another disadvantage of this process is that the high temperatures used in the drying phase may not be suited for the encapsulation of bacterial cells either because they can affect the properties of polymers or the survival of bacteria (Aaftabrouchad and Doelker 1992, Gardiner *et al.* 2000, O'Riordan *et al.* 2001, de Vos *et al.* 2010, Burgain *et al.* 2011, Nazzaro *et al.* 2012). The turmoil caused during atomization can lead to a wide variation of particle size formed. However, a proper control of inlet and outlet temperature in the chamber of atomization can allow getting probiotics encapsulated with the desired dimensions.

In order to improve probiotic survival, protectants can be added to the media prior to drying. Rodrigues *et al.* (2011) studied the survival rates of *L. acidophilus* Ki, *L. paracasei* L26, and *B. animalis* BB-12® after whey protein microencapsulation via spray-drying, with or without L-cysteine-HCl and showed that the effect of Lcysteine-HCl was dependent on the probiotic strain. Trehalose has been shown to enhance the survival rate of *L. salivarius* subjected to spray freeze-drying (Zayed and Roos 2004). Berner and Viernstein (2006) tested the effect of several different protectants on the viability of *Lactococcus lactis* subjected to freeze-drying and found the protectants based on skim milk or MRS-broth (all including sugars) to be the most effective. Sucrose, trehalose, and sorbitol were tested as cryoprotectants in the freeze-drying process of *L. plantarum* and *L. rhamnosus* GG, with sucrose presenting the best results between the three (Siaterlis *et al.* 2009). The addition of polydextrose to reconstituted skim milk (RSM) improved *L. rhamnosus* E800 survival to the spray-drying process, when compared with RSM alone (Corcoran *et al.* 2004). Trehalose and monosodium glutamate were tested, presenting positive results, as a way to preserve viability of two *L. rhamnosus* strains, during spray-drying (Sunny-Roberts and Knorr 2009). Monosodium glutamate, sucrose, and fructooligossacharides in combination with RSM were found to have a protective effect on the viability of two probiotic *L. kefir* strains during spray drying (Golowczyc *et al.* 2011).

5.3.1.1.3 *Emulsification*

The microparticles can also be produced by emulsification. An emulsion is a mixture of two immiscible liquids in which one of them is in small droplets (the dispersed phase, which may contain probiotics) within another liquid (the dispersing phase) to form a stable mixture. Emulsions are thermodynamically unstable and therefore do not form spontaneously, and it is necessary to provide energy to obtain them through agitation. Surfactant agents are mandatory substances added to emulsions to increase its stability.

The simplest method to produce emulsions consists in a reactor with a turbine for agitation (Fig. 5.12). Emulsions can also be obtained using continuous systems with static mixers. These systems consist of tubes wherein elements are inserted in such a way as to cause the fine division of the liquids. These systems allow the production of emulsions in a fraction of seconds at a high liquid flow rate (Poncelet 2006).

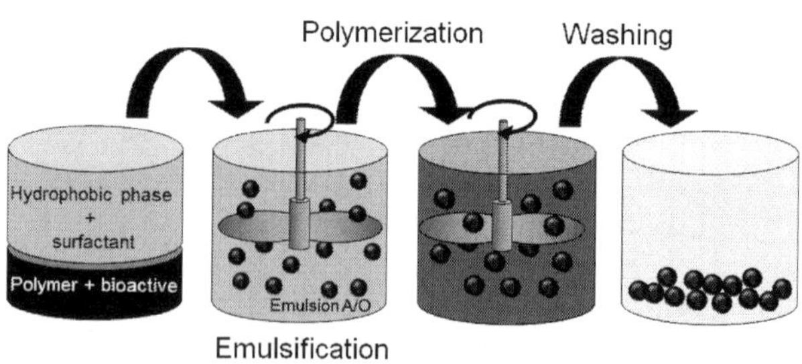

Figure 5.12 Microparticle preparation scheme by simple emulsion technique (hydrophilic active ingredients).

The emulsion technique as a general method for immobilization of sensitive living cells (microbial, algal, plant, and animal cells) was first developed by Nilsson *et al.* (1983).

The smaller the internal phase particle size of the emulsion, the smaller the final microparticles will be. The size of the microparticles is controlled essentially by the agitation rate, and can vary between 25 μm and 2 mm (Krasaekoopt *et al.* 2003). Emulsification allows the production of a wide particle size range from 0.2 to 5000 μm (Burgain *et al.* 2011). Although the obtained microparticles are of small diameter, the main disadvantage of this method is that it provides large size range and shape. For example, alginate microparticles made by the emulsion technique generally vary in size from 20 μm to 2 mm (Rokka and Rantamäki 2010). Using the emulsion technique for the encapsulation of *L. acidophilus* LA1, the diameter of microparticles formed ranged between 100 and 300 μm (Sabikhi *et al.* 2010).

The emulsion technique is easy to scale-up and gives a high survival rate of probiotic bacteria (Chen and Chen 2007, Burgain *et al.* 2011). However, it might be more expensive if vegetable oil has to be removed, and the microparticles have to be washed to eliminate the residual oil on its surface (Zuidam and Shimoni 2010). The emulsion method is one of the techniques most used for probiotic encapsulation aimed at food applications (Heidebach *et al.* 2012).

After the emulsion is formed, it is necessary to stabilize the microparticles obtained by any process. There are various techniques for the stabilization of microparticles, as for example, evaporation of the solvent, solvent extraction, cooling, thermal and chemical cross-linking, and ionic interaction (Kinam and Yoon 2006).

Özer *et al.* (2009) utilized an emulsion technique to encapsulate *B. bifidum* BB-12 and *L. acidophilus* LA-5 in white-brined cheese, verifying a more limited decrease in viability when bacteria were microencapsulated, and no differences in sensory properties were observed. Ding and Shah (2009) tested five different encapsulation materials on the stability of 10 probiotic bacteria, using the emulsion technique. Their results showed that in general, maicroparticles made of alginate, xanthan gum, and carrageenan gum greatly improved the survival of probiotic bacteria when exposed to acidic conditions and bile salts. Shima *et al.* (2007) studied the incorporation of *L. acidophilus* into the inner phase of waterinoilinwater (W/O/W) emulsion, and found that it improved the bacterial survival rate in a model gastric juice.

5.3.1.2 Solid matrix techniques

The division of solid particles can be done by grinding and/or sieving. After that, a solution is sprayed on the microparticles under agitation (air suspension coating or pan coating) until a good and uniform coating is obtained. During these operations, the microparticles can agglomerate, due to same problems. However, if well controlled, the agglomeration may allow the formation of larger particles from fine powders (Poncelet 2006).

5.3.1.2.1 *Air suspension coating*

Air-suspension particle coating (or fluid bed coating) is a process wherein thin coatings are applied to powder particles. This method is different to encapsulation by spray drying, because this last one produces particles consisting of a homogeneously blended matrix of the polymer entrapping the particle, in contrast to the previous method in which a defined film coating is produced over an existing solid core (Werner *et al.* 2007).

Originally developed as a technique for coating pharmaceutical dosage forms, air suspension coating has been increasingly applied in the food industry (Dewettinck and Huyghebaert 1999, Werner *et al.* 2007, Werner *et al.* 2007, Kuang *et al.* 2010). This coating technique was originally developed by Dale Wurster, professor of Pharmacy at the University of Wisconsin, in the 1950s (Wurster 1959) for coating pharmaceutical tablets. The instrument thus created (Bottom Spray or Wurster coating) consists, in general, lines (Kleinbach and Riede 1995, Prista *et al.* 2007, Werner *et al.* 2007) by a vertical tube, a compressor system, a heating system, an adjustable plate system, and one or several atomizers (Fig. 5.13). In the vertical tube, the particles to be coated are introduced; the compressor system launches an air current lift, heated by the heating system, which prevents the deposition of the particulate matter by the action of gravity; the adjustable plate system regulates the speed of the air; the atomizers release the coating liquid onto the particles (Dziezak 1988).

So, this type of coating occurs when an upward flow of air is driven through a bed of particles reaching sufficient speed to suspend them, but not expel them from such air current (Dziezak 1988, Dewettinck and Huyghebaert 1999). In conventional air suspension coating, the basic concept of fluidization depends on balancing the gravity force experienced by the particle by an upward movement of air flow, which ensures the full fluidization of those particles (Gouin 2004). In this type of encapsulation, although the core particles are suspended in the air, the coating material is atomized into the camera, shocking and depositing on the particle's nucleus. As the spraying nozzle is immersed in the airflow and sprays the coating material concurrently into the solid particles, these droplets travel a short distance before contacting it, resulting in a more uniform film (Kinam and Yoon 2006). When the particles strike the top of the camera, their speed becomes slow and by the action of gravity are thrown by a descent column of air that throws them again in the fluidized bed in which they are coated once more and the cycle begins again (Fig. 5.13). The application of a coating to a solid particle is a very complex phenomenon. The uniform coating layer is not formed on a single passage of the randomly oriented microparticles through the atomization zone, but on their successive passages through the zone, ensuring the integrity and uniformity of the coating layer. (Dziezak 1988, Vidhyalakshmi *et al.* 2009).

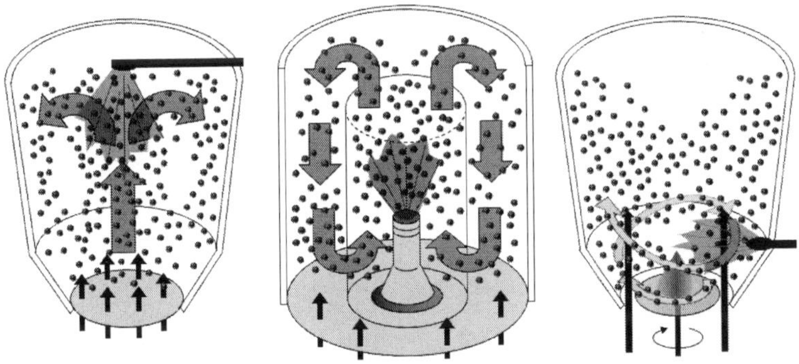

Figure 5.13 Air suspension coating types.

Other air suspension coating systems were also created, namely the Top Spray and Tangential Spray (Kleinbach and Riede 1995, Desai and Park 2005, Kinam and Yoon 2006, Champagne and Fustier

2007, Werner *et al.* 2007). The three technologies illustrated in Fig. 5.13 principally differ in the type of air fluidization employed and the site in the vessel at which the coating material is sprayed. The probiotic bacteria are present in fine powder particles, which are kept in motion in the vessels and are prepared by traditional methods such as fermentation, concentration, freeze-drying, and granulation (Champagne and Fustier 2007).

When the particles are coated by Top Spray system, the microparticles typically have a porous surface and interstitial void spaces; thus, the bulk density of the particles produced is generally lower than that achieved by other methods (Kinam and Yoon 2006).

The Tangential Spray system combines centrifugal, high-density mixing, and the efficiency of fluid-bed drying leading to the formation of a product with a higher bulk density, but it still has some interstitial void spaces (Kinam and Yoon 2006). This method allows to obtain less brittle and more spherical coated particles (Kinam and Yoon 2006).

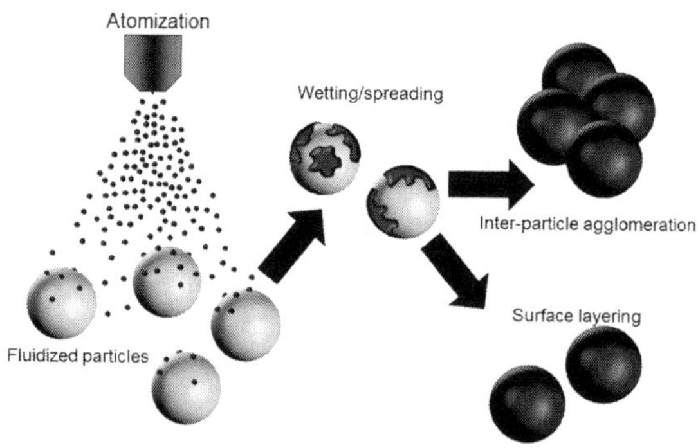

Figure 5.14 Air suspension particle coating. Adapted from Werner *et al.* (2007).

The fluidized bed encapsulation is one of the few technologies that make possible that particles are coated with virtually any type of cover material. In food applications, the coating is mostly lipid-based, but proteins or carbohydrates can also be used (Gouin 2004, Champagne and Fustier 2007, de Vos *et al.* 2010). This technique has been extensively used in the pharmaceutical industry to coat particles from approximately 100 μm up to the size of a few millimeters (Gouin 2004, Desai and Park 2005, Burgess and Hickey 2006, Kuang *et al.*

2010). This technology is especially ideal for aqueous-based coating, as it provides the high energy needed to evaporate the water (Kuang *et al.* 2010).

The advantage of air suspension coating is that it is easy to scale up (Burgain *et al.* 2011). As the food industry requires high volume production with a low cost, this type of coating using the Würster apparatus is still the first choice, whereas the various compromises between particle size and agglomeration can be overcome (Werner *et al.* 2007). Air suspension coating, in food industry, accounts for the second largest commercial production of encapsulated products (Barbosa-Cánovas *et al.* 2005).

5.3.1.2.2 *Pan coating*

Relatively large particles can be encapsulated by pan coating. The size of the solid particle must be greater than 600 μm so as to achieve an effective coating by this method (Kinam and Yoon 2006). This method employs a rotating pan containing the material to be coated on which a liquid containing the coating material is released. The rotation distributes this layer uniformly by the core particles forming a thin layer with a high surface area that favors the evaporation of the solvent (usually water). As the solvent evaporates, the coating hardens and covers the nuclei (Burgess and Hickey 2006, Kinam and Yoon 2006). Often, these pans are pierced (perforated pans) and the coating liquid is atomized in turmoil on the nuclei to be coated. This process is widely used in the pharmaceutical industry and is one of the oldest processes for coating tablets (Vidhyalakshmi *et al.* 2009).

5.3.2 Immobilization/Entrapment Techniques

The third and final step in the preparation of microparticles formed in the previous phase is its stabilization, by chemical (polymerization), physicochemical (coacervation, gelling), or physical processes (evaporation, solidification, coalescence).

5.3.2.1 Solidification

This method consists in the dispersion of the active substance, in this case the living bacteria, in the molten excipient, followed by emulsification of this phase with a heated immiscible solvent at the same temperature. As the formation of this phase requires heating, temperatures a few degrees above the referenced value for the excipients are being used (Kinam and Yoon 2006). The addition of a surfactant agent helps to increase the efficiency of encapsulation, as it increases the wettability of the active substance, which results in a greater incorporation into the microparticles (Passerini 2003). The mixture is then cooled below its melting point until the droplets of internal phase solidify (Burgess and Hickey 2006, Kinam and Yoon 2006).

One of the main advantages of the use of these materials and techniques is that it is not necessary to use organic solvents and the raw materials are well known. One of the main disadvantages is the use of high temperatures.

5.3.2.2 Coacervation

The earliest and one of the most widely used microencapsulation technique involves the separation of phases by coacervation (Kinam and Yoon 2006). This original microencapsulation technique, described by Green (Green 1953), for the production of carbonless copying paper was based on coacervation. It was Tiebackx (Tiebackx 1911) who first reported the phenomenon of coacervation without ever mentioning the word (de Kruif *et al.* 2004). The term coacervation was only introduced in chemistry by Bungenberg de Jong e Kruyt in 1929 (Bungenberg de Jong and Kruyt 1929) to describe the phenomenon of macromolecular aggregation from a liquid system, forming a colloidal system in which two liquid phases separate: one rich in polymers (coacervate) and another low in polymers (supernatant) (Dervichian 1954, Phares and Sperandio 1964, Burgess and Carless 1984, Nixon 1985, Arshady 1990, Sousa e Silva and M. Ferreira 1998). The word derives from Latin "acervus," which means aggregation, and the prefix "co," which means together. So, this word "coacervation" signifies the union of the colloidal particles. The physical and chemical basis behind the coacervation process is now well developed and understood (Bungenberg de Jong and Kruyt 1929, Dervichian 1954, Bakan Joseph 1971, Burgess 1990, Schmitt *et al.* 1998).

The coacervation can be defined to be simple or complex depending on whether it has one or more polymers involved (Nixon 1985, Schmitt *et al.* 1998, Gibbs *et al.* 1999, Burgess and Hickey 2006, Kinam and Yoon 2006, Madene *et al.* 2006, Jyothi *et al.* 2010, Zuidam and Shimoni 2010). The simple coacervation occurs when the conditions are changed, resulting in partial dehydration of macromolecules causing a phase separation. This can be achieved by mixing a polymer with a solvent that is incompatible or which is poorly soluble, by changing the temperature, and so on. In solution, these dehydrating agents promote polymer–polymer interactions through water competition. The complex coacervation occurs when a mixture of two or more polymers and a solvent are put together. In the event that the polymers are highly compatible, for example, two molecules with opposite charges, they interact and concentrate on a poor solvent phase, whereas the solvent forms a phase poor in polymers.

The three basic steps in coacervation are (phase 1) formation of three immiscible phases; (phase 2) deposition of coating; and (phase 3) hardening of coatings (Fig. 5.15). The first step includes the formation of three immiscible phases: the liquid vehicle, the solid core material, and the coating material. The core material is included in a dispersion of polymer coating. The coating material phase, an immiscible polymer in liquid state, can be formed by (i) change of temperature, (ii) adding a salt, (iii) adding a nonsolvent, (iv) adding an incompatible polymer, and (v) inducing polymer–polymer interactions. The second stage includes the deposition of these colloidal particles on the surface of the solid core coating it. Usually, this solid core must be compatible with the polymer and insoluble, or slightly soluble, in the coacervation medium (Arshady 1990, Madene *et al.* 2006). Finally, the micro particles can be stabilized, for example, by cross-linking, desolvation, or heat treatment (Jyothi *et al.* 2010).

This technique is complex, in operational terms, and needs a thorough control of the experimental settings. Many factors, including the type of polymer, pH, ionic strength, concentration, and in the case of two or more polymers, their ratio, affect the strength of the interaction between the polymer and the nature of the complex formed (Augustin and Hemar 2009, de Vos *et al.* 2010). The hydrodynamic conditions play an important role in determining the properties (size) of microparticles prepared by this method (Dobett and Pantaleo 2002).

Although the electrostatic interactions are considered responsible for the interaction between opposite charged polymers, hydrogen bonds and hydrophobic interactions can also contribute significantly to the formation of the complex (Turgeon *et al.* 2007, Augustin and Hemar 2009, de Vos *et al.* 2010).

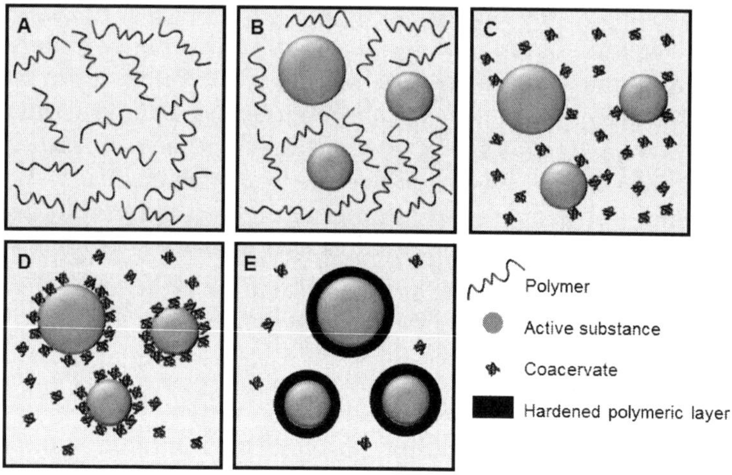

Figure 5.15 Coacervation stages: A and B and C: phase 1; D: phase 2 and E: phase 3; (A) polymer dispersion; (B) inclusion of solid core into polymer dispersion; (C) coacervation; (D) coalescence of colloidal particles at the surface of the solid core; (E) coating hardening. (Adapted from Augustin and Hemar 2009).

A very large number of hydrocolloids systems was evaluated for microencapsulation by coacervation (Gouin 2004), but the most studied and best understood system is probably the arabic gum/gelatine system (Bungenberg de Jong and Kruyt 1929, de Kruif *et al.* 2004, Desai and Park 2005, Kinam and Yoon 2006, Schmitt and Turgeon 2011). However, other coacervation systems present very good properties such as heparin/gelatine, carrageenan, chitosan, soy protein, gelatine/carboxymethylcellulose, β-lactoglobulin/arabic gum, and guar/dextran (Tsung and Burgess 1997, Schmitt *et al.* 2000, de Kruif *et al.* 2004, Gouin 2004).

The coacervation presents some advantages such as a very high payload achievable that is one of the most important characteristic of this method (Gouin 2004, Augustin and Sanguansri 2008). It also presents some problems such as the price and its complexity (Gibbs *et al.* 1999, Gouin 2004, Barbosa-Cánovas *et al.* 2005).

One of the factors that limit the use of coacervates in encapsulation is their sensitivity to pH and ionic strength. To increase the robustness of coacervates, they may be cross-linked using chemical agents, such as glutaraldehyde (an effective cross-linker) that is toxic (Sanchez and Renard 2002, Gouin 2004, Burgess and Hickey

2006, Kinam and Yoon 2006, Madene *et al.* 2006). Heating and adding counter polyions or other cross-linking reagents are alternative cross-linking methods (Kinam and Yoon 2006, Augustin and Sanguansri 2008). Enzymatic crosslinkers are more acceptable in the food industry (Gouin 2004, Augustin and Hemar 2009). Both chemical cross-linking agents and the application of heat may be harmful to the encapsulated materials, such as live cells like probiotic bacteria.

Complex coacervation is mainly used for microencapsulation of oils, but it can also be used for nutrients, vitamins, enzymes, and probiotics (Gouin 2004, Oliveira *et al.* 2007, Rokka and Rantamäki 2010).

5.3.2.3 Gelation

Gelation is one of the most used entrapment techniques to obtain microparticles. The contact of droplets of a gel-forming solution in a gelation bath leads to the formation of these particles. The gelation may be due to ionic bonding between polymer chains or by cooling (Poncelet 2006).

The use of natural polymers in formulating dosage forms containing food and drugs has received much attention because of its excellent biocompatibility and biodegrability. Among them, the alginic acid is a very promising natural polymer and has been widely explored (Gouin 2004, Anal and Singh 2007, Rokka and Rantamäki 2010, Ain Riaz and Masud 2011, Huq *et al.* 2012). It is a linear heteropolysaccharide consisting of β-D-mannuronic acid (M) and α-L-guluronic acid (G) (Anal and Singh 2007, de Vos *et al.* 2010, Draget and Taylor 2011), composed of blocks of homopolymer MM or GG extracted from several species of Brown algae (Aslani and Kennedy 1996, Tonnesen and Karlsen 2002). Figure 5.16 shows the structure of sodium alginate that is the sodium salt of the alginic acid. Depending on the origin, composition and sequence in M and G vary considerably, affecting their functional properties as supporting material (Tonnesen and Karlsen 2002, de Vos *et al.* 2010, Draget and Taylor 2011, Teoh *et al.* 2011).

The alginic acid (or sodium alginate) can react with bivalent cations or with polyvalent cation, as for example calcium, forming cross-links leading to the formation of a gel (Morris *et al.* 1978). Gel formation using calcium cation occurs mainly with GG and therefore blocks (Fig. 5.17) forming a structure called "egg box" (Grant *et al.*

1973) are formed. Even if this model is commonly adopted, it has been questioned several times and is still a subject of debate (Braccini and Pérez 2001). A more realistic coordination pattern supported by molecular modeling has been proposed (Mackie *et al.* 1983).

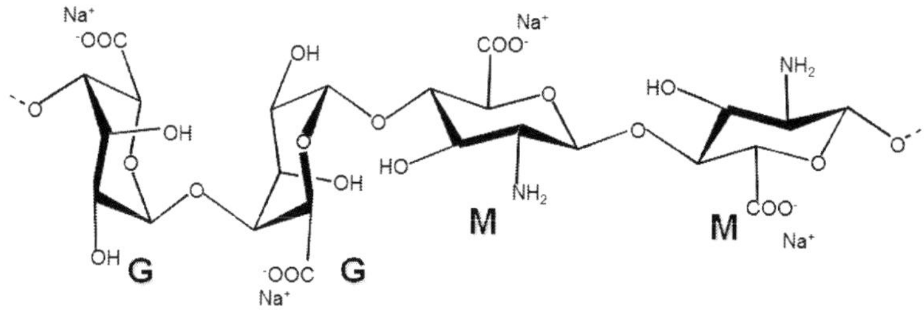

Figure 5.16 Sodium salt of alginic acid: blocks of (1→4)-linked β-D-mannuronate (M) and α-L-guluronate (G) residues.

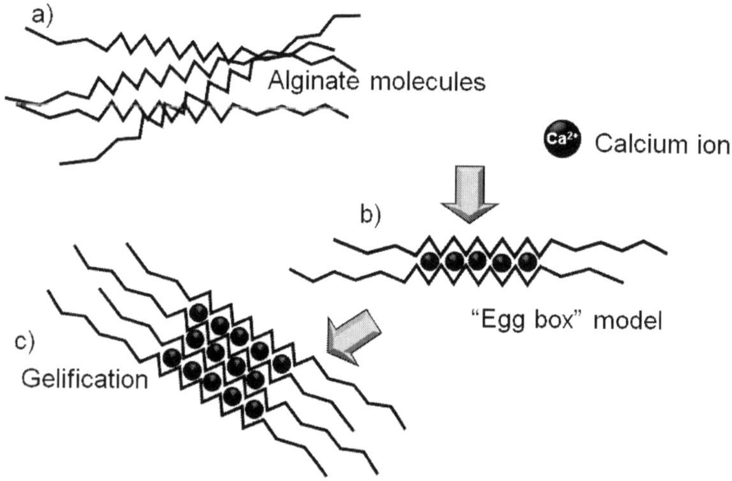

Figure 5.17 Formation of calcium alginate gel: (a) alginic acid molecules dispersed; (b) link between the strings through the groups of guluronic acid and calcium ions; (c) formation of the gel network.

The gelation due to ionic bonding such as an alginate solution dropped in calcium ions bath has been very used. The alginate gel is relatively stable at acidic pH, but easily disintegrates in alkaline conditions (Yoo *et al.* 2006).

Enhanced alginate microspheres as means of oral delivery of bacteriophage for reducing *Staphylococcus aureus* intestinal carriage have been developed (Ma *et al.* 2012). Some other polymer systems that can be used for ionic gelation are chitosan/triphosphate, pectin/calcium, gelan gum/calcium, and carboxymethylcellulose/aluminum (Kinam and Yoon 2006).

Gelation may also be obtained by spraying a thermogel (spray chilling) or, alternatively by the extrusion method, through emulsification followed by cooling or pH change (Poncelet 2006, Nag *et al.* 2011).

The emulsification technique can also be used for the preparation of calcium alginate microparticles. In this technique, an aqueous solution of sodium alginate is dispersed in an immiscible liquid phase and the gel droplets formed react with calcium ions, which are added to the external phase, forming microspheres. It is possible to get a high yield of encapsulation of hydrophilic drugs and particles with size less than 150 μm (Wan *et al.* 1992). Other gelifying agents can be used. Heidebach *et al.* (2009b) obtained microparticles by transglutaminase-catalyzed gelation of casein suspensions containing probiotic cells, namely commercial strains of *L. paracasei* ssp. *paracasei* F19 and *B. lactis* Bb12. *L. casei* cells were successfully entrapped into a gel matrix by a water-in-oil emulsion in which the matrix was formed by sodium caseinate and gellan gum mixture that was gelled by gradually decreasing pH with glucono-δ-lactone (Nag *et al.* 2011). Probiotic cells *L. paracasei* ssp. *paracasei* F19 and *B. lactis* Bb12 were microencapsulated in milk protein matrices by means of an enzymatic induced gelation with rennet (Heidebach *et al.* 2009a).

It is also possible to obtain microparticles of calcium alginate by emulsification-internal gelation (Fig. 5.18). Calcium is dispersed in the form of an insoluble salt (e.g., calcium carbonate or calcium citrate) in sodium alginate solution. This mixture is emulsified in an oily phase in order to obtain a W/O emulsion and the calcium present in the internal phase is released by acidification of the external oily phase causing the gelling of alginic acid (Poncelet *et al.* 1992, Poncelet *et al.* 1995, Poncelet *et al.* 1999).

5.3.2.4 Solvent extraction/evaporation

Solvent extraction technique has often been employed in view of the simplicity of the procedures involved in obtaining the microparticles and the modulation possibilities of physical chemical properties through the choice of components and preparation of the formulation. The origin of this technique can be found in the 1960s (Arshady 1990).

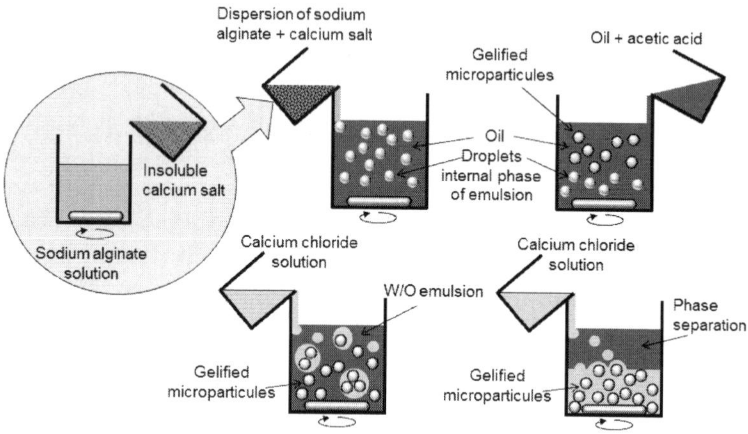

Figure 5.18 Emulsification-internal gelation.

This technique involves the preparation of a solution of a polymer, followed by their emulsification originating droplets. The two main stages of these processes are the formation of an emulsion and the solvent removal. The active is solubilized or dispersed in the polymer dispersion, and this mixture is emulsified in an aqueous solution containing a surfactant. This emulsion is then added to a nonsolvent (liquid medium in which the polymer is insoluble) that causes solvent extraction of the droplets. The resulting emulsion is agitated until the volatile solvent evaporates leading to the formation of solid microparticles (Kinam and Yoon 2006). Solvent removal progressively increases viscosity and decreases the volume, leading to polymer insolubilization (Arshady 1990, Sousa e Silva and M. Ferreira 1998). This method involves the diffusion of polymer solvent from the droplets to the outer space (continuous phase). After this process, the removal of nonsolvent can occur by evaporation, lyophilisation, or atomization (Arshady 1991, Aaftabrouchad and Doelker 1992).

The solvent evaporation technique relies on the high vapor pressure of the solvent that often leads to the use of organic solvents, otherwise the solidification process is slow (Kinam and Yoon 2006). This feature makes this methodology not accessible for encapsulation of probiotics.

In the case of a nonvolatile solvent, it can be removed by extraction into the continuous phase. This case can be done using a solvent that has a higher solubility in the continuous phase, increasing the concentration difference between the dispersed and continuous phase or by the addition of a third solvent into the outer phase to facilitate the solvent extraction (Kinam and Yoon 2006).

In solvent extraction technique, the solvent of the polymer is chosen to be miscible with the nonsolvent (Arshady 1990, Arshady 1991). Solvent extraction leads to microparticles with better characteristics (more regular shape, lower size, smaller variation in diameter) than the solvent evaporation method, but the largest particle porosity due to faster removal of the solvent increases the surface area (greater porosity) (Giunchedi and Conte 1995, Kinam and Yoon 2006), which leads to a faster release of its components.

5.3.2.5 Polymerization

The polymerization can be *in situ* or interfacial, that is, it occurs in the continuous or in the interphase of dispersed system.

In the *in situ* polymerization, no reactive agents are added to the core material, and the polymerization occurs exclusively in the continuous phase and on the side of continuous phase, on the interface with the core dispersed (Jyothi *et al.* 2010). Initially, a prepolymer with low molecular weight will be formed, which with the passage of time will grow in size, and will deposit on the surface of the dispersed core material generating a solid coating (Jyothi *et al.* 2010). The particles obtained are very small, but, typically, have high concentrations of associated monomer. Emulsion polymerization in external organic phase is not so used because it requires large amounts of organic solvents and surfactants and also due to the toxic nature of the monomers used. It is a very fast and easily scale-up technique (Silva *et al.* 2003). The particles obtained have a uniform coating with a size between 0.2 μm and 75 μm (Vidhyalakshmi *et al.* 2009).

In the interfacial polymerization technique, the coating can be formed on the surface of the particle by the polymerization of reactive monomers (Kinam and Yoon 2006, Vidhyalakshmi *et al.* 2009, Jyothi *et al.* 2010). It is characterized by the polymerization of a monomer in two immiscible phases (Nixon 1985, Burgain *et al.* 2011). If the internal phase is a liquid, it is possible to disperse or solubilize the monomer in this phase and emulsify the mixture on the external phase in which the coreagent is added. This starts the polymer formation on the surface of the liquid droplets. This technique can be used to encapsulate microorganisms in order to improve their productivity in fermentation (Yáñez-Fernández *et al.* 2007).

The use of the polymerization technique is limited by toxicity associated with monomers that do not react, by the high permeability of coating, and by the weakness of the membranes obtained (Silva *et al.* 2003).

5.3.3 Other Methods

There are other microencapsulation technologies that, due to their high price, are rarely employed, but for some specific issues can be employed as a solution (Desai and Park 2005, de Vos *et al.* 2010).

One of them is the application of liposomes, which are spherical bilayers vesicles, which can enclose bioactive molecules (Gibbs *et al.* 1999). The liposomes are formed by dispersion of polar lipids (mostly phospholipids) in an aqueous solution and were first described by the British hematologist Alec D. Bangham (Bangham and Horne 1964). Liposomes can be used as carriers for the delivery of nutritional supplements to foods (Shoji and Nakashima 2004, Augustin and Sanguansri 2008). They can range from 25 nm to several micrometers in diameter (Desai and Park 2005).

Another encapsulation method is the usage of cyclodextrins, which can envelop molecular structures by forming molecular inclusion complexes. Cyclodextrins have a hydrophilic exterior and a hydrophobic interior. This hydrophobic interior can be changed by varying the number of glucose units (Del Valle 2004, Brewster and Loftsson 2007, de Vos *et al.* 2010). As the encapsulation in this technique takes place at a molecular level and the internal cavity of cyclodextrins is very small, β-cyclodextrin cavity about 0.60–0.65 nm in diameter (Salústio *et al.* 2012), it cannot be used for the encapsulation of living cells as bacteria. Cyclodextrins have long been used to flavor encapsulation (Barbosa-Cánovas *et al.* 2005).

The microparticle formation technology that uses supercritical fluids has evolved in many different forms during the last years (Yeo and Kiran 2005). A supercritical fluid is any substance at a temperature and pressure above its critical point. The use of supercritical fluids can minimize the use of organic solvents and harsh manufacturing conditions (Kinam and Yoon 2006). Supercritical fluids can be used for the production of bioactive loaded microparticles (Augustin and Sanguansri 2008). Moolman *et al.* (2006) developed a method to encapsulate *B. longum* in an interpolymer complex formation between poly-(vinylpyrrolidone) (PVP) and poly-(vinylacetate-co-crotonic acid) in supercritical carbon dioxide.

In a micromolding technique, very small molds can be used to create microparticles with well-defined sizes and morphologies. In this technique, polymer solution is poured into a mold with a specific size and shape followed by adjustment of solution or environmental conditions to promote the gelation (Fukuda *et al.* 2006, Khademhosseini *et al.* 2006, Qiu *et al.* 2007, Dang *et al.* 2009, Matalanis *et al.* 2011). This micromolding technique offers the ability to prepare controlled shape microscale particles, even nonspherical ones, although batch process is difficult to scale up for food industry (Rabanel *et al.* 2009, Matalanis *et al.* 2011).

The electrostatic microencapsulation technique (electrostatic coagulation) is a dry process in which core particles can be coated with fine particles of different materials forming a highly porous encapsulating shell (De *et al.* 2002). Due to the characteristics of this technique, it cannot be used to encapsulate living cells such as bacteria.

The potential use of compression coating is also an alternative method for the encapsulation of probiotic bacteria (Chan and Zhang 2002, Calinescu *et al.* 2005, Vidhyalakshmi *et al.* 2009, Teoh *et al.* 2011). Previous works have demonstrated that compression coating significantly improved the storage stability and protection in an acidic medium of *L. acidophilus* (Chan and Zhang 2002, Chan and Zhang 2005). In another work, succinylated β-lactoglobulin revealed to be a suitable natural excipient to form tablets containing *B. longum* and promoted their survival against gastric conditions (Poulin *et al.* 2011). Carboxymethyl high-amylose starch was proposed as an excipient for oral tablet formulation of *Escherichia coli* ensuring its protection in the stomach and delivery in the intestine (Calinescu *et al.* 2005). Carboxymethyl high-amylose starch and chitosan were proposed as excipients for probiotic colon delivery of *L. rhamnosus* (Calinescu and Mateescu 2008). The effects on bacterial survival in tablets containing *L. fermentum* were investigated concerning compression force, matrix-forming excipients, such as hydroxypropyl methylcellulose phthalate (HPMCP), or other swelling agents, such as sodium alginate, apple pectin, and hydroxypropyl methylcellulose (HPMC) replacing partly HPMCP (Klayraung *et al.* 2009). This strategy will be further developed in the next chapter of this book.

5.4 Microparticle Characterization

Physical properties, the release behavior, and probiotics stability depend on the intrinsic characteristics of microparticles and the conditions used for storage. The characterization of microparticles is essential to ensure the encapsulation effectiveness, as well as to predict *in vivo* behavior.

The properties of the microparticles that should be considered in their characterization are general structure of the particle; fine structure; size and granulometric distribution; composition of the shell and the core; production yield; and release behavior and activity.

The quality of the materials used for the encapsulation is an important factor to obtain products with appropriate characteristics and batch-to-batch reproducibility. In cases in which polymers are used, these must be well characterized in terms of purity and molecular weight. The film-forming characteristics of encapsulation materials must be well known and controlled (Burgess and Hickey 2006).

The techniques used for microparticles characterization are diversified (Burgess and Hickey 2006, Graff *et al.* 2008, Alli 2011, Doherty *et al.* 2011, Mamvura *et al.* 2011, Lee *et al.* 2012). For external and internal structure, optical, electronic, and confocal microscopy can be used. The fine structure of the microparticles can be determined using X-ray diffraction and thermal analysis. For the size and granulometric distribution, optical, electron microscopy, and particle size analyzer can be used. For the composition of the shell and the core thermal analysis, chemistry, chromatography, and spectroscopic methods can be used. The production yield can be determined by assay. In terms of probiotics survival and activity, several microbiological analyses can be performed to assess the number of viable cells and their metabolic state. The release behavior can be verified using release tests.

The rate of release of probiotics from the microparticles will in many cases dictate their therapeutic action. This release is generally governed by the type of microparticles present, by the molecular structure of the encapsulant material, the resistance of this material to erosion or degradation, and surface area and porosity of the microparticles (Barbosa-Cánovas *et al.* 2005, Burgess and Hickey 2006, Kinam and Yoon 2006).

For the characterization of the microparticles, the probiotics release profile should be tested *in vitro* and whenever possible *in vivo*. In the pharmaceutical industry, *in vitro* dissolution testing is one of the most important tools in drug development and quality control. To assure the survival during the gastric transit, the dissolution studies may be performed in simulated gastric fluid (SGF) or/and simulated intestinal fluid (SIF) (Lee and Heo 2000, Stadler and Viernstein 2003, Graff *et al.* 2008, Sabikhi *et al.* 2010, Alli 2011, Rodrigues *et al.* 2011, Heidebach *et al.* 2012).

The release behavior of the probiotics can also be tested *in vivo* (Heidebach *et al.* 2012). Unfortunately, only a few *in vivo* studies were experimented and they used animals such as rats or mice (Kushal *et al.* 2006, Graff, Hussain *et al.* 2008, Heidebach *et al.* 2012).

5.5 Conclusions and Future Trends

The use of microencapsulated ingredients for the release control inside the human body is a promising alternative to solve some problems that the food industry has been facing. Some of these problems are related to low stability, poor absorption, poor organoleptic characteristics, low viability, and so on.

Often, the greatest challenge is to select the appropriate microencapsulation technique and the most appropriate encapsulating material. Despite the wide range of encapsulated products that have been developed, manufactured and marketed successfully in cosmetic and pharmaceutical industries, the microencapsulation has found a comparatively limited market in the food industry (Gouin 2004). With regard to the different methods of encapsulation, consumer health and safety are factors that should be taken into account, and then only approved food materials can be used in these techniques of encapsulation. Environmental consciousness of the consumers also deserves special attention in the design of future products and technology, because some of them might not be environment-friendly.

For a successful implementation of probiotics microparticles in food products, some important demands must be met. Therefore, they should be generated by processes that do not decrease the living cell count or induce sublethal damages, should not alter the sensory properties of the food, and should provide protection against adverse conditions caused by food processing and/or the environment of the food matrix. They also should protect the probiotic cells against stress induced by the acidic gastric conditions and should release the cells in the intestine at a high level of activity (Heidebach and Kulozik 2010).

The microencapsulation of probiotics raises some specific problems. The survival of probiotic bacteria during processing, storage, and in gastric conditions is highly dependent on the strain used. Stability of the strain is thus one of the main criteria in selecting suitable probiotics (Rokka and Rantamäki 2010). The encapsulation process must therefore contribute to an increased stability of probiotics. Food matrix environment has to be taken into account when selecting the materials for the encapsulation.

Probiotic encapsulation was previously developed from the technology involved in cell culture (ICT). The majority of microparticles produced for ICT applications in dairy systems were produced by two main methods, the extrusion and the emulsion method, and consequently, in most of the studies on probiotic encapsulation for food applications, these methods were also applied. More recently, spray drying has been also utilized to encapsulate probiotic cells as an alternative to the encapsulation methods previously referred based on ICT (Heidebach *et al.* 2012). Today, the vast majority of probiotic microparticles are produced by these three methods: the extrusion technique, the emulsion technique, and the spray drying technique (Heidebach and Kulozik 2010, Rokka and Rantamäki 2010, Heidebach *et al.* 2012).

The development time of a microencapsulated product is quite long and requires specific equipment and a multidisciplinary cooperation. Often, the complex transition from the laboratory scale to the large production scale has led to difficulties in the marketing of the final product. The low-profit margins, usually reached in food ingredients, are an impediment to the development and implementation of new technologies that could result in truly unique food products (Gouin 2004, Desai and Park 2005). New developments in the area of probiotics encapsulation are thus expected in upcoming years at the level of new encapsulation techniques, new encapsulant materials, and/or new commercial applications containing these bioactive agents.

References

Aaftabrouchad, C. and E. Doelker (1992). "Preparation methods for biodegradable microparticles loaded with water-soluble drugs." *STP Pharma Sciences* **2**: 365–380.

Acosta, E. (2009). "Bioavailability of nanoparticles in nutrient and nutraceutical delivery." *Current Opinion in Colloid & Interface Science* **14**(1): 3–15.

Alli, S. M. (2011). "Preparation and characterization of a coacervate extended-release microparticulate delivery system for Lactobacillus rhamnosus." *International Journal of Nanomedicine* **6**: 1699–1707.

Amsden, B. G. and M. F. A. Goosen (1997). "An examination of factors affecting the size, distribution and release characteristics of polymer microbeads made using electrostatics." *Journal of Controlled Release* **43**(2–3): 183–196.

Anal, A. K. and H. Singh (2007). "Recent advances in microencapsulation of probiotics for industrial applications and targeted delivery." *Trends in Food Science & Technology* **18**(5): 240–251.

Ananta, E., M. Volkert and D. Knorr (2005). "Cellular injuries and storage stability of spray-dried Lactobacillus rhamnosus GG." *International Dairy Journal* **15**(4): 399–409.

Anantachoke, N., M. Makha, C. L. Raston, V. Reutrakul, N. C. Smith and M. Saunders (2006). "Fine tuning the production of nanosized beta-carotene particles using spinning disk processing." *Journal of the American Chemical Society* **128**(42): 13847–13853.

Annan, N. T., A. Borza, D. L. Moreau, P. M. Allan-Wojtas and L. T. Hansen (2007). "Effect of process variables on particle size and viability of Bifidobacterium lactis Bb-12 in genipin-gelatin microspheres." *Journal of Microencapsulation* **24**(2): 152–162.

Arshady, R. (1989). "Microspheres and microcapsules: a survey of manufacturing techniques. Part 1: Suspension cross-linking." *Polymer Engineering and Science* **29**(24): 1746–1758.

Arshady, R. (1990). "Microspheres and microcapsules, a survey of manufacturing techniques Part II: Coacervation." *Polymer Engineering and Science* **30**(15): 905–914.

Arshady, R. (1990). "Microspheres and microcapsules, a survey of manufacturing techniques: Part III: Solvent evaporation." *Polymer Engineering and Science* **30**(15): 915–924.

Arshady, R. (1991). "Preparation of biodegradable microspheres and microcapsules." *Controlled Release Society* **17**: 1–21.

Arshady, R. (1991). "Preparation of biodegradable microspheres and microcapsules. 2. Polyactides and related polyesters." *Journal of Controlled Release* **17**(1): 1–21.

Arumuganathar, S., N. Suter, P. Walzel and S. N. Jayasinghe (2009). "Aerodynamically assisted jetting and threading for processing concentrated suspensions containing advanced structural, functional and biological materials." *Biotechnology Journal* **4**(1): 64–72.

Aslani, P. and R. A. Kennedy (1996). "Studies on diffusion in alginate gels .1. Effect of cross-linking with calcium or zinc ions on diffusion of acetaminophen." *Journal of Controlled Release* **42**(1): 75–82.

Augustin, M. A. and Y. Hemar (2009). "Nano- and micro-structured assemblies for encapsulation of food ingredients." *Chemical Society Reviews* **38**(4): 902–912.

Augustin, M. A. and L. Sanguansri (2008). Encapsulation of bioactives. In: *Food Materials Science*. Aguilera, J. M. and P. J. Lillford (eds), Springer, New York: 577–601.

Bakan Joseph, A. (1971). Method of making microscopic capsules. United States Patent Office. U. S. P. Office: US Patent 3,567,650.

Bangham, A. D. and R. W. Horne (1964). "Negative staining of phospholipids and their structural modification by surface-active agents as observed in the electron microscope." *Journal of Molecular Biology* **8**(5): 660-IN610.

Barbosa-Cánovas, G. V., E. Ortega-Rivas, P. Juliano and H. Yan (2005). *Encapsulation Processes. Food Powders Physical Properties, Processing, and Functionality*. Kluwer Academic/Plenum Publishers, New York: 199–219.

Bégin, A., F. Castaigne and J. Goulet (1991). "Production of alginate beads by a rotative atomizer." *Biotechnology Techniques* **5**(6): 459–464.

Berkland, C., K. Kim and D. W. Pack (2001). "Fabrication of PLG microspheres with precisely controlled and monodisperse size distributions." *Journal of Controlled Release* **73**(1): 59–74.

Berner, D. and H. Viernstein (2006). "Effect of protective agents on the viability of Lactococcus lactis subjected to freeze-thawing and freeze-drying." *Scientia Pharmaceutica* **74**: 137–149.

Braccini, I. and S. Pérez (2001). "Molecular basis of Ca2+-induced gelation in alginates and pectins: the egg-box model revisited." *Biomacromolecules* **2**(4): 1089–1096.

Brewster, M. E. and T. Loftsson (2007). "Cyclodextrins as pharmaceutical solubilizers." *Advanced Drug Delivery Reviews* **59**(7): 645–666.

Bungenberg de Jong, H. and H. Kruyt (1929). "Coacervation (partial miscibility in colloid systems)." *Proceedings of the Koninklijke Nederlandse Akademie van Wetenschappen, Series A* **32**: 849–856.

Burgain, J., C. Gaiani, M. Linder and J. Scher (2011). "Encapsulation of probiotic living cells: From laboratory scale to industrial applications." *Journal of Food Engineering* **104**(4): 467–483.

Burgess, D. J. (1990). "Practical analysis of complex coacervate systems." *Journal of Colloid and Interface Science* **140**(1): 227–238.

Burgess, D. J. and J. E. Carless (1984). "Microelectrophoretic studies of gelatin and acacia for the prediction of complex coacervation." *Journal of Colloid and Interface Science* **98**(1): 1–8.

Burgess, D. J. and A. J. Hickey (2006). Microsphere technology and applications. *Encyclopedia of pharmaceutical technology, Third Edition*: 2328–2338.

Calinescu, C. and M. A. Mateescu (2008). "Carboxymethyl high amylose starch: chitosan self-stabilized matrix for probiotic colon delivery." *European Journal of Pharmaceutics and Biopharmaceutics 70(2): 582–*589.

Calinescu, C., J. Mulhbacher, E. Nadeau, J. M. Fairbrother and M. A. Mateescu (2005). "Carboxymethyl high amylose starch (CM-HAS) as excipient for Escherichia coli oral formulations." *European Journal of Pharmaceutics and Biopharmaceutics* **60**(1): 53–60.

Cerini, A. (2001). *Estudo in vitro da liberação de vancomicina encapsulada em blendas de poli(ácido lático)/poli(óxido de etileno).* Universidade Estadual de Campinas.

Champagne, C. P. and P. Fustier (2007). "Microencapsulation for the improved delivery of bioactive compounds into foods." *Current Opinion in Biotechnology* **18**(2): 184–190.

Chan, E. S. and Z. Zhang (2002). "Encapsulation of probiotic bacteria Lactobacillus acidophilus by direct compression." *Food and Bioproducts Processing* **80**(C2): 78–82.

Chan, E. S. and Z. Zhang (2005). "Bioencapsulation by compression coating of probiotic bacteria for their protection in an acidic medium." *Process Biochemistry* **40**(10): 3346–3351.

Chen, M.-J. and K.-N. Chen (2007). Applications of probiotic encapsulation in dairy products. *Encapsulation and Controlled Release Technologies in Food Systems*, Blackwell Publishing: 83–112.

Corcoran, B. M., R. P. Ross, G. F. Fitzgerald and C. Stanton (2004). "Comparative survival of probiotic lactobacilli spray-dried in the presence of prebiotic substances." *Journal of Applied Microbiology* **96**(5): 1024–1039.

Dang, T. T., Q. Xu, K. M. Bratlie, E. S. O'Sullivan, X. Y. Chen, R. Langer and D. G. Anderson (2009). "Microfabrication of homogenous, asymmetric cell-laden hydrogel capsules." *Biomaterials* **30**(36): 6896–6902.

de Kruif, C. G., F. Weinbreck and R. de Vries (2004). "Complex coacervation of proteins and anionic polysaccharides." *Current Opinion in Colloid & Interface Science* **9**(5): 340–349.

De, S., M. Pritchett, M. K. Mazumder, C. U. Yurteri and P. Egorov (2002). "Electrostatic microencapsulation technique for producing composite particles." *Particulate Science and Technology* **20**(3): 169–185.

de Vos, P., M. M. Faas, M. Spasojevic and J. Sikkema (2010). "Encapsulation for preservation of functionality and targeted delivery of bioactive food components." *International Dairy Journal* **20**(4): 292–302.

Del Valle, E. M. M. (2004). "Cyclodextrins and their uses: a review." *Process Biochemistry* **39**(9): 1033-1046.

Dervichian, D. G. (1954). "A comparative study of the flocculation and coacervation of different systems." *Discussions of the Faraday Society* **18**(18): 231–239.

Desai, K. G. H. and H. J. Park (2005). "Recent developments in microencapsulation of food ingredients." *Drying Technology* **23**(7): 1361–1394.

Dewettinck, K. and A. Huyghebaert (1999). "Fluidized bed coating in food technology." *Trends in Food Science & Technology* **10**(4-5): 163–168.

Ding, W. K. and N. P. Shah (2009). "Effect of various encapsulating materials on the stability of probiotic bacteria." *Journal of Food Science* **74**(2): M100–M107.

Dobett, L. and V. Pantaleo (2002). "Application of a hydrodynamic model to microencapsulation by coacervation." *Journal of Microencapsulation* **19**(2): 139–151.

Doherty, S. B., V. L. Gee, R. P. Ross, C. Stanton, G. F. Fitzgerald and A. Brodkorb (2011). "Development and characterisation of whey protein micro-beads as potential matrices for probiotic protection." *Food Hydrocolloids* **25**(6): 1604–1617.

Draget, K. I. and C. Taylor (2011). "Chemical, physical and biological properties of alginates and their biomedical implications." *Food Hydrocolloids* **25**(2): 251–256.

Dulieu, C., D. Poncelet and R. J. Neufeld (1999). *Encapsulation and immobilization techniques*. Boston, MA, USA, Birkhauser.

Dziezak, J. D. (1988). "Microencapsulation and encapsulated ingredients." *Food Technology* **42**(4): 136-&.

Favaro-Trindade, C., S. Pinho and G. Rocha (2008). "Revisão: Microencapsulação de ingredientes alimentícios." *Brazilian Journal of Food Technology* **11**(2): 103–112.

Franjione, J. and N. Vasishtha (1995). "The art and science of microencapsulation." *Technology Today*.

Fukuda, J., A. Khademhosseini, Y. Yeo, X. Yang, J. Yeh, G. Eng, J. Blumling, C. F. Wang, D. S. Kohane and R. Langer (2006). "Micromolding of photocrosslinkable chitosan hydrogel for spheroid microarray and co-cultures." *Biomaterials* **27**(30): 5259–5267.

Gañán-Calvo, A. M. and A. Barrero (1999). "A novel pneumatic technique to generate steady capillary microjets." *Journal of Aerosol Science* **30**(1): 117–125.

Gardiner, G. E., E. O'Sullivan, J. Kelly, M. A. Auty, G. F. Fitzgerald, J. K. Collins, R. P. Ross and C. Stanton (2000). "Comparative survival rates of human-derived probiotic Lactobacillus paracasei and L. salivarius strains during heat treatment and spray drying." *Applied and Environmental Microbiology* **66**(6): 2605–2612.

Gharsallaoui, A., G. Roudaut, O. Chambin, A. Voilley and R. Saurel (2007). "Applications of spray-drying in microencapsulation of food ingredients: An overview." *Food Research International* **40**(9): 1107–1121.

Gibbs, B. F., S. Kermasha, I. Alli and C. N. Mulligan (1999). "Encapsulation in the food industry: a review." *International Journal of Food Sciences and Nutrition* **50**(3): 213–224.

Giunchedi, P. and U. Conte (1995). "Spray-drying as a preparation method of microparticulate drug-delivery systems: an overview." *STP Pharma Sciences* **5**(4): 276–290.

Gölker, C. (1993). Final recovery steps: Lyophilisation, spray-drying. In: *Biotechnology*, Vol. 3, H. J. Rehm, G. Reed and G. Stephanopoulos (eds), Weinheim, VCH: pp. 695–714.

Golowczyc, M. A., C. L. Gerez, J. Silva, A. G. Abraham, G. L. De Antoni and P. Teixeira (2011). "Survival of spray-dried Lactobacillus kefir is affected by different protectants and storage conditions." *Biotechnology Letters* **33**(4): 681–686.

Gouin, S. (2004). "Microencapsulation: industrial appraisal of existing technologies and trends." *Trends in Food Science & Technology* **15**(7–8): 330–347.

Graff, S., S. Hussain, J. C. Chaumeil and C. Charrueau (2008). "Increased intestinal delivery of viable Saccharomyces boulardii by encapsulation in microspheres." *Pharmaceutical Research* **25**(6): 1290–1296.

Grant, G. T., E. R. Morris, D. A. Rees, P. J. C. Smith and D. Thom (1973). "Biological interactions between polysaccharides and divalent cations: the egg-box model." *FEBS Letters* **32**(1): 195–198.

Green, B. K. (1953). "Carbonless paper production." NCR Corporation, Ohio.

Green, B. K. (1955). Pressure sensitive record material. United States Patent Office. U. S. P. Office. US Patent 2,712,507.

Heidebach, T., P. Forst and U. Kulozik (2009a). "Microencapsulation of probiotic cells by means of rennet-gelation of milk proteins." *Food Hydrocolloids* **23**(7): 1670–1677.

Heidebach, T., P. Forst and U. Kulozik (2009b). "Transglutaminase-induced caseinate gelation for the microencapsulation of probiotic cells." *International Dairy Journal* **19**(2): 77–84.

Heidebach, T., P. Forst and U. Kulozik (2012). "Microencapsulation of probiotic cells for food applications." *Critical Reviews in Food Science and Nutrition* **52**(4): 291–311.

Heidebach, T. and U. Kulozik. (2010). "Microencapsulation of microbial cells." *SciTopics* Retrieved February 20, 2012, from http://www.scitopics.com/Microencapsulation_of_microbial_cells.html.

Heinzen, C. (2002). Microencapsulation by prilling and coextrusion. *Nutraceuticals and Probiotics.* Technology training centre, Basil, Germany: 26–28.

Heinzen, C., I. Marison, A. Berger and U. von Stockar (2002). "Use of vibration technology for jet break-up for encapsulation of cells, microbes and liquids in monodisperse microcapsules." *Practical Aspects of Encapsulation Technologies*(241): 19–25.

Huang, K. S., T. H. Lai and Y. C. Lin (2007). "Using a microfluidic chip and internal gelation reaction for monodisperse calcium alginate microparticles generation." *Frontiers in Bioscience* **12**: 3061–3067.

Huq, T., A. Khan, R. A. Khan, B. Riedl and M. Lacroix (2012). "Encapsulation of probiotic bacteria in biopolymeric system." *Critical Reviews in Food Science and Nutrition.*

Hyun-Jik, O., K. So-Hyun, B. Ju-Yeoul, S. Gi-Hun and L. Sang-Hoon (2006). "Hydrodynamic micro-encapsulation of aqueous fluids and cells via ' on the fly ' photopolymerization." *Journal of Micromechanics and Microengineering* **16**(2): 285.

Jayasinghe, S. N. and N. Suter (2006). "Aerodynamically assisted jetting: a pressure driven approach for processing nanomaterials." *Micro & Nano Letters* **1**(1): 35–38.

Johnson, J. A. C. and M. R. Etzel (1995). "Properties of Lactobacillus helveticus CNRZ-32 attenuated by spray-drying, freeze-drying, or freezing." *Journal of Dairy Science* **78**(4): 761–768.

Jyothi, N. V., P. M. Prasanna, S. N. Sakarkar, K. S. Prabha, P. S. Ramaiah and G. Y. Srawan (2010). "Microencapsulation techniques, factors influencing encapsulation efficiency." *Journal of Microencapsulation* **27**(3): 187–197.

Kailasapathy, K. (2002). "Microencapsulation of probiotic bacteria: technology and potential applications." *Current Issues in Intestinal Microbiology* **3**(2): 39–48.

Kas, H. and L. Oner, Microencapsulation using coacervation/phase separation: an overview of the technique and applications, in *Handbook of Pharmaceutical Controlled Release Technology*, D. Wise, editor (2000), Marcel-Dekker: New York. p. 301–328.

Khademhosseini, A., G. Eng, J. Yeh, J. Fukuda, J. Blumling, 3rd, R. Langer and J. A. Burdick (2006). "Micromolding of photocrosslinkable hyaluronic acid for cell encapsulation and entrapment." *Journal of Biomedical Materials Research Part A* **79**(3): 522–532.

Kim, K. K. and D. W. Pack, Microspheres for Drug Delivery, in Biological and Biomedical Nanotechnology, M. Ferrari, A. P. Lee, and L. J. Lee, editors (2006), Springer: New York. p. 19–50.

Kinam, P. and Y. Yoon (2006). Microencapsulation technology. *Encyclopedia of pharmaceutical technology, Third Edition*, Informa Healthcare: 2315–2327.

King Alan, H. (1995). Encapsulation of food ingredients. *Encapsulation and controlled release of food ingredients*, American Chemical Society. **590:** 26–39.

Klayraung, S., H. Viernstein and S. Okonogi (2009). "Development of tablets containing probiotics: effects of formulation and processing parameters on bacterial viability." *International Journal of Pharmaceutics* **370**(1–2): 54–60.

Kleinbach, E. and T. Riede (1995). "Coating of solids." *Chemical Engineering and Processing* **34**(3): 329–337.

Knorr, D. (1998). "Technology aspects related to microorganisms In functional foods." *Trends in Food Science & Technology* **9**(8–9): 295–306.

Krasaekoopt, W., B. Bhandari and H. Deeth (2003). "Evaluation of encapsulation techniques of probiotics for yoghurt." *International Dairy Journal* **13**(1): 3–13.

Kuang, S. S., J. C. Oliveira and A. M. Crean (2010). "Microencapsulation as a tool for incorporating bioactive ingredients into food." *Critical Reviews in Food Science and Nutrition* **50**(10): 951–968.

Kushal, R., S. K. Anand and H. Chander (2006). "In vivo demonstration of enhanced probiotic effect of co-immobilized Lactobacillus acidophilus and Bifidobacterium bifidum." *International Journal of Dairy Technology* **59**(4): 265–271.

Lee, K. Y. and T. R. Heo (2000). "Survival of Bifidobacterium longum immobilized in calcium alginate beads in simulated gastric juices and bile salt solution." *Applied and Environmental Microbiology* **66**(2): 869–873.

Lee, W. L., Y. C. Seh, E. Widjaja, H. C. Chong, N. S. Tan and S. C. Loo (2012). "Fabrication and drug release study of double-layered microparticles of various sizes." *Journal of Pharmaceutical Sciences* **101**(8): 2787–2797.

Leimann, F. V. (2008). *Microencapsulação de óleo essencial de capim limão utilizando o processo de coacervação simples*, MSc dissertation, Universidade Federal de Santa Catarina.

Ma, Y. S., J. C. Pacan, Q. Wang, P. M. Sabour, X. Q. Huang and Y. P. Xu (2012). "Enhanced alginate microspheres as means of oral delivery of bacteriophage for reducing Staphylococcus aureus intestinal carriage." *Food Hydrocolloids* **26**(2): 434–440.

Mackie, W., S. Perez, R. Rizzo, F. Taravel and M. Vignon (1983). "Aspects of the Conformation of Polyguluronate in the Solid-State and in Solution." *International Journal of Biological Macromolecules* **5**(6): 329–341.

Madene, A., M. Jacquot, J. Scher and S. Desobry (2006). "Flavour encapsulation and controlled release: a review." *International Journal of Food Science and Technology* **41**(1): 1–21.

Mamvura, C. I., F. S. Moolman, L. Kalombo, A. N. Hall and M. S. Thantsha (2011). "Characterisation of the Poly-(Vinylpyrrolidone)-Poly-(Vinylacetate-Co-Crotonic Acid) (PVP:PVAc-CA) interpolymer complex matrix microparticles encapsulating a Bifidobacterium lactis Bb12 probiotic strain." *Probiotics and Antimicrobial Proteins* **3**(2): 97–102.

Manojlovic, V., J. Djonlagic, B. Obradovic, V. Nedovic and B. Bugarski (2006). "Immobilization of cells by electrostatic droplet generation: a model system for potential application in medicine." *International Journal of Nanomedicine* **1**(2): 163–171.

Matalanis, A., O. G. Jones and D. J. McClements (2011). "Structured biopolymer-based delivery systems for encapsulation, protection, and release of lipophilic compounds." *Food Hydrocolloids* **25**(8): 1865–1880.

Mattheus, G., B. Branko, O. Bojana and N. Viktor (2005). Electrostatic droplet generation technique for cell immobilization. *Finely Dispersed Particles*, CRC Press: 869–886.

Mattila-Sandholm, T., P. Myllarinen, R. Crittenden, G. Mogensen, R. Fonden and M. Saarela (2002). "Technological challenges for future probiotic foods." *International Dairy Journal* **12**(2–3): 173–182.

McCuan, J. (1997). "Retardation of Plateau-Rayleigh instability: a distinguishing characteristic among perfectly wetting fluids." *Arxiv preprint math/9701214*.

Meiners, J. A. (2009). "Micro-Encapsulation of Probiotics." In: *Prebiotics and Probiotics Science and Technology,* Charalampopoulos, Dimitris; Rastall, Robert A. (eds), ISBN 978-0-387-79057-2. Springer-Verlag New York, 2009, **1**: 805.

Moolman, F. S., P. W. Labuschagne, M. S. Thantsa, T. L. van der Merwe, H. Rolfes and T. E. Cloete (2006). "Encapsulating probiotics with an interpolymer complex in supercritical carbon dioxide." *South African Journal of Science* **102**(7–8): 349–354.

Morris, E. R., D. A. Rees, D. Thom and J. Boyd (1978). "Chiroptical and stoichiometric evidence of a specific, primary dimerization process in alginate gelation." *Carbohydrate Research* **66**(Oct): 145–154.

Nag, A., K.-S. Han and H. Singh (2011). "Microencapsulation of probiotic bacteria using pH-induced gelation of sodium caseinate and gellan gum." *International Dairy Journal* **21**(4): 247–253.

Nazzaro, F., P. Orlando, F. Fratianni and R. Coppola (2012). "Microencapsulation in food science and biotechnology." *Current Opinion in Biotechnology* **23**(2): 182–186.

Nie, Z., S. Xu, M. Seo, P. C. Lewis and E. Kumacheva (2005). "Polymer particles with various shapes and morphologies produced in continuous microfluidic reactors." *Journal of the American Chemical Society* **127**(22): 8058–8063.

Nilsson, K., S. Birnbaum, S. Flygare, L. Linse, U. Schroder, U. Jeppsson, P. O. Larsson, K. Mosbach and P. Brodelius (1983). "A general-method for the immobilization of cells with preserved viability." *European Journal of Applied Microbiology and Biotechnology* **17**(6): 319–326.

Nisco J1, N. E. A. V. (2009–2011). "Coaxial airflow induced dripping VAR J1." Retrieved September 21st, 2011, from http://www.nisco.ch/working_principle_coaxial_air_flow_driven.htm.

Nisco J30, N. E. A. V. (2009–2011). "Aerodynamically assisted spraying VAR J30." Retrieved September 21, 2011, from http://www.nisco.ch/working_principle_airdynamic_driven.htm.

Nisco V1, N. E. A. V. (2009–2011). "Electrostatically assisted spraying VAR V1." Retrieved September 21, 2011, from http://www.nisco.ch/working_principle_electrostatically_driven.htm.

Nixon, J. R. (1985). "Preparation of microcapsules with possible pharmaceutical use." *Endeavour* **9**(3): 123–128.

O'Riordan, K., D. Andrews, K. Buckle and P. Conway (2001). "Evaluation of microencapsulation of a Bifidobacterium strain with starch as an approach to prolonging viability during storage." *Journal of Applied Microbiology* **91**(6): 1059–1066.

Oh, J. K., R. Drumright, D. J. Siegwart and K. Matyjaszewski (2008). "The development of microgels/nanogels for drug delivery applications." *Progress in Polymer Science* **33**(4): 448–477.

Oliveira, A. C., T. S. Moretti, C. Boschini, J. C. Baliero, O. Freitas and C. S. Favaro-Trindade (2007). "Stability of microencapsulated B. lactis (BI 01) and L. acidophilus (LAC 4) by complex coacervation followed by spray drying." *Journal of Microencapsulation* **24**(7): 673–681.

Oxley, P., C. Brechtelsbauer, F. Ricard, N. Lewis and C. Ramshaw (2000). "Evaluation of spinning disk reactor technology for the manufacture of pharmaceuticals." *Industrial & Engineering Chemistry Research* **39**(7): 2175–2182.

Ozer, B., H. A. Kirmaci, E. Senel, M. Atamer and A. Hayaloglu (2009). "Improving the viability of Bifidobacterium bifidum BB-12 and Lactobacillus acidophilus LA-5 in white-brined cheese by microencapsulation." *International Dairy Journal* **19**(1): 22–29.

Passerini, N. (2003). "Controlled realease of verapamil hydrochloride from waxy microparticles prepared by spray congealing." *Journal of Controlled Release* **88**: 263–275.

Pedroso, D. D., M. Thomazini, R. J. B. Heinemann and C. S. Favaro-Trindade (2012). "Protection of Bifidobacterium lactis and Lactobacillus acidophilus by microencapsulation using spray-chilling." *International Dairy Journal* **26**(2): 127–132.

Peighambardoust, S. H., A. G. Tafti and J. Hesari (2011). "Application of spray drying for preservation of lactic acid starter cultures: a review." *Trends in Food Science & Technology* **22**(5): 215–224.

Phares, R. E., Jr. and G. J. Sperandio (1964). "Coating Pharmaceuticals by Coacervation." *Journal of Pharmaceutical Sciences* **53**(5): 515–518.

Picot, A. and C. Lacroix (2004). "Encapsulation of bifidobacteria in whey protein-based microcapsules and survival in simulated gastrointestinal conditions and in yoghurt." *International Dairy Journal* **14**(6): 505–515.

Plateau, J. (1873). Experimental and theoretical statics of liquids subject only to molecular forces, Gauthier-Villars: Paris. Accessed 20 January 2014 from http://www.susqu.edu/brakke/aux/downloads/plateau-eng.pdf.

Poncelet, D. (2006). Microencapsulation: fundamentals, methods and applications. In: *Surface Chemistry in Biomedical and Environmental Science*, J. Blitz and V. Gun'ko (eds), Springer, Netherlands: 23–34.

Poncelet, D., V. Babak, C. Dulieu and A. Picot (1999). "A physico-chemical approach to production of alginate beads by emulsification-internal ionotropic gelation." *Colloids and Surfaces a-Physicochemical and Engineering Aspects* **155**(2–3): 171–176.

Poncelet, D., V. G. Babak, R. J. Neufeld, M. F. A. Goosen and B. Burgarski (1999). "Theory of electrostatic dispersion of polymer solutions in the production of microgel beads containing biocatalyst." *Advances in Colloid and Interface Science* **79**(2–3): 213–228.

Poncelet, D., R. Lencki, C. Beaulieu, J. P. Halle, R. J. Neufeld and A. Fournier (1992). "Production of alginate beads by emulsification/internal gelation. I. Methodology." *Applied Microbiology and Biotechnology* **38**(1): 39–45.

Poncelet, D., R. J. Neufeld, M. F. A. Goosen, B. Burgarski and V. Babak (1999). "Formation of microgel beads by electric dispersion of polymer solutions." *Aiche Journal* **45**(9): 2018–2023.

Poncelet, D., B. Poncelet De Smet, C. Beaulieu, M. L. Huguet, A. Fournier and R. J. Neufeld (1995). "Production of alginate beads by emulsification/internal gelation. II. Physicochemistry." *Applied Microbiology and Biotechnology* **43**(4): 644–650.

Porubcan, R. S. and R. L. Sellars (1979). Lactic starter culture concentrates. IN: *Microbial Technology*, H. J. Peppler and D. Perlman (eds). Academic Press, New York **1:** 59–92.

Poulin, J. F., R. Caillard and M. Subirade (2011). "beta-Lactoglobulin tablets as a suitable vehicle for protection and intestinal delivery of probiotic bacteria." *International Journal of Pharmaceutics* **405**(1–2): 47–54.

Prista, L. N., A. C. Alves, R. Morgado and J. M. Sousa Lobo (2011). Granulação. *Tecnologia Farmacêutica*. L. N. Prista, A. C. Alves, R. Morgado and J. M. Sousa Lobo. Lisboa, Fundação Calouste Gulbenkian. **1**: 361–380.

Prüsse, U., L. Bilancetti, M. Bučko, B. Bugarski, J. Bukowski, P. Gemeiner, D. Lewińska, V. Manojlovic, B. Massart, C. Nastruzzi, V. Nedovic, D. Poncelet, S. Siebenhaar, L. Tobler, A. Tosi, A. Vikartovská and K.-D. Vorlop (2008). "Comparison of different technologies for alginate beads production." *Chemical Papers* **62**(4): 364–374.

Prüsse, U., J. Dalluhn, J. Breford and K. D. Vorlop (2000). "Production of Spherical Beads by JetCutting." *Chemical Engineering & Technology* **23**(12): 1105–1110.

Prüsse, U., B. Fox, M. Kirchhoff, F. Bruske, J. Breford and K.-D. Vorlop (1998). "New process (Jet Cutting Method) for the production of spherical beads from highly viscous polymer solutions." *Chemical Engineering & Technology* **21**(1): 29–33.

Prüsse, U., B. Fox, M. Kirchhoff, F. Bruske, J. Breford and K. D. Vorlop (1998). "The jet cutting method as a new immobilization technique." *Biotechnology Techniques* **12**(2): 105–108.

Qiu, C., M. Chen, H. Yan and H. Wu (2007). "Generation of uniformly sized alginate microparticles for cell encapsulation by using a soft-lithography approach." *Advanced Materials* **19**(12): 1603–1607.

Rabanel, J. M., X. Banquy, H. Zouaoui, M. Mokhtar and P. Hildgen (2009). "Progress technology in microencapsulation methods for cell therapy." *Biotechnology Progress* **25**(4): 946–963.

Rayleigh, L. (1878). "On the instability of jets." *Proceedings of the London Mathematical Society* **1**(1): 4.

Riaz, Q. U. and T. Masud (2013). "Recent trends and applications of encapsulating materials for probiotic stability." *Critical Reviews in Food Science and Nutrition* **53**(3): 231–244.

Rodrigues, D., S. Sousa, T. Rocha-Santos, J. P. Silva, J. M. Sousa Lobo, P. Costa, M. H. Amaral, M. M. Pintado, A. M. Gomes, F. X. Malcata and A. C. Freitas (2011). "Influence of L-cysteine, oxygen and relative humidity upon survival throughout storage of probiotic bacteria in whey protein-based microcapsules." *International Dairy Journal* **21**(11): 869–876.

Rokka, S. and P. Rantamäki (2010). "Protecting probiotic bacteria by microencapsulation: challenges for industrial applications." *European Food Research and Technology* **231**(1): 1–12.

Sabikhi, L., R. Babu, D. Thompkinson and S. Kapila (2010). "Resistance of microencapsulated Lactobacillus acidophilus LA1 to processing treatments and simulated gut conditions." *Food and Bioprocess Technology* **3**(4): 586–593.

Salústio, P. J., J. F. Pinto, P. C. Costa and H. M. Cabral-Marques (2012). "Release profiles of indometacin in β-cyclodextrin complexes from HPMC capsules." *Journal of Inclusion Phenomena and Macrocyclic Chemistry*: 1–9.

Sanchez, C. and D. Renard (2002). "Stability and structure of protein-polysaccharide coacervates in the presence of protein aggregates." *International Journal of Pharmaceutics* **242**(1–2): 319–324.

Schmitt, C., C. Sanchez, S. Desobry-Banon and J. Hardy (1998). "Structure and technofunctional properties of protein-polysaccharide complexes: a review." *Critical Reviews in Food Science and Nutrition* **38**(8): 689–753.

Schmitt, C., C. Sanchez, S. Despond, D. Renard, F. Thomas and J. Hardy (2000). "Effect of protein aggregates on the complex coacervation between β-lactoglobulin and acacia gum at pH 4.2." *Food Hydrocolloids* **14**(4): 403–413.

Schmitt, C. and S. L. Turgeon (2011). "Protein/polysaccharide complexes and coacervates in food systems." *Advances in Colloid and Interface Science* **167**(1-2): 63-70.

Schultz, T. H., K. P. Dimick and B. Makower (1956). "Incorporation of natural fruit flavors into fruit juice powders .1. Locking of citrus oils in sucrose and dextrose." *Food Technology* **10**(1): 57–60.

Semyonov, D., O. Ramon, Z. Kaplun, L. Levin-Brener, N. Gurevich and E. Shimoni (2010). "Microencapsulation of Lactobacillus paracasei by spray freeze drying." *Food Research International* **43**(1): 193–202.

Senuma, Y., C. Lowe, Y. Zweifel, J. G. Hilborn and I. Marison (2000). "Alginate hydrogel microspheres and microcapsules prepared by spinning disk atomization." *Biotechnology and Bioengineering* **67**(5): 616–622.

Seo, M., Z. Nie, S. Xu, M. Mok, P. C. Lewis, R. Graham and E. Kumacheva (2005). "Continuous microfluidic reactors for polymer particles." *Langmuir* **21**(25): 11614–11622.

Shahidi, F. and X. Q. Han (1993). "Encapsulation of food ingredients." *Critical Reviews in Food Science and Nutrition* **33**(6): 501–547.

Shima, M., T. Matsuo and S. Adachi (2007). "Effects of inner-phase components of water-in-oil-in-water emulsion on low-pH tolerance of Lactobacillus acidophilus incorporated into inner-water phase." *Journal of Bioscience and Bioengineering* **103**(3): 278–281.

Shoji, Y. and H. Nakashima (2004). "Nutraceutics and delivery systems." *Journal of Drug Targeting* **12**(6): 385–391.

Siaterlis, A., G. Deepika and D. Charalampopoulos (2009). "Effect of culture medium and cryoprotectants on the growth and survival of probiotic lactobacilli during freeze drying." *Letters in Applied Microbiology* **48**(3): 295–301.

Silva, C., A. Ribeiro, D. Ferreira and F. Veiga (2003). "Administração oral de peptídeos e proteínas: II. Aplicação de métodos de microencapsulação." *Revista Brasileira de Ciências Farmacêuticas* **39**: 1–20.

Silva, J., A. S. Carvalho, P. Teixeira and P. A. Gibbs (2002). "Bacteriocin production by spray-dried lactic acid bacteria." *Letters in Applied Microbiology* **34**(2): 77–81.

Sousa e Silva, J. P. and J. P. M. Ferreira (1998). "Microencapsulação: técnicas e aplicações." *Revista Portuguesa de Farmácia* **48**(3): 97–104.

Sousa, S., A. M. Gomes, M. M. Pintado, F. X. Malcata, J. P. Silva, J. M. Sousa, P. Costa, M. H. Amaral, D. Rodrigues, T. A. P. Rocha-Santos and A. C. Freitas (2012). "Encapsulation of probiotic strains in plain or cysteine-supplemented alginate improves viability at storage below freezing temperatures." *Engineering in Life Sciences* **12**(4): 457–465.

Stadler, M. and H. Viernstein (2003). "Optimization of a formulation containing viable lactic acid bacteria." *International Journal of Pharmaceutics* **256**(1–2): 117–122.

Suave, J., E. C. Dall'agnol, A. P. T. Pezzin, D. A. K. Silva, M. M. Meier, V. Soldi and Libecon (2006). "Microencapsulação: Inovação em diferentes áreas." *Revista Saúde e Ambiente / Health and Environment Journal* **7**: 12–20.

Sun, W. and M. W. Griffiths (2000). "Survival of bifidobacteria in yogurt and simulated gastric juice following immobilization in gellan–xanthan beads." *International Journal of Food Microbiology* **61**(1): 17–25.

Sunny-Roberts, E. O. and D. Knorr (2009). "The protective effect of monosodium glutamate on survival of Lactobacillus rhamnosus GG and Lactobacillus rhamnosus E-97800 (E800) strains during spray-drying and storage in trehalose-containing powders." *International Dairy Journal* **19**(4): 209–214.

Swisher, H. E. (1957). Solid flavouring composition and method of preparing same. US Patent no. 2, 895., Sunkist Growers Inc., Sherman Oaks, CA.

Teoh, P. L., H. Mirhosseini, S. Mustafa, A. S. M. Hussin and M. Y. A. Manap (2011). "Recent approaches in the development of encapsulated delivery systems for probiotics." *Food Biotechnology* **25**(1): 77–101.

Teunou, E. and D. Poncelet (2005). "Rotary disc atomisation for microencapsulation applications—prediction of the particle trajectories." *Journal of Food Engineering* **71**(4): 345–353.

Tiebackx, F. W. (1911). "Gleichzeitige Ausflockung zweier Kolloide." *Colloid & Polymer Science* **8**(4): 198–201.

Tonnesen, H. H. and J. Karlsen (2002). "Alginate in drug delivery systems." *Drug Development and Industrial Pharmacy* **28**(6): 621–630.

Tsung, M. and D. J. Burgess (1997). "Preparation and stabilization of heparin/gelatin complex coacervate microcapsules." *Journal of Pharmaceutical Sciences* **86**(5): 603–607.

Turgeon, S. L., C. Schmitt and C. Sanchez (2007). "Protein–polysaccharide complexes and coacervates." *Current Opinion in Colloid & Interface Science* **12**(4–5): 166–178.

Utada, A. S., E. Lorenceau, D. R. Link, P. D. Kaplan, H. A. Stone and D. A. Weitz (2005). "Monodisperse double emulsions generated from a microcapillary device." *Science* **308**(5721): 537-541.

Vidhyalakshmi, R., R. Bhakyaraj and R. Subhasree (2009). "Encapsulation "The future of probiotics"-A review." *Adv Biol Research* **3**: 96–103.

Wan, L. S., P. W. Heng and L. W. Chan (1992). "Drug encapsulation in alginate microspheres by emulsification." *Journal of Microencapsulation* **9**: 309–316.

Wang, Z. L., W. H. Finlay, M. S. Peppler and L. G. Sweeney (2006). "Powder formation by atmospheric spray-freeze-drying." *Powder Technology* **170**(1): 45–52.

Werner, S. R. L., J. R. Jones, A. H. J. Paterson, R. H. Archer and D. L. Pearce (2007). "Air-suspension coating in the food industry: Part II—micro-level process approach." *Powder Technology* **171**(1): 34–45.

Werner, S. R. L., J. R. Jones, A. H. J. Paterson, R. H. Archer and D. L. Pearce (2007). "Air-suspension particle coating in the food industry: Part I - state of the art." *Powder Technology* **171**(1): 25–33.

Wurster, D. E. (1959). "Air-suspension technique of coating drug particles. A preliminary report." *Journal of the American Pharmaceutical Association* **48**(8): 451–454.

Yáñez-Fernández, J., E. G. Ramos-Ramírez and J. A. Salazar-Montoya (2007). "Rheological characterization of dispersions and emulsions used in the preparation of microcapsules obtained by interfacial polymerization containing Lactobacillus sp." *European Food Research and Technology* **226**(5): 957–966.

Yeo, S.-D. and E. Kiran (2005). "Formation of polymer particles with supercritical fluids: A review." *The Journal of Supercritical Fluids* **34**(3): 287–308.

Yoo, S.-H., Y.-B. Song, P.-S. Chang and H. G. Lee (2006). "Microencapsulation of α-tocopherol using sodium alginate and its controlled release properties." *International Journal of Biological Macromolecules* **38**(1): 25–30.

Yoshizawa, H. (2004). "Trends in microencapsulation research." *Kona* **22**: 23–31.

Zayed, G. and Y. H. Roos (2004). "Influence of trehalose and moisture content on survival of Lactobacillus salivarius subjected to freeze-drying and storage." *Process Biochemistry* **39**(9): 1081–1086.

Zhang, H., E. Tumarkin, R. M. A. Sullan, G. C. Walker and E. Kumacheva (2007). "Exploring microfluidic routes to microgels of biological polymers." *Macromolecular Rapid Communications* **28**(5): 527–538.

Zuidam, N. J. and E. Shimoni (2010). Overview of microencapsulates for use in food products or processes and methods to make them. In: *Encapsulation Technologies for Active Food Ingredients and Food Processing,* N. J. Zuidam and V. Nedovic (eds.), Springer, New York: 3–29.

Chapter 6

Development of Probiotic Dosage Forms

Maria H. Amaral,[a] J. Paulo Sousa e Silva,[a] Paulo J. C. Costa,[a] and Ana M. Gomes[b]
[a]*Faculty of Pharmacy, University of Porto, Rua de Jorge Viterbo Ferreira, 228, 4050-313 Porto, Portugal*
[b]*CBQF, Biotechnology School of Portuguese Catholic University, Rua Dr. António Bernardino Almeida, 4200-072 Porto, Portugal*
hamral@ff.up.pt

6.1 Introduction

The use of health-beneficial microorganisms was first introduced in the beginning of the 20th century. As reported in the previous chapters, probiotics represent alternative therapeutic agents. In order to improve the clinical efficacy of probiotics, optimization will still be achieved by the application of new approaches (Sleator and Hill 2008). Several European Union projects have shown that with coordinated efforts toward a scientific approach to the selection and application of probiotics, effective functional products can be developed with health benefits for consumers (Saarela *et al.* 2000).

This chapter is concerned with formulated preparations to administer probiotics (medicines or dietary/food supplement).

Probiotic Bacteria: Fundamentals, Therapy, and Technological Aspects
Edited by J. Paulo Sousa e Silva and Ana C. Freitas

ISBN 978-981-4411-62-2 (Hardcover), 978-981-4411-63-9 (eBook)
www.panstanford.com

Dosage forms as dietary/food supplement may be capsules, tablets, powders (in sachets), or liquids in measured doses, and as pharmaceutical dosage forms, which also include suppositories gels or eye drops apart from the already mentioned. Dosage forms are products designed for the administration of bioactive agents and should have a high potential of acceptability by the patients. For this, special attention should be given to the steps of pre-formulation and formulation of a probiotic product and the integration of diverse knowledge from areas of microbiology, chemistry, and pharmaceutical technology.

Under current FDA guidelines (FDA 2006), probiotics, as therapeutic agents, may fit within the live biotherapeutic products (LBPs) concept. LBPs are biological products (nonrecombinant) that:

(1) Contain live microorganisms, such as bacteria or yeast;
(2) Are applicable to the prevention, treatment, or cure of a disease;
(3) Are not vaccines.

To confer health benefits to the host, probiotics taken orally must survive the adverse gastrointestinal (GI) conditions and maintain the viability when they reach their site of action. Therefore, there is a need for formulations that protect the bacteria from the harsh conditions of the stomach. The oral administration of probiotics, and the technology associated with it, has been mainly studied by the food industry. However, the stability (shelf life) required for a nutritional product is much lower than that required for a pharmaceutical product. The stability of an active substance within a dosage form is a critical parameter to be taken into account in the development of pharmaceutical products. The stability within a dosage form and the viability after release is also applied to the administration of probiotic bacteria.

The development of formulations containing probiotics needs the selection and characterization of strains with proven therapeutic properties, the selection of excipients, and the processes suitable for large-scale production of the final dosage form. Before the marketing of probiotics as medicinal products, it is necessary to evaluate the safety and efficacy of the final products, first with laboratory tests, then with animal models, and finally testing in humans. After this whole process is completed, probiotics can then be commercialized as medicinal products. However, the dose–response relationships of probiotic products should be further characterized, in addition to ways of optimizing the administration of these products (Hoffman *et al.* 2008).

Several studies have been conducted to develop products containing probiotics; however, there are not many pharmaceutical dosage forms in the market. Table 6.1 present some examples of pharmaceutical dosage forms containing probiotics marketed in several countries of Europe (Sweetman 2009).

Table 6.1 Pharmaceutical dosage forms containing probiotics marketed in Europe

Probiotic product	Country
Antibiophilus® Bioflorin® Doederlein® Symbioflor®	Austrich
Bioflorin® Lacteol®	Belgium
Antibiophilus® Diarlac® Lacteol® Lyobifidus® UL-250®	France
Antibiophilus® Hamadin® Hylac N® Omnisept® Symbioflor® Vagiflor®	Germany
Lacteol® Lactofilus® Lactoliofil® Ultra Levura®	Spain
Bio Acidophilus® Biodophilus®	U.K.
Lacteol® Antibiophilus® UL-250®	Portugal

Source: Adapted from Sweetman (2009)

Probiotic strains must be able to grow under industrial conditions and survive and retain their functionality during storage. The reduction of viable cells during storage, processing, and passage through the GI tract is a significant challenge in formulating dosage forms containing probiotics. Several studies have reported that oral doses higher than 10^9 colony forming units (cfu) per day are required to restore and maintain the bacterial flora (Zárate and Nader-Macias 2006).

Because several pharmaceutical industrial processes may induce an increase in the temperature of the handled material and may expose it to moisture variations, the viability of probiotics must be studied at different conditions of temperature and relative humidity (RH). These temperatures and moisture conditions should be selected according to the guidelines of the International Conference Harmonization of Technical Requirements for the Registration of Pharmaceuticals for Human Use (ICH 2002). Temperature and RH conditions for climatic zones I—Temperate (e.g., Japan, Northern Europe, United States, Canada, Russia) and II—Mediterranean subtropical (United States, Japan, Southern Europe) are for real-time test conditions 25 ± 2°C and 60 ± 5 % and for accelerated test conditions 40 ± 2°C and 75 ± 5% (ICH, 2002, USP).

The first probiotic products available were mostly liquid formulations that showed low cell viability after oral administration, mainly because bacteria did not survive in the stomach conditions. Nowadays, the development of suitable solid dosage forms allows obtaining higher levels of bacterial survival.

6.2 Manufacturing of Dosage Forms Containing Probiotics

A critical aspect of product development is the implementation of a manufacturing process that assures that a product can be produced in a reproducible manner (Ross and Boucher 2012). Expectations for product development of an LBP do not differ from other regulated products that consist of live microorganisms, such as live vaccines or microbial vectors for gene therapy. The development and manufacturing of dietary/food supplement dosage forms is similar to medicines; nevertheless, they do not need to follow the stringent guidelines used in a medicinal product.

Safe and effective use of an LBP depends on consistent manufacture according to valid specifications. Probiotic formulations should include selected microorganisms with the ability to survive during the technological process and remain viable afterward with unaltered properties for long periods of storage (Zárate and Nader-Macias 2006).

Probiotic products often utilize lyophilizates of microorganisms in order to produce dosage forms. Lyophilization is a process extensively used for preservation of biological samples. However, during freeze-drying, the cells experience extreme environmental conditions such as low temperature and low humidity that may produce structural and physiological damage to the bacterial cells resulting in the loss of viability. To reduce these undesirable effects, protective agents are usually added to the samples before freezing or freeze-drying (Zárate and Nader-Macias 2006).

Sutton (2008) suggested that the early development of probiotic products should include the following steps:

1. Select and characterize a strain;
2. Document the production batches for nonclinical studies and establish working specifications;
3. Repeat the production with few or even no modifications to the product clinical lots;
4. Confirm or modify the specifications on the basis of clinical results;
5. Begin stability studies.

The active ingredient of a biotherapeutic is the microorganism that should be administered in a dosage form suitable to ensure accurate dosing and good stability (Sutton 2008). Generally, concentrated cultures of microorganisms are adjusted by dilution, dry preparations are mixed with dry ingredients such as stabilizers or diluents, and powders may be supplied with pre-packaged buffer solutions for reconstitution. (Sutton 2008).

The reactivation of dried cultures is a critical parameter in obtaining active and effective probiotic strains (Muller *et al.* 2010). Muller *et al.* studied the effect of several rehydration conditions on the viability of *B. longum NCC3001* and *L. Johnsonii* La1. These authors concluded that the reactivation conditions are a vital step to obtain maximal viability counts. Furthermore, a variation can be found between species and strains and, as a consequence, any universal proceeding suitable for reactivation of bacteria cannot be designed. The reactivation conditions should be optimized for each strain used in order to achieve accurate numbers of viable probiotics.

Probiotic formulations in the form of solid dosage forms often require some type of other ingredients (also termed excipients in the pharmaceutical field) such as diluents (to increase to the volume), binders (to give adhesiveness), lubricants (to reduce adhesion), glidants (to improve powder flow), or even disintegrants (to facilitate deaggregation).

The release of probiotics from dosage forms may be modified. In pharmaceutical field, modified-release dosage forms are preparations in which the release of the drug has been deliberately changed, regarding the rate and/or the place where it occurs, resulting from a specific process of formulation and/or a special manufacturing method, and is therefore different from that achieved with an immediately-release form (*Eur. Pharmacopeia* 2008).

Modified-release dosage forms include prolonged or extended-release (special type of modified-release dosage form showing a slower release of the drug than that achieved with an immediate or conventional-release administered by the same route), delayedrelease (special type of modified-release dosage form showing a release of the drug that is delayed), and pulsatile-release (special type of modified-release dosage form showing a sequential release of the drug) dosage forms (Figure 6.1) (*Eur. Pharmacopeia* 2008).

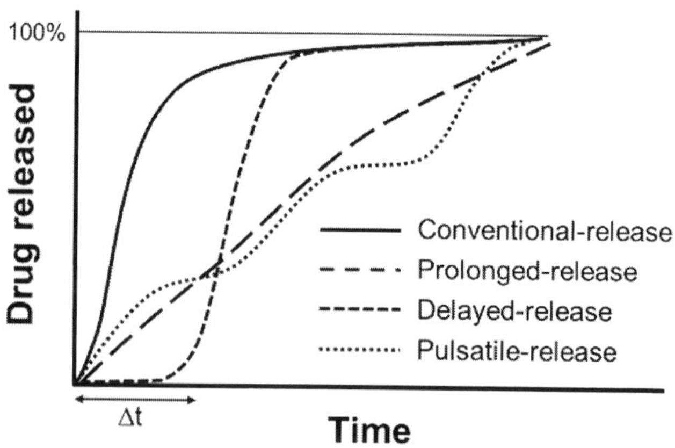

Figure 6.1 Several types of modified drug release.

Solid dosage forms may be enteric protected to ensure passage through the adverse conditions of the stomach and the release of probiotics in the intestine. They are called gastro-resistant (GR) forms and can be prepared with excipients, in which the therapeutic agents are homogeneously dispersed, preventing the entrance of the gastric fluid (enteric-matrix) or cover the dosage form (enteric-coated). In this GR case, the release of probiotics is delayed until the dosage form reaches the intestinal fluid. The main principle of probiotics release is to the change the gastric pH to enteric pH, which activates its release from the solid dosage form.

With a proper selection of a solid-forming matrix, entrapped bacteria can be more easily protected against the low pH of the stomach. Suitable functional polymers have been studied to produce solid dosage forms having the ability to maintain their physical integrity in gastric fluid, minimize the penetration of solvent at acidic pH values, and increase the bacteria survival.

Several probiotic products containing specific probiotic strains have been developed in formulations such as powders (Ying *et al.* 2010), capsules (Bruno and Shah 2003), tablets (Stadler and Viernstein 2003; Klayraung *et al.* 2009), vaginal suppositories (Kale *et al.* 2005), and other dosage forms (Kouimtzi *et al.* 1997; Çaglar *et al.* 2007; Iovieno *et al.* 2008)

6.2.1 Powders

Oral powders are dosage forms consisting of solid, loose, dry, finely divided particles that are intended for internal use (Eur. Pharmacopeia 2008; USP31 2008). They may contain bioactive compounds and/or other excipients such as coloring, flavoring, and sweetening agents. In general, oral powders are limited to relatively nonpotent drugs or dietary/food supplements. The administration of oral powders could overcome the difficulty in swallowing tablets experienced by children or even some adults. In the production of oral powders, measures are taken to ensure an adequate particle size, which is generally done by milling and/or sieving.

Powders containing probiotics are frequently used to disperse in water (extemporaneous oral suspensions). Some examples of marketed powders for oral suspension containing probiotics are presented in Table 6.2.

Table 6.2 Marketed powders for oral suspensions containing probiotics

Probiotic product	Composition
UL-250®	*Sacharomyces boulardii*
Bacilor®	*Lactobacillus acidophilus*
Antibiophilus®	*Lactobacillus casei*
Lyobifidus®	*Bifidobacterium bifidum*

In the studies of Ying *et al.* (2010), a commercial lyophilized powder was encapsulated in a oil-in-water emulsion, stabilized by whey protein and modified resistant starch, and dried into powders by freeze-drying or spray drying. The results of this study showed that when the same encapsulating matrix and probiotic preparation were used, the probiotics survival after manufacturing was similar using freeze-drying or spray drying.

6.2.2 Capsules

Capsules are solid dosage forms with hard or soft container or shell made from gelatin or, less often, from other suitable material (Eur. Pharmacopeia 2008; USP31 2008). There are two types of capsules, hard and soft (one-piece). Hard capsules are generally preferred in order to administer probiotics.

The hard capsules, which consist of two cylindrical pieces (body and cap) closed at one end, are typically used to contain powders. These capsules are produced by a process based in a patent dated from 1846 (Jones 2004). Empty standard size hard capsules are supplied in bulk containers.

The filling of hard capsules may employ machines that form powder plugs and eject them into the capsule bodies after having separated the cap of the shell.

Hard capsule sizes are standard, generally ranging from n° 5 (0.13 ml), the smallest, to n° 000 (1.37 ml), although for human administration the largest size used is n° 00 (0.95 or 0.93 ml depending on the manufacturing). Gelatin capsules are readily soluble in water at 37°C.

Probiotics in the form of powders are also used to fill capsules. The powder formulations often require some type of excipients such as fillers, glidants, or even disintegrants. It is also possible to prepare

GR capsules that typically use GR-coated granules or in certain cases coated shells.

As probiotic preparations include different excipients, apart from the probiotic strains, it is technologically valuable to evaluate the effect of these compounds on the physiology of the selected microorganisms. For this reason, Zárate and Nader-Macias (2006) evaluated the survival rates and probiotic properties of three human vaginal lactobacilli lyophilized with different excipients (lactose, skim milk, and ascorbic acid), and stored in gelatin capsules placed in glass flasks at 5°C under darkness during 15 months. This study demonstrated that the *Lactobacillus* spp. tested maintained high viability up to 12 months in capsules containing ascorbic acid used individually or combined with lactose, milk, or both, whereas lyophilization and storage with only lactose or skim milk significantly decreased their survival.

A study by Reid and Bruce (2006) demonstrated that daily oral intake for 2 months of gelatin capsules containing *L. rhamnosus* GR-1 and *L. fermentum* RC-14 resulted in a significant increase in the number of vaginal lactobacillus, combined with a decrease of coliforms and fungi.

Ya *et al.* (2010) studied the effectiveness of vaginal probiotic capsules for recurrent bacterial vaginosis (BV) prevention and concluded that the short-term probiotic prophylaxis was well tolerated and reduced BV recurrence and *G. vaginalis* risk through 11 months after treatment.

Table 6.3 presents some examples of marketed capsules containing probiotics.

Table 6.3 Marketed capsules containing probiotics

Probiotic product	Composition
Bactilsubtil®	*Bacillus subtilis*
Activecomplex Flora®	*Lactobacillus acidophilus* and *Bifidobacterium bifidum*
Infloran Berna®	*Lactobacillus acidophilus* and *Bifidobacterium bifidum*
Lacteol®	*Lactobacillus acidophilus*
Antibiophilus®	*Lactobacillus casei*
UL-250®	*Saccharomyces boulardii*

6.2.3 Tablets

Tablets are solid dosage forms usually obtained by compressing uniform volumes of particles (powders or particles aggregates) (*Eur. Pharmacopeia* 2008). Tablets are the most widely used pharmaceutical dosage form. The first tablets comparable to those used today have their roots in the invention of William Brockedon, in the 19th century. In 1843, Brockedon obtained a patent for "Shaping Pills, Lozenges and Black Lead by Pressure in Dies." It is believed that John Wyeth and his brother Frank were the first to use the term "compressed tablet" and register it in 1877 to protect and restrict its use (Troy 2005).

Tablets are prepared by the application of a high pressure to uniform volumes of powders (direct compression) or granules (obtained by wet or dry granulation) using tablet presses (Fig. 6.2). Tablets may be coated in order to facilitate its administration, to protect its bioactive content, or to modify its release.

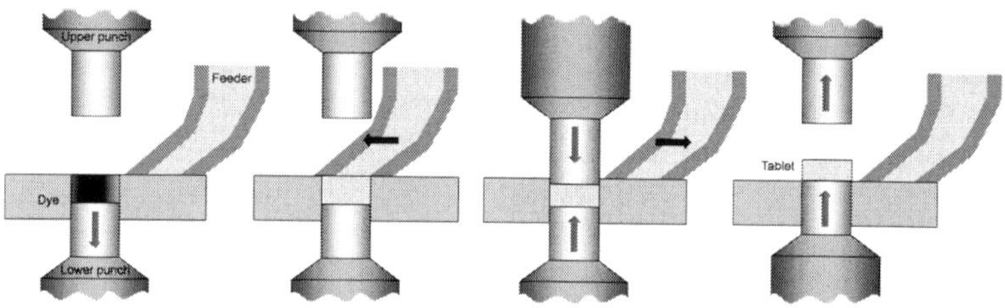

Figure 6.2 Compression of tablets.

To obtain a tablet, it is usually necessary to use some type of excipients such as diluents, binders, disintegrants, lubricants, and glidants. The design of tablets using functional polymers improves the stability of probiotics, contributes to accurate dosing and ease of administration, and provides the ability to produce dosage forms containing probiotics at a large scale (Klayraung *et al.* 2009).

Generally, tablets containing probiotics are produced by direct compression of mixtures of excipients and freeze-dried probiotics. In the studies of Graff *et al.* (2008), matrix tablets containing freeze-dried probiotics were prepared by direct compression using hydroxypropylmethylcellulose (HPMC), which is one of the most used hydrophilic polymers for the production of modified release systems. HPMC has the ability to form a gelling barrier limiting the release of viable probiotics.

In the studies carried out by Klayraung *et al.* (2009) to evaluate the effects of formulation and processing parameters on bacterial viability, tablets were also prepared by direct compression. In this study, an exactly weighed amount of powder mixture containing LAB powder and HPMC phthalate was filled into a die and tablets were formed under a determined force ranging from 2 to 20 kN.

Tablets can be designed to modify the release and enhance the adhesion and colonization of the probiotic microorganisms to the epithelial mucosa of human host by using suitable kinds of tablet excipients (Maggi *et al.* 2000).

Different polymers have been studied to form the protective matrix. For example, Rodrigues *et al.* (2011) studied the viability of five probiotic strains (*L. casei 01, L. acidophilus La-5*®, *L. acidophilus Ki, B. animalis BB-12*®, and *B. lactis Bo*) immobilized on various polymers [sodium alginate, xanthan gum, L-carrageenan, cellulose acetate phthalate (CAP), chitosan/sodium alginate, and whey protein concentrate] at various concentrations and concluded that alginate and whey proteins were the most suitable polymers, except for *L. acidophilus Ki* and *L. casei 01* at 2% (m/v) alginate.

Some examples of polymers used in the production of GR tablets containing probiotics are summarized in Table 6.4.

Table 6.4 Examples of polymers used in the production of GR tablets containing probiotics

Polymers	Reference
Sodium alginate in combination with hydroxypropylcellulose	Chan and Zhang, 2002, 2005
HPMC acetate succinate	Stadler and Vernstein, 2003
Carboxymethyl high amylase starch	Calinescu *et al.*, 2005
Carboxymethyl high amylase starch in combination with chitosan	Calinescu and Mateescu, 2008
HPMC phthalate	Klayraung *et al.*, 2009

Chan and Zhang (2005) developed tablets with a core of *L. acidophilus ATCC 4356* cells surrounded with sodium alginate and obtained a higher stability than the powders containing the same bacteria after 30 days of storage at 25°C.

GR tablet formulations of lactic acid bacteria (LAB) were developed by Stadler and Viernstein (2003) using HPMC acetate succinate (HPMCAS) as well as alginates, apple pectin, and Metolose™ (methylcellulose/hydroxypropyl methylcellulose) as matrix-forming agents. The results of this study demonstrated that a high content of HPMCAS as well as medium or high compaction force (5 or 10 kN, respectively) are needed to achieve gastric juice resistance. When tablets were prepared with low amounts of HPMCAS, the addition of sodium alginate was necessary to ensure protection against artificial gastric juice.

Novel excipients were tested for the protection and intestinal delivery of probiotic bacteria. Calinescu *et al.* (2005) proposed three variants of carboxymethyl high-amylase starch (CM-HAS) as new excipients for the formulation of oral tablets containing lyophilized *E. coli*. These authors also developed a new hydrophilic dosage system on the basis of an ionic self-stabilization of CM-HAS and chitosan for probiotic colon delivery and found that the increase of percentage and molecular weight of chitosan caused a decrease of bacteria release rate. The CMHAS dry-coated monolithic tablets changed the effect of chitosan molecular weight on bacteria release and improved the percentage of delivered bacteria in simulated intestinal conditions.

The use of succinylated β-lactoglobulin (S β-LG) as a novel functional tablet excipient was studied by Poulin *et al.* (2011). These studies showed that tablets produced by direct compression of a mixture of *B. longum* HA-135 and S β-LG enhanced bacteria survival in gastric conditions and showed good stability after storage at 4°C during 3 months.

Particular attention should be given to the design and production of pharmaceutical dosage forms, intended for the vaginal administration of living cells, as bacterial suspensions show poor stability and are easily cleared after vaginal application. Different types of formulations for vaginal delivery of probiotics are nowadays commercialized in the international market. However, the largest group of probiotic vaginal formulations consists of freeze-dried probiotics compressed into tablets or encapsulated in a gelatin base (Santiago *et al.* 2009).

A significant proportion of tablets containing probiotics are designed for vaginal administration aiming the treatment of vulvo-vaginal disorders. Throughout the production process and storage, cell viability of probiotic strains should be maintained and a strict quality control should ensure the safety and efficacy of the final product. Thus, a probiotic vaginal formulation should (Santiago *et al.* 2009) provide a long retention time to maximize the release of probiotics and present a suitable release, so that colonization occurs in different parts of the vagina, does not damage the vaginal mucosa and vaginal microflora, provides an easy form of administration, and do not cause discomfort to the patient.

Lactobacilli are the predominant microorganisms in the healthy human vaginal ecosystem (Lepargneur and Rousseau 2002). Therefore, is important to know the properties of lactobacilli and their capacity to proliferate or to maintain their viability in the vaginal medium.

Several studies of probiotics for vaginal infections have been reported (Falagas *et al.* 2006; Dover *et al.* 2008; Gil *et al.* 2010). Most probiotic preparations for vaginal use include one or more lactobacillus species (Elmer 2001). For example, studies using vaginally administered *L. rhamnosus* GR1 in association with either *L. reuteri* B54 or RC 14 have shown that vaginal colonization can be achieved (Reid and Bruce 2006).

Mastromarino *et al.* (2009) determined the effectiveness of vaginal tablets containing *Lactobacillus* spp. in the treatment of BV and in the restoration of a healthy vaginal flora showing that intravaginal administration of exogenous selected strains of lactobacilli can restore a normal vaginal microbiota and be used in the treatment of BV.

Fazeli *et al.* (2006) evaluated the viability and release of *L. acidophilus* from slow-release vaginal tablets prepared using six different retarding polymers and from two effervescent fast-release tablets prepared using citric or adipic acid. Although fast-release formulations produced a fast bacterial release in comparison to polymer-based slow-release tablets, they were less stable upon storage. All the slow-release polymers showed a high bacterial release except carbomers with poor bacterial shedding probably due to their high viscosity characteristics.

Maggi *et al.* (2000) formulated single and double-layer tablets containing four types of lactobacilli for vaginal administration (*L. brevis, L. salivarius, L. crispatus,* and *L. gasseri*). In this study, double-layer tablets containing an effervescent layer for the fast release of a percentage of bacteria and a slow-release layer to sustain probiotics in vaginal environment were prepared. Three types of polymers (HPMC-HV, HPMC-LV, and Carbopol 934 PH) were studied, and formulations were tested regarding technological processing, cell adhesion properties of the microorganisms, and bacterial viability and stability. These studies showed that both fast and slow-release tablets maintained a good stability after storage in plastic containers at 4°C–6°C during 18 months, however, lower than the stability showed by the freeze-dried powder.

6.2.4 Vaginal Suppositories

A suppository is a solid drug delivery system of various weights and shapes adapted for introduction into the rectum (rectal suppository), vagina (vaginal suppository), or urethra (urethral suppository). Suppositories usually melt, soften, or dissolve at body temperature (USP31 2008; Sweetman 2009).

The word suppository derives from the Latin term *suppositorium* that in turn seems to come from the union of the words *supositum* (low position) + *torus* (torus), hence its etymological roots suggest a solid pharmaceutical form for administration into the lower body cavities (rectum, vagina, urethra) (Prista *et al.* 1990). This broad concept, although followed in North America, is not followed in some countries. So, the name suppository in Europe designates only the solid preparations for rectal administration, while the solid formulations for vaginal administration are called pessaries (Eur. Pharmacopeia 2008).

The suppositories are frequently obtained by compression or molding (sometimes referred as fusion) techniques. The molding technique is the most used method for the preparation of supositories and consists in the melting of excipients, addition of probiotics at lower temperatures, and pouring the mixture into appropriate molds. Suppository bases usually employed are hard fat, cocoa butter, mixtures of polyethylene glycols (PEGs), and various gelatinous mixtures. The vaginal suppositories have certain advantages over other dosage forms, including the fact that the uniformity of mass can be maintained, are easy to apply into the vagina without irritation, and does not require a large volume of dissolution medium for the release of the active substance (Kale *et al.* 2005).

The earlier studies involving the use of vaginal probiotics date from 1990s of the 20th century. Reid *et al.* (1992) examined the recurrence of urinary tract infections (UTIs) in women who were administered vaginal suppositories containing probiotics, and after administration of the vaginal suppositories, only 21% of women had recurrences of UTI, compared with 47% that were observed in women who were given placebo. However, later studies proved that the opposite and one of the possible causes for these results may have been the fact that these authors used *L. casei* in the formulation of vaginal suppositories, which would not be the most suitable strain for vaginal administration (Baerheim *et al.* 1994).

On the contrary, more recent studies have demonstrated the efficacy and safety of such treatments. In a study by Uehara *et al.* (2006), it was shown that vaginal suppositories with *L. crispatus* GAI 98332 can significantly reduce the recurrence of UTI, without causing adverse complications during treatment. In this study, vaginal suppositories containing 1×10^8 cfu were administered to each patient, twice a day, during 1 year. The reason why this study has proved to be so promising is related to the selection of a more stable strain, isolated from the vagina of healthy women, known for their ability to produce hydrogen peroxide, as well as their ability to adhere to the vaginal epithelium.

To further evaluate the safety and efficacy of vaginal suppositories containing *L. crispatus* CTV-05 for prevention of recurrent UTI, Czaja *et al.* (2007) performed a randomized, double-blind study in premenopausal women with a history of recurrent UTI and concluded that vaginal suppositories containing this probiotic were well tolerated and mild inflammation of the urinary tract was only detected in some women.

Kale *et al.* (2005) developed formulations of vaginal suppositories containing freeze-dried *L. sporogenes*, and then studied the *in vivo* performance of the formulations developed. Three vaginal suppositories formulations were prepared using the molding technique, containing cocoa butter, glycerinated gelatin, and PEG 1000, respectively. Glycerinated gelatin vaginal suppositories had the most satisfactory physical properties. Similarly, studies with different formulations of vaginal tablets containing different bacterial strains have shown to be promising in the transport of probiotics (Mastromarino *et al.* 2002).

Kaewsrichan *et al.* (2007) prepared two vaginal formulations, namely effervescent tablets and hollow-type PEG-based suppositories, containing lactobacillus, aiming to maintain as high as possible the live cells with proper probiotic properties. In this study, suppositories were prepared by melting the PEG 4000 at 60°C before the addition of PEG 400. After cooling, the mixture of PEGs was poured into suppository molds, and a hollow centered to the mold was made by pressing sterile stirring rod into the mixed base prior setting. Bacterial powder was filled into the hollow followed by capping with the mixed PEG, in order to avoid the exposure of probiotics to wetting steps and excessive manipulation techniques. The results of this study showed that effervescent tablets promptly released the microorganisms and the abilities on bacteriocin and H_2O_2 productions were not deteriorated by the suppositories manipulation.

Kaewnopparat and Kaewnopparat (2009) also undertook the development of vaginal suppositories with a mixture of PEG and Witepsol H15, using different methods of preparation, in order to compare the viability of *L. casei*. These authors prepared vaginal suppositories by the conventional method and by the hollow-type method. The hollow-type method (Fig. 6.3) was developed by Watanabe and Matsumoto (1986) in order to study the effectiveness of active substances when administered by rectal route. The vaginal suppositories whose base excipient used was a mixture of PEGs and whose method of preparation was the hollow-type method proved to be the most suitable for the administration of vaginal lactobacillus, regarding the quick release and microbiological stability. The hollow-type method can eliminate the disadvantage of the heating process on the survival of lactobacillus during preparation and also the interactions between these microorganisms and the suppository excipients.

More recently, Rodrigues (2011) developed two formulations of vaginal suppositories with PEGs and Witepsol H12 for the administration of vaginal *L. acidophilus*. The results of this study showed that the incorporation of freeze-dried bacteria on these excipients did not result in significant losses of viable bacteria, giving rise to the idea that these vaginal suppositories possess good properties to promote the replacement of the vaginal flora in situations of UTI.

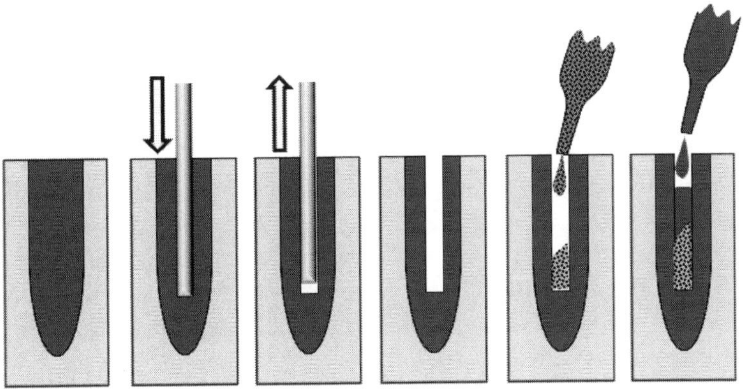

Figure 6.3 Suppositories prepared by the hollow-type method. Adapted from Kaewnopparat *et al.* (2009).

Some examples of vaginal suppositories available in the international market are presented in Table 6.5 (Nader-Macias 2008).

Table 6.5 Examples of vaginal suppositories available in the international market (Nader-Macias 2008)

Product	Probiotic composition
Vagiflor® (Germany)	*L. acidophilus*
Lactinex® (Argentina)	*L. acidophilus*
Tropivag®(Argentina)	*L. rhamnosus Lcr35®*
HLC Candaclear®(Canada)	*L. acidophilus*
Intrafresh® (UK)	*L. acidophilus*

6.2.5 Other Pharmaceutical Dosage Forms

6.2.5.1 Chewing gums and lozenges

Chewing gums are an ancient and widely popular form of confection that recently came to be used as a drug delivery system (Sweetman 2009). Chewing gums are solid preparations with a base consisting mainly of gum that is intended to be chewed but not swallowed (Eur. Pharmacopeia 2008). Their active substance is released by chewing, followed by dissolution or dispersion in saliva for local or systemic treatment. Chewing gums can be made by compression or other processes.

Lozenges are solid preparations, usually in flavored, sweetened base, which are intended to dissolve or disintegrate slowly in the mouth (USP31 2008; Sweetman 2009). They can be prepared by molding (sometimes referred as pastilles) or by compression (sometimes referred as troches) (USP31 2008).

Oral research related to the beneficial effects of probiotics has shown that one strain with a proven intestinal effect may not be beneficial to health in the oral environment. Recent clinical trials have demonstrated a decrease in the prevalence of moderate or severe gingival inflammation in adults who frequently use chewing gums containing probiotics.

Saliva plays an important role in propagating oral biofilms. However, sometimes, the role of saliva on bacterial survival can be contradictory (Stamatova and Meurman 2009). Some probiotic bacteria may be beneficial for periodontal health if they are able to attach to the oral biofilm inhibiting the pathogen growth and metabolism. Dental caries are formed due to interaction between acid-producing bacteria and fermentable carbohydrates. It has been demonstrated that probiotics in dairy products may change oral ecology. For example, Çaglar *et al.* (2006) investigated the effect of two oral delivery systems containing *L. reuteri* ATCC 55730 on the levels of salivary mutans streptococci (MS) and lactobacilli (LB) and concluded that the daily ingestion of straws or lozenges containing lactobacilli-derived probiotics reduced the levels of salivary bacteria.

In another study, Çaglar *et al.* (2007) investigated whether the association of potential anticarie agents, such as probiotic bacteria and xylitol, would increase the suppressive effect on dental caries caused by bacteria in saliva. These authors evaluated the effect of xylitol and probiotic chewing gums taken by healthy human volunteers, three times daily after meals, on salivary MS and LB. Chewing gums contained two strains of *L. reuteri* (ATCC 55730 and ATCC PTA 5289), and each pellet of the xylitol gum contained approximately 1.0 g of xylitol as single sweetener. The results of this study demonstrated that chewing gums containing probiotic bacteria or xylitol may decrease significantly the levels of salivary MS. However, the association of probiotic and xylitol chewing gums did not appear to be advantageous.

Twetman *et al.* (2009) investigated the effect of short-term use of probiotic chewing gums containing two strains of *L. reuteri* (ATCC 55730 and ATCCPTA 5289) at a dose of 10^8 cfu/gum. The results of this study demonstrated the significant dosedependent modulating effect of a short-term intake of probiotics on the oral immune response. In another study, Mayanagi *et al.* (2009) studied the effect of the oral administration of lactobacilli on the bacterial population in supra/subgingival plaque. Healthy volunteers without severe periodontitis were randomized into two groups to receive *L. salivarius* WB21 (2.01×10^9 cfu/day) and xylitol in tablets or placebo with xylitol for 8 weeks. These authors concluded that the oral administration of probiotic lactobacilli decreased the number of five selected periodontopathic bacteria and contributed to the beneficial effects on periodontal conditions.

For the prevention and treatment of halitosis, the replacement of bacteria involved in halitosis by colonization with probiotic strains from the indigenous oral microbiota of healthy humans may have potential application. The use of probiotics in the treatment of halitosis has been reported in several studies. For example, it was shown that *S. salivarius* K12 taken in a lozenge after a mouthwash could reduce the oral volatile sulfur compounds levels in 85% of the volunteers submitted to the test (Stamatova and Meurman 2009).

Iwamoto *et al.* (2010) also studied the influence of probiotics on halitosis and oral health. These authors postulated that with the administration of *L. salivarius* WB21, the amount of periodontopathic bacteria, which produce H_2S and CH_3SH, in the saliva of the patients with halitosis would decrease. However, this study emphasizes the need for better understanding of probiotic functions in the oral cavity.

6.2.5.2 Gels

Gels are semisolid systems consisting of either suspensions made up of small inorganic particles, forming a network of small discrete particles (two phase gel), or large organic molecules interpenetrated by a liquid in such a manner that no apparent boundaries exist between them (single phase gel) (USP31 2008). In Europe, gels are defined in a slightly different manner as "liquids gelled by means of suitable gelling agents" (*Eur. Pharmacopeia* 2008).

Gels can be used to administer drugs topically, into body cavities or orally. Few commercialized vaginal gels containing probiotics are available. For example, as described before, two vaginal gels containing *L. acidophilus* are marketed in France (*Trophigil*® and *Florgynal*®).

Ahmad *et al.* (2008) developed a bioadhesive vaginal gel for the treatment of vaginal infections using guar gum, xanthan gum, and HPMC K4M as bioadhesive polymers and monosodium citrate as an acid-buffering agent to provide a pH of 4.4. To treat vaginal infections, clotrimazole and metronidazole were used in the formulation along with lactobacillus spores. The results of this study showed that the bioadhesive gel developed had better antimicrobial action than intravaginal drug delivery systems commercially available.

6.2.5.3 Eye drops

Eye drops are sterile aqueous or oily solutions or suspensions intended for instillation into the eye (*Eur. Pharmacopeia* 2008).

Iovieno *et al.* (2008) evaluated the efficacy of *L. acidophilus* eye drops in controlling the symptoms of vernal keratoconjunctivite (VKC). In this study, eye drops containing *L. acidophilus* diluted in a saline solution (2×10^8 cfu/ml) were applied in both eyes of seven patients with mild to moderate VKC, four times a day, during 4 weeks. The results of this study showed that probiotic eye drops improved symptoms of VKC. However, the authors of this study concluded that to confirm the effects of Lactobacilli on VKC, additional double-blind studies are needed.

6.2.5.4 Pellets

Pellets can be defined as small, free-flowing, spherical, or semi-spherical solid units, typically from about 0.5 mm to 1.5 mm, usually intended for oral administration and generally manufactured by the process of extrusion-spheronization (process usually used in the pharmaceutical industry to produce spheroids with uniform size) (Troy 2005). The death of intestinal microflora by antibiotic or radiation treatment can lead to overgrowth of pathogenic microorganisms. Reintroduction of a normal flora into the "sterilized" gut may help to resolve this problem. Pellets containing bacteria have been prepared by extrusion-spheronization to assess the effects of processing on bacterial survival. Gram-negative aerobic (*Escherichia coli*), gram-positive aerobic (*Staphylococcus saprophyticus* and *B. subtilis*), and gram-positive anaerobic (*B.

angulatum) vegetative bacteria, together with spores of *B. subtilis*, were introduced separately into a formulation, which was extruded, spheronized, and dried to produce pellets. Samples were taken at each stage of the pellet production process and checked for bacterial survival. The results showed that spores survived all stages of the process. Survival levels of the gram-positive organisms after extrusion, spheronization, and drying were significantly higher than the gram-negative *E. coli*, with 5% *B. angulatum* remaining viable in the final dried pellets. The effects of extrusion speed, extrusion die length-to-radius ratio, and extrusion pressure on the viability of the more sensitive *E. coli* were investigated. The level of death was not affected by extrusion speed or die length-to-radius ratio. However, survival was inversely proportional to extrusion pressure over the range 1–8000 kPa (Kouimtzi *et al.* 1997).

6.3 Dosage Forms Characterization

To orientate the development of the pharmaceutical dosage forms, some pharmacopeial tests may be used. These tests that are fully described in pharmacopeias were primarily developed to confirm the quality of the medicines or probiotic dosage forms. Pharmacopeias are official compendia that publish quality standards for pharmaceutical substances and products (monographs containing directions for their identification, characterization, and assay). There are three large pharmacopeias in the world, the European Pharmacopoeia (Ph. Eur.), the United States Pharmacopeia (USP), and the Japanese Pharmacopoeia (JP).

Uniformity of mass test (or more recently the Uniformity of Dosage Unit test), disintegration tests, and dissolution/release studies are some of the tests that should be performed in order to ensure the quality of solid dosage forms. The uniformity of dosage test can be made by two methods, namely, content uniformity (assay of the individual content in a number of individual dosage units) or weight variation (consists in individually weighing a number of individual units and determining their average mass). The disintegration test determines whether solid dosage forms disintegrate within a prescribed time when placed in an immersion fluid at a temperature of 37 ± 0.5°C. The time for disintegration is registered when the dosage form is completely disintegrated or dissolved in the medium and the mean values are calculated from six parallel measurements. The dissolution test is used to determine the dissolution rate of the active ingredients of dosage forms placed in an immersion fluid at 37 ± 0.5°C. The basket (apparatus 1), the paddle (apparatus 2), the reciprocating cylinder (apparatus 3), or the flow-through cell (apparatus 4) may be used (Fig. 6.4). At specified time, samples of the dissolution liquid are withdrawn, filtered, and the amount of bioactive ingredient released is evaluated by suitable analytical methods (USP31 2008). In the case of dosage forms containing probiotics, the enumeration of viable cells released should be done.

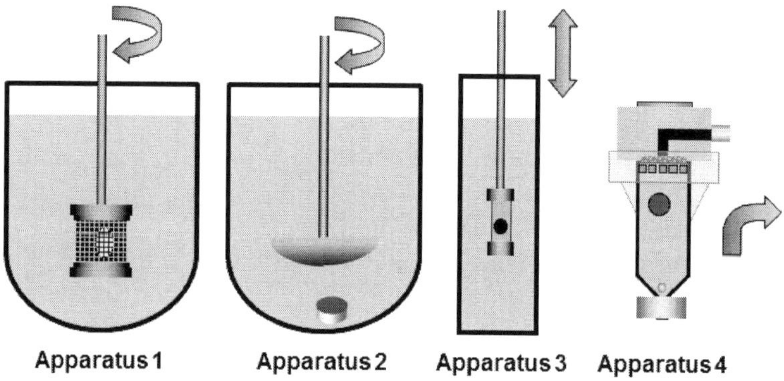

Figure 6.4 USP dissolution test apparatus.

In the pharmaceutical industry, dissolution testing is one of the most important tools in drug development and quality control. Dissolution studies of oral tablets may be performed in simulated gastric fluid (SGF) or/and simulated intestinal fluid (SIF). In the studies reported by Poulin *et al.* (2011), the dissolution of tablets was performed in SGF and in SIF without the addition of pancreatin because preliminary studies had demonstrated that this enzyme did not influence probiotics viability.

Vaginal tablets unless intended for prolonged local action can be evaluated with the test for disintegration of suppositories with modifications (Eur. Pharmacopeia 2008). In the case of dissolution studies for vaginal tablets, they should be performed in simulated vaginal fluid. The understanding of the interactions of probiotic microorganisms with the vaginal fluid can help to design improved vaginal probiotic formulations. For this purpose, *in vitro* conditions similar to those *in vivo* are needed (Tomás and Nader-Macías 2007).

In order to achieve a close *in vitro/in vivo* correlation for tablets containing probiotics for oral or vaginal administration, some parameters that must be considered when designing a dissolution apparatus include the volume and composition of the dissolution medium. Taking this into account, Kale *et al.* (2005) developed a dissolution apparatus that could simulate the vaginal environmental for vaginal tablets containing a probiotic agent (lactobacillus). These tablets are a special type of dosage form in which the released bacteria attach to the vaginal membrane in such a way that they colonize to form a protective environment against the vaginal pathogens. The design of the apparatus was a modified form of a model by Setnikar and Fantelli (1962). With this study Kale *et al.* (2005) concluded that the apparatus developed presented several advantages such as the minimization of the dissolution fluid volume and elimination of exposure of the vaginal formulation to agitation and sampling devices, being a very promising method to be adopted for routine quality control testing.

In the case of suppositories, it may be necessary to perform a proper test to demonstrate that the release of the active substances is satisfactory as, for example, the dissolution test. For hydrophilic suppositories, the basket, paddle, or flow-through cell (already referred) can be used (Fig. 6.5). For lipophilic suppositories, a modified basket method, a paddle method with a wired screen and a sinker, and a modified flow-through cell with a specific dual chamber suppository cell (Eur. Pharmacopeia 2008) (Fig. 6.5) have been recommended (Siewert *et al.* 2003).

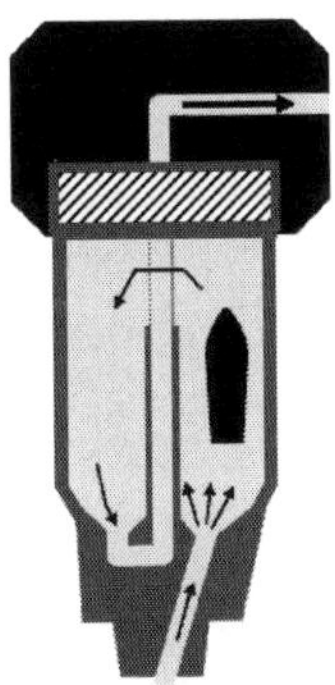

Figure 6.5 Dual chamber suppository cell.

Biologic products are not heat sterilized because active ingredients are heat labile. An important concern is related with the prevention of cross-contamination with other products manufactured in the same area and, as a consequence, product contact equipment should be sterilized.

One of the key parameters indicating the effectiveness of dosage forms to protect cells originating long shelf life is the stability of probiotic cells. In quality control in addition to technological properties, functional properties must also be taken into account. Properties such as bile and acid stability, adhesiveness, survival during the manufacturing process, and colonization properties must be monitored and optimized (Forssten *et al.* 2011).

It is important to consider that probiotics are living organisms, and as a consequence, their number undergoes a decrease with time. Stability is a crucial parameter that provides the capability of a probiotic to induce health benefices. Thus, the probiotics should be able to withstand the processing conditions and to survive during storage. Probiotic stability is related to factors such as gender, species, strain biotype, and composition of other ingredients of the dosage form. The stability is also influenced by other factors such as water, temperature, pH, osmotic pressure, and oxygen (Del Piano *et al.* 2006).

The tests of stability are performed to guarantee that the product continues to be safe and effective throughout the expiration date stated on the label. Stability studies should be performed using the same storage conditions that characterize commercial life of the product. The dosage form should be tested in the respective container intended for marketing and should be stored at the recommended temperature (Sutton 2008).

Special attention is required in all steps of the formulation development (fermentation, concentration, cell washing, cryoprotection, freeze-drying, grinding, mixing, and packaging) in order to guarantee probiotic cultures viability. It is important to specify the conditions under which the bacteria are produced and stored to minimize variability from batch to batch, improving the efficiency of probiotic strains in the final products (Del Piano *et al.* 2006).

For those final products that are dried or lyophilized, the moisture content is a critical parameter that may affect the viability of microorganisms and quality of product throughout its useful life, so for this type of products, the moisture content must be controlled. Final specifications for the final dosage forms are established on the basis of clinical data and manufacturing performance (Sutton 2008).

As stated above, the stability and viability of probiotics in dry state are affected by the surrounding temperature and water activity. Using temperatures below 30°C and water activities lower than 0.20, it is possible to maintain the probiotic viability by preserving the integrity of microbial cell membrane. Solid dosage forms such as powders, tablets, and capsules have a very low water activity, and as a consequence, their storage time is longer (Forssten *et al.* 2011).

Klayraung *et al.* (2009) studied the stability of tablets containing probiotics when stored at temperatures of 10°C and 30°C. These authors reported that tablets stored at 10°C during 6 months showed very good stability with almost full preservation of the number of viable cells.

The addition of excipients that act as protecting agents of probiotics during storage must be taken into account in the development of a probiotic formulation with a stable shelf-life (Zárate and Nader-Macias 2006). For example, Champagne *et al.* (1996) reported the effect of the addition of gelatin, xanthan gum, or maltodextrins on the survival during freeze-drying and stability during storage of four LAB. The results of these studies showed that gelatin improved the storage stability of freeze-dried *L. casei*, *L. rhamnosus* RO11, and *B. longum* RO23 cultures kept at 20°C and 4°C. In general, the additives had a detrimental effect on the stability of *S. thermophilus* RO57 during storage at 20°C.

Bora *et al.* (2009) studied the effect of buffering agents, encapsulating agents, diluents, disintegrants, glidants, and lubricants on the survival of *B. coagulans* spores under isothermal stress conditions at 40 ± 2°C under 75 ± 5% RH. The results of this study demonstrated the detrimental effect of RH conditions of 75% on the viability of the spores of *B. coagulans* and these probiotics were found to be compatible with the excipients studied, with the exception of citric acid monohydrate meglumine and sodium starch glycolate. In another study, Brachkova (2010) studied the influence of the incorporation of *Lactobacillus* spp. into different dosage forms keeping their viability and antibacterial activity. In order to achieve this aim, the survival of probiotic microorganisms in freeze-dried powders, tablets, pellets, calcium alginate beads, and films was investigated. In this study, two strategies were used: (i) the direct incorporation of bacterial suspensions into pellets, sodium alginate beads, and films, and (ii) the mixture of freeze-dried bacteria with tabletting excipients to produce tablets. The vegetative forms of *L. plantarum*, *L. rhamnosus* GG, *L. lactis*, and *L. bulgaricus* and spore form of *B. subtilis* were considered as model bacterial strains. With this study, the successful production of various dosage forms for the delivery of viable lactobacilli with an antibacterial activity against multi-resistant bacteria was demonstrated.

As stated above, probiotics viability should also be maintained after the manufacture of dosage forms. For example, one of the methods described to evaluate the relationship between the applied pressure during tablets manufacturing and bacterial viability consisted in producing tablets using different compression forces. After compression, the tablets are dissolved/disintegrated in an accurate volume of SIF, and the resulting suspension is diluted and plated in MRS (Man, Rogosa and Sharpe) agar. After incubation for 48 h at 37°C, the number of viable cells was determined. The initial number of viable cells in the individual tablet doses of probiotics should be also evaluated following the same procedure without compressing the powder mixture.

In the studies of Stadler and Viernstein (2003), the degradation of lyophilized viable LAB cells during the tablets formulation and preparation as well as the survival in artificial gastric juice were evaluated. The loss of bacteria due to the compression of tablets was evaluated by calculation from the number of viable cells in the mixed powders before compression and in the tablets resulting from the compression. The results of these studies showed that for achieving the resistance of the gastric juice, high content of HPMCAS as well as a compaction force of high or medium intensity are required.

Klayraung *et al.* (2009) also studied the influence of matrix-forming excipients and compression forces on the viability of probiotics. The results of these studies showed that the percentage of matrix-forming agents and the compression forces can significantly influence the tensile strength and disintegration of tablets containing probiotics and also the survival of bacteria. These studies also demonstrated that the tablets produced with high compression forces exhibited a slow disintegration time and a bacterial viability greater than 80%. Furthermore, the addition of sodium alginate resulted in higher cell survival in simulated GI fluid and a disintegration time of approximately 5 hours.

Saccharomyces boulardii is a nonpathogenic yeast with proven health benefits; however, the living yeast is sensitive to environmental conditions and its viability is less than 1% in the feces after oral administration. Thus, the studies of Graff *et al.* (2008) aimed to formulate dosage forms able to protect the probiotic *S. boulardii* from degradation in acidic conditions. Alginate microspheres and tablets (50.80% of Flowlac® 100 and 13.35% of Methocel® K4M) enabled to protect the yeast from degradation in acidic conditions and to release viable cells at pH 6.8. However, despite similar release profile from both dosage forms, the compression led to a significant decrease in the viability of the freeze-dried yeast. These investigators concluded that although both formulations were efficient in protecting *S. boulardii* in acidic conditions, microspheres provided higher entrapment efficiency and a faster release of the viable probiotic in intestinal conditions than matrix tablets.

It has been reported that to improve probiotic survival, it is necessary to induce a stresstolerance response achieved by pre-exposing cells to sublethal stresses, such as salt, heat, bile, and low pH. This pre-exposure can significantly increase probiotic survival following subsequent exposure to lethal stress. Other strategies, including cell immobilization technology and microencapsulation, have also been demonstrated to improve the stress-tolerance profiles of certain probiotic strains (Sleator and Hill 2008). Borges *et al.* (2012) studied the effects of encapsulation on the viability of probiotic strains (*L. casei, L. paracasei, L. acidophilus Ki,* and *B. animalis BB-12*) during exposure to lethal conditions (25% NaCl, pH 3.0 and 55–60°C). The results of this study showed that with the exception of exposure to 25% (w/v) NaCl, *L. acidophilus Ki* (free and encapsulated cells) demonstrated the highest survival rates through exposure to lethal conditions of temperature and pH.

6.4 Packaging and Storage of Dosage Forms Containing Probiotics

The packaging materials used and the storage conditions are important for the quality and shelf-life of products containing probiotic bacteria (Saarela *et al.* 2000).

The methods of packaging and storage must avoid moisture, oxygen, light, microbial contamination, and high temperatures. Generally, probiotic dosage forms contain microorganisms in the freeze-dried form. Freeze-dried products are stored within sealed glass ampoules, or glass vials, and for dried products, there are other options such as high barrier plastic bags and blister packs (Morgan *et al.* 2006).

Customized probiotic stick packs are also one of the best ways to ensure that the probiotic products are sufficiently protected from the detrimental effects of humidity and oxygen. For example, several lactobacillus strains are packaged in aluminum triple-foil, thermo-closed packs.

There are few studies on packaging and storage, as manufacturers are charged to establish how their products will be packaged, labeled, and marketed. Currently, oral powders are often stored in heat-sealable laminated sachets (individual doses) and in glass or plastic flasks. For example, for the treatment of acute diarrhea, probiotics are combined with oral rehydration salts. The salts and the probiotic strain can be packed in separate sachets, or salt solution can be put in a carton and the bacteria in a straw (i.e., suspended in oil and dried inside the straw) (Saxelin 2008). Powdered products may be supplied with pre-packaged buffered reconstituting solutions. Hard capsules are generally stored in blisters (container consisting of two layers in which one is shaped to contain the capsule) and in glass or plastic flasks. Tablets are generally stored in blisters, strips (container consisting of two layers, usually provided with perforations, suited for containing one tablet), and in glass or plastic flasks. In the case of probiotic products, the materials used in the container should have low water-vapor transmission rate.

6.5 Conclusions and Future Trends

The use of probiotics as therapeutic agents is currently widespread. Probiotic strains should be incorporated into suitable dosage forms in which they can retain their viability and functionality. In addition, probiotics should be packaged in suitable conditions that can ensure adequate quality standards.

Highly reproducible probiotic products are required for clinical use and, as a consequence, validation of each step of the manufacturing process is a fundamental means of controlling product reproducibility. For these products, formulation and packaging constitute significant challenges to maintain stability and to ensure microorganisms viability.

Generally, for probiotics administration, solid dosage forms such as powders, capsules, and tablets represent the best delivery systems, as they provide higher stability. Tablets have several advantages above other dosage forms and, as a consequence, these delivery systems have been widely studied for probiotics administration. Novel functional polymers used to improve the stability and survival of probiotics in gastric conditions are also gaining attention. Furthermore, the study of the best manufacturing conditions is also important to maintain the microorganisms viability. For example, some studies (Stadler and Viernstein 2003; Klayraung *et al.* 2009) have demonstrated that probiotic tablets should be prepared with suitable amounts of excipients and high compression forces in order to prolong the tablet disintegration, maintaining the viability of bacteria.

For vaginal administration of probiotics, suppositories have also been extensively studied and developed because these dosage forms are easy to apply into the vagina without irritation. In order to maintain viability of probiotics, hollow-type suppositories have been prepared. The advantage of using the hollow-type method is that it can minimize the effect of the heating process on the survival of bacteria during preparation. However, the industrial production of this type of suppositories has not yet been implemented.

Although there are currently hundreds of products marketed and labeled as containing probiotics, many of the strains they contain have not been evaluated in scientific trials involving humans (Saxelin 2008). It is also important to note that a higher dose does not always mean a better effect, and health claims that are being considered for approval should be connected to an effective daily intake and a recommended frequency of administration of the dosage forms containing probiotics (Hoffman 2008).

One approach that should be more investigated in the future is a combination of probiotics and prebiotics (symbiotic action), which can result in improved health beneficial products. However, although the trend is to combine different types of probiotics, it is important to know the potential antagonistic interactions between strains. Moreover, the research and production of genetically modified therapeutic microorganisms and their incorporation in dosage forms will allow the production of medicinal products tailored to the individual needs of each patient.

References

Ahmad, F., M. Alam, *et al.* (2008). "Development and *in vitro* evaluation of an acid buffering bioadhesive vaginal gel for mixed vaginal infections." *Acta Pharmaceutica* **58**(4): 407–419.

Baerheim, A., E. Larsen, *et al.* (1994). "Vaginal application of lactobacilli in the prophylaxis of recurrent lower urinary tract infection in women." *Scandinavian Journal of Primary Health Care* **14**(1): 11–16.

Bora, P., V. Puri, *et al.* (2009). "Physicochemical properties and excipient compatibility studies of probiotic Bacillus coagulans spores." *Scientia Pharmaceutica* **77**: 625–637.

Borges, S., J. Barbosa, *et al.* (2012). "Effects of encapsulation on the viability of probiotic strains exposed to lethal conditions." *International Journal of Food Science & Technology* **47**(2): 416–421.

Brachkova, M. I. (2010). *Evaluation of the Viability of Lactobacillus spp. in Different Dosage Forms.* PhD, University of Lisbon.

Bruno, F. A. and N. P. Shah (2003). "Viability of two freeze-dried strains of Bifidobacterium and of commercial preparations at various temperatures during prolonged storage." *Journal of Food Science* **68**(7): 2336–2339.

Çaglar, E., S. Kavaloglu Cildir, *et al.* (2006). "Salivary mutans streptococci and lactobacilli levels after ingestion of the probiotic bacterium Lactobacillus reuteri ATCC 55730 by straws or tablets." *Acta Odontologica Scandinavica* **64**(5): 314–318.

Çaglar, E., S. Kavaloglu, *et al.* (2007). "Effect of chewing gums containing xylitol or probiotic bacteria on salivary mutans streptococci and lactobacilli." *Clinical Oral Investigations* **11**(4): 425–429.

Calinescu, C., J. Mulhbacher, *et al.* (2005). "Carboxymethyl high amylose starch (CM-HAS) as excipient for Escherichia coli oral formulations." *European Journal of Pharmaceutics and Biopharmaceutics* **60**(1): 53–60.

Champagne, C. P., F. Mondou, *et al.* (1996). "Effect of polymers and storage temperature on the stability of freeze-dried lactic acid bacteria." *Food Research International* **29**(5–6): 555–562.

Chan, E. S. and Z. Zhang (2005). "Bioencapsulation by compression coating of probiotic bacteria for their protection in an acidic medium." *Process Biochemistry* **40**(10): 3346-3351.

Czaja, C., A. Stapleton, *et al.* (2007). "Phase I trial of a Lactobacillus crispatus vaginal suppository for prevention of recurrent urinary tract infection in women." *Infections Diseases in Obstetrics and Gynecology*, doi: 10.1155/2007/35387.

Del Piano, M., L. Morelli, *et al.* (2006). "Probiotics: from research to consumer." *Digestive and Liver Disease* **38**(2): S248–S255.

Dover, S., A. Aroutcheva, *et al.* (2008). "Natural antimicrobials and their role in vaginal health: a short review." *International Journal of Probiotics and Prebiotics* **3**(4): 219–230.

Elmer, G. W. (2001). "Probiotics: living drugs." *American Journal of Health-System Pharmacy* **58**(12): 1101–1109.

Eur. Pharmacopeia (2008). Strasbourg, EDQM.

Falagas, M. E., G. I. Betsi, *et al.* (2006). "Probiotics for prevention of recurrent vulvovaginal candidiasis: a review." *Journal of Antimicrobial Chemotherapy* **58**(2): 266–272.

Fazeli, M. R., T. Toliyat, *et al.* (2006). "Viability of lactobacillus acidophilus in various vaginal tablet formulations." *DARU* **14**(4): 172–177.

FDA (2006). Guidance for industry: complementary and alternative medicine products and their regulation by the Food and Drug Administration.

Forssten, S. D., C. W. Sindelar, *et al.* (2011). "Probiotics from an industrial perspective." *Anaerobe* **17**(6): 410–413.

Gil, N., R. Martinez, *et al.* (2010). "Vaginal lactobacilli as potential probiotics against Candida spp." *Brazilian Journal of Microbiology* (41): 6–14.

Graff, S., J.-C. Chaumeil, *et al.* (2008). "Formulations for protecting the probiotic Saccharomyces boulardii from degradation in acidic condition." *Biological & Pharmaceutical Bulletin* **31**(2): 266–272.

Hoffman, F. A. (2008). "Business considerations in the development of probiotics." *Clinical Infectious Diseases* **46**(Supplement 2): S141–S143.

Hoffman, F. A., J. T. Heimbach, *et al.* (2008). "Executive summary: scientific and regulatory challenges of development of probiotics as foods and drugs." *Clinical Infectious Diseases* **46**(Supplement 2): S53–S57.

ICH (2002). International Conference Harmonization of Technical Requirements for the Registration of Pharmaceuticals for Human Use.

Iovieno, A., A. Lambiase, *et al.* (2008). "Preliminary evidence of the efficacy of probiotic eye-drop treatment in patients with vernal keratoconjunctivitis." *Graefe's Archive for Clinical and Experimental Ophthalmology* **246**(3): 435–441.

Iwamoto, T., N. Suzuki, *et al.* (2010). "Effects of probiotic Lactobacillus salivarius WB21 on halitosis and oral health: an open-label pilot trial." *Oral Surgery, Oral Medicine, Oral Pathology, Oral Radiology, and Endodontology* **110**(2): 201–208.

Jones, B. E. (2004). Pharmaceutical Capsules. *The History of the Medicinal Capsule*_B. E. J. Fridrun Podczeck. London, Pharmaceutical Press.

Kaewnopparat, S. and N. Kaewnopparat (2009). "Formulation and evaluation of vaginal suppositories containing lactobacillus." *World Academy of Science, Engineering and Technology* **55**: 25–28.

Kaewsrichan, J., K. Chandajoti, *et al.* (2007). "Evaluation of lactobacilli containing suppository formulation for probiotic use." *Mahidol University Journal of Pharmaceutical Sciences* **34**(1–4): 1–8.

Kale, V. V., R. V. Trivedi, *et al.* (2005). "Development and evaluation of a suppository formulation containing lactobacillus and its application in vaginal diseases." *Annals of the New York Academy of Sciences* **1056**(1): 359–365.

Klayraung, S., H. Viernstein, *et al.* (2009). "Development of tablets containing probiotics: Effects of formulation and processing parameters on bacterial viability." *International Journal of Pharmaceutics* **370**(1–2): 54–60.

Kouimtzi, M., R. J. Pinney, *et al.* (1997). "Survival of bacteria during extrusion-spheronization." *Pharmacy and Pharmacology Communications* **3**(7): 347–351.

Lepargneur, J. P. and V. Rousseau (2002). "Protective role of the Doderlein flora." *Journal of Gynécologie Obstétrique et Biologie de la Reproduction* **31**(5): 485–494.

Maggi, L., P. Mastromarino, *et al.* (2000). "Technological and biological evaluation of tablets containing different strains of lactobacilli for vaginal administration." *European Journal of Pharmaceutics and Biopharmaceutics* **50**(3): 389–395.

Mastromarino, P., P. Brigidi, *et al.* (2002). "Characterization and selection of vaginal Lactobacillus strains for the preparation of vaginal tablets." *Journal of Applied Microbiology* **93**(5): 884–893.

Mastromarino, P., S. Macchia, *et al.* (2009). "Effectiveness of Lactobacillus-containing vaginal tablets in the treatment of symptomatic bacterial vaginosis." *Clinical Microbiology and Infection* **15**(1): 67–74.

Mayanagi, G., M. Kimura, *et al.* (2009). "Probiotic effects of orally administered Lactobacillus salivarius WB21-containing tablets on periodontopathic bacteria: a double-blinded, placebo-controlled, randomized clinical trial." *Journal of Clinical Periodontology* **36**(6): 506–513.

Morgan, C. A., N. Herman, *et al.* (2006). "Preservation of micro-organisms by drying; A review." *Journal of Microbiological Methods* **66**(2): 183–193.

Muller, J. A., C. Stanton, *et al.* (2010). "Reconstitution conditions for dried probiotic powders represent a critical step in determining cell viability." *Journal of Applied Microbiology* **108**(4): 1369–1379.

Nader-Macias, M. E. (2008). "Advances in the knowledge and clinical applications of lactic acid bacteria as probiotics in the urogenital tract." *Current Womens Health Reviews* **4**: 240–257.

Poulin, J.-F., R. Caillard, *et al.* (2011). "β-Lactoglobulin tablets as a suitable vehicle for protection and intestinal delivery of probiotic bacteria." *International Journal of Pharmaceutics* **405**(1–2): 47–54.

Prista, L. N., A. C. Alves, *et al.* (1990). Técnica Farmacêutica e Farmácia Galénica. Lisboa, Fundação Calouste Gulbenkian. **III**.

Reid, G. and A. Bruce (2006). "Probiotics to prevent urinary tract infections: the rationale and evidence." *World Journal of Urology* **24**(1): 28–32.

Reid, G., A. W. Bruce, *et al.* (1992). "Recurrence of urinary tract infections (UTI) in women who were administered vaginal suppositories on recurrence of urinary tract infections." *Clinical Therapeutics* **14**(1): 11–16.

Rodrigues, D., T. Rocha-Santos, *et al.* (2011). "On the viability of five probiotic strains when immobilised on various polymers." *International Journal of Dairy Technology* **64**(1): 137–144.

Rodrigues, F. (2011). *Desenvolvimento e caracterização de óvulos de Lactobacillus acidophilus*. MsD, Porto.

Ross, J. and P. Boucher (2012). "Considerations in the development of live biotherapeutic products for clinical use." *Current Issues Molecular Biology* **10**: 13–16.

Saarela, M., G. Mogensen, *et al.* (2000). "Probiotic bacteria: safety, functional and technological properties." *Journal of Biotechnology* **84**(3): 197–215.

Santiago, G. L. d. S., H. Verstraelen, *et al.* (2009). "A pilot study evaluating the safety of vaginal administration of a multi-particulate pellet formulation." *European Journal of Pharmaceutics and Biopharmaceutics* **73**(3): 399–403.

Saxelin, M. (2008). "Probiotic formulations and applications, the current probiotics market, and changes in the marketplace: a European perspective." *Clinical Infectious Diseases* **46**(Supplement 2): S76–S79.

Setnikar, I. and S. Fantelli (1962). "Liquefaction time of rectal suppositories." *Journal of Pharmaceutical Sciences* **51**(6): 566–571.

Siewert, M., J., C. Dressman, *et al.* (2003). "FIP/AAPS guidelines to dissolution/*in vitro* release testing of novel/special dosage forms." *AAPS PharmSciTech* **4**(1): E7.

Sleator, R. D. and C. Hill (2008). "New frontiers in probiotic research." *Letters in Applied Microbiology* **46**(2): 143–147.

Stadler, M. and H. Viernstein (2003). "Optimization of a formulation containing viable lactic acid bacteria." *International Journal of Pharmaceutics* **256**(1–2): 117–122.

Stamatova, I. and J. Meurman (2009). "Probiotics: health benefits in the mouth." *American Journal of Dentistry* **22**(6): 329–338.

Sutton, A. (2008). "Product development of probiotics as biological drugs." *Clinical Infectious Diseases* **46**(Supplement 2): S128–S132.

Sweetman, S. C. (2009). *Martindale: The Complete Drug Reference*, Pharmaceutical Press.

Tomás, M. S. and M. E. Nader-Macías (2007). Effect of a medium simulating vaginal fluid on the growth and expression of beneficial characteristics of potentially probiotic lactobacilli. A. Méndez-Vilas: 732–739.

Troy, D. B. (2005). Remington, the science and practice of pharmacy. USA, Lippincott Williams & Wilkins.

Twetman, S., B. Derawi, *et al.* (2009). "Short-term effect of chewing gums containing probiotic Lactobacillus reuteri on the levels of inflammatory mediators in gingival crevicular fluid." *Acta Odontologica Scandinavica* **67**(1): 19–24.

Uehara, S., K. Monden, *et al.* (2006). "A pilot study evaluating the safety and effectiveness of Lactobacillus vaginal suppositories in patients with recurrent urinary tract infection." *International Journal of Antimicrobial Agents* **28,** Supplement 1(0): 30–34.

USP31 (2008). The United States Pharmacopeia US Pharmacopeia.

Watanabe, Y. and M. Matsumoto (1986). "Pharmaceutical evaluation of hollow type suppositories. IV. Improvement of viability of propanolol in rabbits after rectal administration." *Journal of Pharmacobio-dynamics* **9**(6): 526–531.

Ya, W., C. Reifer, *et al.* (2010). "Efficacy of vaginal probiotic capsules for recurrent bacterial vaginosis: a double-blind, randomized, placebo-controlled study." *American Journal of Obstetrics and Gynecology* **203**(2): 120.e121–120.e126.

Ying, D. Y., M. C. Phoon, *et al.* (2010). "Microencapsulated Lactobacillus rhamnosus GG powders: relationship of powder physical properties to probiotic survival during storage." *Journal of Food Science* **75**(9): E588–E595.

Zárate, G. and M. E. Nader-Macias (2006). "Viability and biological properties of probiotic vaginal lactobacilli after lyophilization and refrigerated storage into gelatin capsules." *Process Biochemistry* **41**(8): 1779–1785.

Chapter 7

Guidelines and Regulations

J. Paulo Sousa e Silva[a] and Ana M. Gomes[b]
[a]*Faculty of Pharmacy, University of Porto, Rua de Jorge Viterbo Ferreira, 228, 4050-313 Porto, Portugal*
[b]*CBQF, Biotechnology School of Portuguese Catholic University, Rua Dr. António Bernardino Almeida, 4200-072 Porto, Portugal*
paulo.silva@ff.up.pt

7.1 Introduction

To better understand the regional or country-specific regulations, this chapter will first provide a broad overview of the global legal framework concerning probiotics.

There is no universal definition of probiotics that can be considered generically either as a food (including food additives and dietary supplements) or as a drug (medicines). Nevertheless, the definition of probiotics by a joint Food and Agriculture Organization of the United Nations (FAO)/World Health Organization (WHO) expert consultation in October of 2001 (already mentioned in Chapter 1) has been widely used. These experts produced a report on *Evaluation of Health and Nutritional Properties of Probiotics in Food Including Powder Milk with Live Lactic Acid Bacteria*. This report,

Probiotic Bacteria: Fundamentals, Therapy, and Technological Aspects
Edited by J. Paulo Sousa e Silva and Ana C. Freitas

ISBN 978-981-4411-62-2 (Hardcover), 978-981-4411-63-9 (eBook)
www.panstanford.com

together with another on *Drafting Guidelines for the Evaluation of Probiotics in Food* developed by a joint FAO/WHO expert working group in 2002, provides scientific advice on the methodology for evaluation of probiotics in food, addressing methods for strain identification, safety assessment and functional characterization as well indication of what data are required to accurately substantiate health claims. The problems associated with probiotic product selection also become more understandable by application of guidelines established by the International Scientific Association for Probiotics and Prebiotics (ISAPP, 2009). These guidelines will be detailed in Section 7.2.

7.1.1 Food Standards

The Codex Alimentarius commission, created by FAO and WHO in 1963, is responsible for compiling the Codex Alimentarius, which is a collection of standards, codes of practice, guidelines, and other recommendations developed under the joint FAO/WHO Programme. Among other objectives, this program aims to protect the health of the consumers and ensure fair trade practices in the food market. Independently of the type of codex documents, they are generally designated as standards. These standards could be general or sometimes very precise with detailed specifications related to foods, such as practice guides concerning operation or managing operation process. For example, Codex Standard for Fermented Milks (CODEX STAN 243-2003) is an international standard with implications in probiotic products.

Codex Alimentarius or food code has become a global reference to face emerging challenges and codex standards are used in trade disputes at the World Trade Organization (WTO) (Lähteenmäki-Uutela 2009; WHO 2012). WTO was created after The Uruguay Round of General Agreement on Tariffs and Trade (GATT) negotiations (1986–1994) and begun its work in 1995. WTO aims to ensure free (as possible) trade among nations by the establishment of international agreements, and dispute resolutions between its 155 members (10 May 2012). Codex standards are specifically referred to in the WTO agreements on Technical Barriers to Trade (TBT) and on the Agreement on Sanitary and Phytosanitary Measures (SPS) (Lähteenmäki-Uutela 2009). The TBT agreement includes technical regulations, standards, testing, and certification procedures. The SPS agreement defines how nations can regulate food safety and apply animal and plant health measures. The goal of these agreements is that technical measures and health concerns do not create artificial obstacles to trade.

Codex Alimentarius also contributes directly to probiotics and all related issues from a legal point of view via the Nutrition and Health Claims standard developed and revised in the beginning of the 21st century (Codex Alimentarius: www.codexalimentarius.net)

7.1.2 Drug Standards

Although probiotics could be regulated as a drug, based on their physiological roles, it is more difficult and expensive to choose this approach due to stringent legislation.

WHO supports member states in the development of medicine policies and guidelines to implement marketing authorization system for pharmaceutical products [*Marketing Authorization of Pharmaceutical Products with Special Reference to Multisource (Generic) Products: A Manual for National Medicines Regulatory Authorities (NMRAs)*, 2nd edition].

The International Conference on Harmonisation of Technical Requirements for Registration of Pharmaceuticals for Human Use (ICH) was established in 1990 with the goal of harmonizing testing of medicines and promoting the international coordination of the authorization procedures. ICH, which brings together the regulatory authorities and research-based pharmaceutical industry in the European Union, Japan, and the United States of America, meets twice a year with the aim of reducing the cost of research by avoiding unnecessary work duplication. It consists of six organizations: European Union (EU), the European Federation of Pharmaceutical Industries and Associations, Ministry of Health, Labour and Welfare (MHLW), Japan Pharmaceutical Manufacturers Association, Food and Drug Administration (FDA), and the Pharmaceutical Research and Manufacturers of America. Although ICH guidelines are not global, they are generally accepted worldwide.

7.2 Guidelines for Probiotic Selection

It is important that probiotic bacteria selected for commercial use in foods and medicines maintain the characteristics for which they were originally selected and that justify their health-promoting effects. These include growth and viability during processing and storage as well as during transit through the gastrointestinal transit upon consumption. Consequently, it is necessary to constantly control strain properties, their stability during manufacture and storage, and to ensure that they are retained in different types of foods as well as maintained when assessed in relation to expected clinical effects (Gueimonde, 2011). Establishment and implementation of guidelines contributes to product safety, quality, reliability, and level playing for all companies introducing and producing probiotic products.

7.2.1 Safety Criteria

Regulating safety and efficacy of probiotic products is basic "consumer protection law," specifically if one considers that product safety is defined as "physical safety, protecting the consumer's body." Safety is a relative term implying absence of negative health effects.

In general, microbial food cultures (MFC) with a technological role (starter cultures), be it acidification or flavor/texture enhancement, have a long, safe history of use in food, and have generally been considered safe, and suitable for myriad uses. According to the U. S. standards, these cultures hold a GRAS (generally recognized as safe) status, which is based on either a history of presence in food prior to 1958 or by scientific procedures. Cultures used for traditional fermentation with controlled metabolism and effect on food substrate are associated with a reasonable expectation of safety. However, with respect to probiotic strains, these not only perform technological functionality but also promote added health benefits to consumers, and as science and clinical relevance advances, manufacturers need to ensure that these MFC are totally safe and reveal a safe history of use in food. Historical data indicate that probiotic lactobacilli and bifidobacteria associated with food have been considered to be safe, yet clinical evidences suggesting the need for high doses (order of magnitude around 10^{10} colony-forming unit (cfu)) and the development of improved fermentation and formulation techniques have led to emerging high-dose preparations on the market that may eventually impact negatively on the host. In this context, three areas of safety concern have been addressed as far as probiotic authorization is concerned: (i) potential for transmigration (accepted safety for long-used probiotic isolates regarding translocation, yet rare reports on bacteremia alert the need for continued surveillance, especially in immunocompromised individuals); (ii) potential negative impact of physiological and metabolic properties on the physiology, immunology, and microbiology of the gastrointestinal tract (deconjugated bile acid, D-lactate, need for absence of haemolytic activity); and (iii) absence of antibiotic resistance (negative data concerning antibiotic/gene transfer are required for each strain under each circumstance) (Henriksson *et al.*, 2005). An important highlight is that special care must be taken with those individuals presenting defective immunity, abnormal gut structure, and/or metabolic defects with respect to safe use of probiotics (Henriksson *et al.*, 2005). Safety issues have been on the agenda of many food industry committees as well as government regulatory authorities. Sets of guidelines have been drawn up and tentatively implemented by both probiotic manufacturers and scientific bodies. According to Joint FAO/WHO expert committee guidelines, strains to be used as probiotics must be characterized with a set of tests that evaluate antibiotic resistance patterns and horizontal transfer capacity, certain metabolic activities, eventual side effects, and potential virulence factors (more details are listed in the next section in Table 7.2).

The European Food Safety Authority (EFSA) has developed a list of microbial cultures with a Qualified Presumption of Safety (QPS), which need no further safety determination for the purposes of registration in the European Union (EFSA, 2010). The QPS is a well-designed concept that lists probiotic organisms, among other biological agents, by genus/species level and is based upon the scientific literature and the long history of safe use of many of the organisms in human food. The list is annually revised and updated, and following the most recent review, no modifications were made to the QPS recommended biological agents list, although modifications concerning antimicrobial susceptibility qualifications were included (EFSA, 2010). Very recently, the bacterial species *L. paracasei* was considered by EFSA to be suitable for the QPS approach (EFSA 2011). More details on the QPS system and its principles can be found on the EFSA Web site (http://www.efsa.europa.eu/EFSA/efsa_locale_1178620753812_1178667590178.htm, Accessed August 2012). The FDA also lists organisms by genus and species in its partial list of organisms used in food (FDA, 2001). A comparison of the assessment schemes of the FDA and EFSA is given in Table 7.1.

Table 7.1 Comparison between assessment schemes for dietary/food supplements in the United States (FDA GRAS system) and proposed scheme in the EU (EFSA QPS system)

GRAS guidelines	QPS guidelines
Applies to food additives, in general	Applies to microorganisms only
Determination of GRAS status by FDA and/or external experts	Determination of QPS status by EFSA
Open list	Positive list
Based on common use	Based on history of use and adverse effects
Describes specific substance or microorganism	Describes taxonomic unit (e.g., genus, species, or strain)
Case-by-case assessment	General assessment

Source: Adapted from Wassenaar and Klein (2008)

The International Food Additives Council in its position paper considers the MFC listed in the International Dairy Federation Inventory (http://www.effca.org/content/inventory-microorganisms) and those having a QPS status as GRAS. It is important to note that compared with the GRAS system used in the United States, the QPS system seems to be more flexible and considers additional emerging safety risks, such as acquisition of antibiotic resistance or virulence determinants, an important aspect that gains strength with advances in science (Wassenaar and Klein, 2008).

7.2.2 Functionality, Technological, and Labeling Criteria

The rational use of probiotics to improve physiological functions of the host has as basis (i) functional characterization and identification of bacteria and viability maintenance at consumption; (ii) required dose and enumeration techniques (influenced by strain type, alone or combined with other strains, food vector, and industrial form of presentation); (iii) health benefits for the host and their definition; and (iv) safety of use (supported by the two FAO/WHO documents of

2001 and 2002 and of the concept of QPS for the safety assessment of bacteria, recently introduced by EFSA, as previously mentioned). These documents together with other information published in the meantime, identify essential steps needed to select and validate a probiotic strain (Table 7.2). Then according to each country's

Table 7.2 Guidelines for development of a probiotic food based on Joint Expert FAO/WHO committee guidelines (2001 and 2002) combined with the need to include the impact of the food delivery vector—such matrix specifically contributes to probiotic physiology, gene expression, stability, and efficacy

Factor	Information required for substantiation
Thorough identification of the test product	Genus and species determination based on most current genetic methods. Generation of strain-specific identification, with patterns from appropriate molecular techniques. Reproducible genetic methods such as pulsed-field gel electrophoresis or randomly amplified polymorphic DNA analysis are important tools. Polyphasic characterization combining phenotypic, biochemical, genotypic, and sequencing results is suggested as a reliable strategy to identify bacteria to the strain level. Description of the food product vector for probiotic. Understand how the food matrix may affect probiotic function including, if applicable, the impact on functionality of any food transformation that results from probiotic growth.
Probiotic strain must be deposited in an international culture collection—guarantee historical reference substance is available and enables research to be repeated by independent researchers	Stock cultures must be maintained under appropriate conditions to ensure that the given culture maintains its beneficial properties.

(*Continued*)

Table 7.2 (*Continued*)

Factor	Information required for substantiation
Extensive safety assessment	Description of use (dose, format, stability). Verification that the product is manufactured under good manufacturing practices specific for the product category. Survey of literature to determine to what extent the strain, species, or genus was involved in adverse events. Description of physiological and genetic capacity for toxic activity: toxin producer, haemolytic activity. Description of physiological and genetic capacity for pathogenic/opportunistic pathogenic activity. Genetic stability of the probiotic. Presence of transferable antibiotic resistance markers. Review of the above information by regulatory authority or a panel of experts qualified in the field to evaluate the safety of the substance for its intended use, depending on the product category and requirements.
Efficacy assessment. This will be specific for the particular effects being targeted.[a] Only *in vitro* characteristics that are confirmed to be related to *in vivo* functionality are useful. Minimum daily amount required to confer the purported health benefits is to be defined explicitly on the basis of *in vitro* and *in vivo* studies on cell lines and animal models as well as human clinical trials.	Valid *in vitro* assessments, as dictated by specific probiotic strain and intent of use. Valid animal studies using test product, which might be useful for safety assessment, mechanistic studies, and suggestions of endpoints to confirm in human studies. Human efficacy studies using test product, which provide the basis for substantiation of health benefits and the rationale for the dose being delivered in the product—RDBPC[b] human trials by enrolling adequate number of subjects to achieve statistical significance. Note: dose may vary in terms of strain, food vector and the host (age, sex, target specific, healthy, and/or immunocompromised).

Factor	Information required for substantiation
Product labeling (on product label or in accompanying information on product website)	Genus, species, and strain designation for each probiotic included in the product. Minimum viable numbers of each probiotic strain at the end of the shelf-life—important that product delivers the declared level in a serving of stated size throughout product shelf-life. Expiration date. Serving size required to deliver effective dose for onset of labeled effects. Health benefits description. Identification of proper storage conditions. Corporate contact details for consumer information. Product website URL.
Post-market surveillance	All stake holders need to develop some form of system to monitor the health outcome of long-term probiotic administration. Potential side effects and long-term benefits to be recorded and documented. Proper trace back system—a pre-requisite for surveillance of probiotic products.

Source: Adapted from Sanders and Marco (2010)

[a]The traditional assertion that probiotics possess certain traits such as specific source of isolation (human, animal, environmental, food), acid resistance, bile resistance, and other such traits may not be relevant for specific applications, and therefore cannot be considered essential.

[b]Randomized, double blind, placebo controlled.

specifications, an authorization dossier needs to be submitted. As discussed later on, in the case of a dossier submitted to EFSA, this has to include a clear identification and characterization of the probiotic strain, a clear statement of the claimed health benefit, flawless evidence supporting the claimed benefit, and justification for why the benefit is substantiated by the evidence (Sanders and Marco, 2010).

7.3 Probiotics Legal Status

Regulatory standards and guidelines are crucial to prevent possibility of products on the market that are unreliable in content and contain strains with unvalidated scientific efficacy. The consumer needs to be confident that launched probiotic products are effective and fulfil all standards and recommendations through evidence-based studies. All the leading nations have a different regulatory framework for probiotics and products containing probiotics. The following sections will give an overview of regulatory bodies and issues of probiotics in different countries.

7.3.1 Asia–Pacific

7.3.1.1 Australia and New Zealand

The Australia and New Zealand food regulation system is a cooperative arrangement between the Australian States and Territories (including mainland—Western Australia, Northern territory, South Australia, Queensland, Victoria, New South Wales, Australian Capital Territory, and islands—Tasmania) and New Zealand to develop and implement uniform food standards.

The food regulatory system is underpinned by a number of agreements and legislative instruments, listed as follows:

- The Australia New Zealand Joint Food Standards Agreement between Australia and New Zealand, otherwise known as The Treaty, provides for New Zealand's involvement in the food regulatory system.
- The Food Regulation Agreement, initially signed by the Council of Australian Governments in November 2000 and amended in December 2002, is an intergovernmental agreement signed by the Australian Government, States, and Territories, and commits these signatories to a cooperative national system of food regulation. This agreement establishes the Ministerial Council, which sets food policy and considers food standards for Australia and New Zealand.
- The Food Standards Australia New Zealand Act 1991 (FSANZ Act) came into effect on 1 July 2002, and is the legislative basis for the binational statutory authority, FSANZ. The objective

of the FSANZ Act is to ensure a high standard of public health protection throughout Australia and New Zealand by maintaining a safe food supply. All food sold in Australia and New Zealand must be safe.

- FSANZ is the independent statutory authority in Australia that develops (i) food standards for primary production, processing, and food hygiene; and (ii) set residue limits for agricultural and veterinary products. The Legislative and Governance Forum on Food Regulation (formerly the Australia and New Zealand Food Regulation Ministerial Council) sets policy guidelines for the development of food standards by FSANZ. In New Zealand, these activities are undertaken by the New Zealand Ministry for Primary Industries.
- Once approved, the Standards are incorporated into the Australia New Zealand Food Standards Code (the Food Standards Code). Australian States and Territories adopt the Food Standards Code under State and Territory Food or Health Acts. New Zealand adopts the Food Standards Code under the Food Act 1981.
- Enforcement of the Food Standards Code occurs through State and Territory health departments and local councils. New Zealand enforces the Food Standards Code through its national enforcement body, the New Zealand Food Safety Authority.
- The Fair Trading Acts in New Zealand and the States and Territories of Australia apply to the supply of food in trade and commerce relating to any conduct that is considered false, misleading, or deceptive.

With respect to probiotics, probiotic products in Australia and New Zealand are considered either functional foods and are regulated by FSANZ, or complementary medicine and regulated by the Therapeutic Goods Administration (TGA). Under the Food Standards Code, fermented milk beverages and yoghurts that claim to be probiotic should have a minimum of 1 million live bacteria per gram. The number of probiotic bacteria should be maintained to the end of a product's shelf-life to be of any health benefit.

In what concerns FSANZ and the TGA proof of efficacy for complementary medicines (which include dietary supplements), these are only required if the product is making high-level health claims or is randomly audited; nevertheless, it is advisable that evidence for claim be held by food manufacturers for other eventual claims required. In fact, Australia has a registration system for dietary supplements that uses a convenient electronic application system and a validation process. Products eligible for registration in the Australian Register of Therapeutic Goods (ARTG) contain low-risk ingredients in acceptable amounts that have been evaluated and accepted by the TGA and manufactured under GMP principles, for example, probiotics. A manufacturer must submit qualitative formulation/ingredient information and finished good specifications. The label may carry indications (i.e., claims about therapeutic use of the product) only for health maintenance and health enhancement or certain indications for nonserious, self-limiting conditions. If high-level health claims are intended, the manufacturer must also certify that, according to the applicable guidelines, it holds substantiation for claims and shelf-life. The government reviews the registration in 2–4 weeks, after which time the product can appear on the market with an "Aust L" number that must be included on the label. There were approximately 69.487 products on the ARTG as at May 2012 including up to 122 probiotic products containing either *Bifidobacterium* (9 authorized strains) and/or *Lactobacillus* (26 authorized strains) probiotic strains. FSANZ is currently working on a new Nutrition, Health and Related Claims Standard to replace the transitional standard, in practice since 2002 that has banned the making of most health claims. The proposed framework classifies as health claims (i) General Level Claims that refer to the presence of a nutrient or substance in a food and to its effect on a health function; and (ii) High Level that implies a health claim that directly or indirectly refers to a serious disease or a biomarker. Nutrient content claims are not to be classified as health claims.

7.3.1.1.1 *Regulations*

http://www.comlaw.gov.au/ Australian Government Law site containing all standards included in Australian New Zealand Food Standards Code

7.3.1.1.2 *Web pages*

https://www.ebs.tga.gov.au/ Australian register of therapeutic goods

http://www.health.gov.au/ Australian Government Department of Health and Ageing http://www.tga.gov.au/index.htm Therapeutic Goods Administration

http://www.foodstandards.gov.au/ Food Standards Australia New Zealand

http://www.comlaw.gov.au/Details/F2009C00878 Australian New Zealand Food Standards Code - Standard 1.1A.2 - Transitional Standard - Health Claims

7.3.1.2 China

In China, probiotics tend to be considered a foodstuff either as a novel food or as a health food, if health claims are invoked. The central government authority with jurisdiction over food and health food (as well as medicines and cosmetics) is the State Food and Drug Administration (SFDA) but the Ministry of Health and other entities such as the General Administration of Quality Supervision, Inspection and Quarantine, the State Administration for Industry and Commerce, and so on are also in charge of the regulation of food, drug and cosmetic products. (http://www.chinafdc-law.com/glossary.html Accessed January 2012)

The first Food and Hygiene Law of the People's Republic of China was promulgated in 1995 (Kaushik and Kaushik, 2010) and the current basic food law is Food Safety Law, which entered into force in 1 June 2009; they both define food as any finished product or raw materials provided for people to eat or drink, and articles that are traditionally food and medicine, excluding articles that are used for the purpose of medical treatment.

Novel food has been regulated by the regulation by "Administrative Measures on Novel Food 2007" and included four types (article 2). Type 1 refers specifically microorganisms that are not traditionally consumed in China. Types 2 and 3 also refer microorganisms, which are not traditionally consumed in China or new varieties, as raw food materials derived (type 2) or as food processing. According to the regulation, production and import of novel food are subject to pre-market approval by China's Ministry of Health. Probiotic strains have already been approved by the current regulation (*Lactobacillus paracasei* GM-080 and *L. paracasei* GMNL-33 by GenMont in 2008) http://www.genmont.com.tw/englishwebsite/company.html Accessed December 2011.

Novel food cannot bear health claims; therefore, to make this kind of claim, the health food registration process must be followed (Patel *et al.* 2008; Lähteenmäki-Uutela 2011).

Health food is defined in the interims Provisions for Health Food Registration (SFDA Order No. 19) issued by the SFDA on 30 April 2005 as a "food claiming that it has certain health improving functions or is able to supply vitamins and minerals. It is good for a particular group of people and able to adjust body functions. But, it is not used to cure certain diseases." All health food must be approved and registered with the SFDA, which will assess and examine the safety, efficacy, quality, and labeling of products.

In accordance with the Provisions for Health Food Registration, there is a particular document about Requirements for Probiotic Microflora Health Food Application and Reviewing (interim) formulated and issued by SFDA.

The permitted probiotics are included in a list, and to add a new one, it is necessary to fulfil an SFDA application. The following probiotics are allowed: *Bifidobacterium bifidum, Bifidobacterium infantis, Bifidobacterium longum, Bifidobacterium breve, Bifidobacterium adolescentis, Lactobacillus delbrueckii* subspecies *bulgaricus, Lactobacillus acidophilus, Lactobacillus casei* subspecies *casei, Lactobacillus reuteri, and Streptococcus thermophilus.* (Lähteenmäki-Uutela 2011). There is also a list of 27 categories of health claims allowed (Patel *et al.* 2008), some of them can be applied to probiotics such as enhancing immune systems, regulating gastrointestinal flora, alleviating constipation, or facilitating digestion. However, other new claims may be invoked if can be proved by testing on humans and/or animals.

In the Chinese Health registration process, the applicant must submit the product to SFDA authorized testing laboratories and cannot apply for more than two health claims.

7.3.1.2.1 *Regulations*

Food Safety Law of the People's Republic of China. June 1 2009. (Food Safety Law)

Ministry of Health. Administrative Regulations for Health Food. Order No. 46; 1996-06-01. (Health Food Regulation)

Ministry of Health: Technical Standards for Testing and Assessment of Health Food. Order No. 42; 2003

Ministry of Health. Administrative Regulation for Novel Food. 2007. (Novel food regulation 2007)
Food Hygiene Law of the People's Republic of China. October 1995. (Food Hygiene Law. Not in force)

7.3.1.2.2 *Web pages*

http://english.gov.cn/ Central People's Government of the People's Republic of China

http://www.sfda.gov.cn SFDA

http://www.most.gov.cn Ministry of Science and Technology

http://www.fehd.gov.hk The Government of the Hong Kong Special Administrative Region of the People's Republic of China: Food and Environmental Hygiene Department

7.3.1.3 Japan

Japan is a key player in probiotic-based functional foods accounting for more than half of global probiotic foods market. These probiotic products have different applications, including immunity, allergy, cold-like symptoms, gastrointestinal health, blood pressure levels, cholesterol levels, and so on (Amagase, 2008; He and Benno, 2011).

In terms of food regulation, Japan began a systematic research on health benefits of foods in 1984. As a consequence, a definition for functional food was provided by the Japanese scientific academic community involved. In this context, functional foods were defined as those foods with three functions: apart from nutrient provision and a sensory function, functional foods also have additional physiological functions contributing to health maintenance (Shimizu, 2003).

Dynamic changes began in 1991 when the Japanese Ministry of Health, Labour and Welfare established the regulatory system "Foods for Specified Health Use" (FOSHU) in which foods wishing to bear health claims on the label have to be examined and approved, prior to use, by the Council of Pharmaceutical Affairs and Food Hygiene (practical minimum period required for approval is approximately one year) in terms of specific safety and efficacy requirements including:

(i) Proven scientific effectiveness on the human body functions;

(ii) Total safety (animal toxicity, identification of effects in case of excess intake among others);

(iii) Adequate nutrient profiles (e.g., no excessive use of sugar, saturated fat, salt);

(iv) Product specifications must be present at time of consumption—recommended dose of the functional food ingredient;

(v) Quality control methods, including product specifications, production procedure, and methods of analysis need to be well documented.

In 2001, the regulatory range of FOSHU was broadened in order to include pharmaceutical vehicles such as tablets and capsules, apart from conventional foods. At that time, the MHLW established a new regulatory system "Foods with Health Claims," which included the already existing FOSHU system and a second newly created "Foods with Nutrient Function Claims" (FNFC). In this second system, the government has set the range of nutrition and mineral content levels and labeling standards; more precisely, 12 vitamins (vitamins A, complex B, C, E, D) and two minerals (Ca, Fe) are standardized. Both regulations are under the jurisdiction of Health Promotion Law, section of Foods with Health Claims Act of 2001. These regulations differ mainly in their target specificity: the FOSHU system is a product-specific (not ingredient-specific) approval system, whereas the FNFC counterpart enables any product that meets the standards to make a standardized health claim without official approval (He and Benno, 2011). The FOSHU system has helped greatly in leading consumers in their food choices; the FOSHU-approved logo and the health claim statements clarify the relationship between food and health.

By March 2009, there were 847 existing approved FOSHU products with health claims classified into eight groups, including gastrointestinal conditions, mineral absorption, blood pressure, blood cholesterol, bone health, dental health, and blood glucose levels. In the FOSHU, product category targeting gastrointestinal health probiotics are undoubtedly the most important ingredient. Among the approved FOSHU products (with health claim), 76 were probiotic products containing one of the 16 approved bacterial strains (He and Benno, 2011). The approved strains include *Lactobacillus rhamnosus* GG, *Bifidobacterium longum* BB536,

Lactobacillus delbrueckii subsp. *Bulgaricus* 2038, *Streptococcus salivarius* subsp. *Thermophilus* 1131, *Lactobacillus casei* Shirota, *Bifidobacterium breve* Yakult, *Bifidobacterium lactis* FK120, *B. lactis* LKM512, *Lactobacillus acidophilus* CK92, *Lactobacillus herbeticus* CK60, *L. casei* SBR1202, *Lactobacillus gaseeri* SP, *Bifidobacterium* SP, *L. casei* NY1301, *Lactobacillus* LC1, and *B. lactis* Bb-12.

It is important to note that the current FOSHU approval system includes three categories, namely, standardized FOSHU, qualified FOSHU, and reduction of disease FOSHU (Fig. 7.1), yet approved probiotics only fall under standardized FOSHU (He and Benno, 2011).

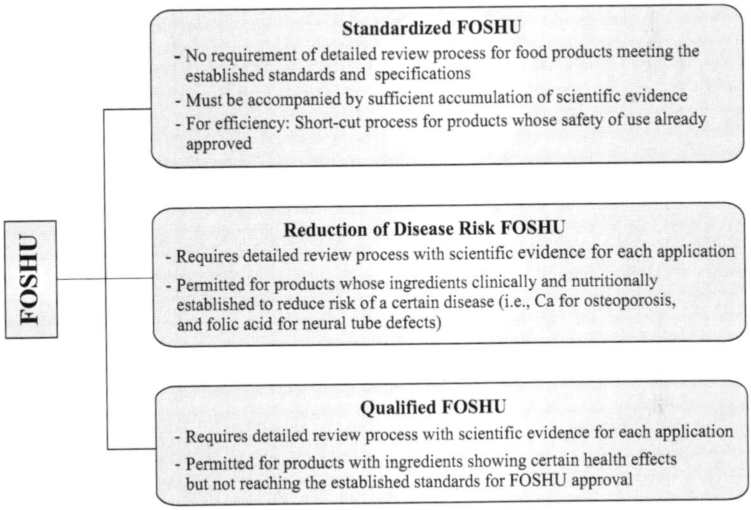

Figure 7.1 Categories of food for specified uses for regulation purposes.

As previously mentioned, FOSHU health claims for probiotic products are focused mainly on gastrointestinal conditions so the scientific evidence gathered consists mainly of data demonstrating improvement in intestinal microflora balance, increase in local beneficial bacteria in detriment of decrease of pathogenic species (*Clostridium perfringens*), lower bacteria metabolite production, and increased defecation frequency in human studies (Amagase, 2008; He and Benno, 2011). On the basis of these criteria, the approved FOSHU health claims for probiotics include:

- reaches the intestine alive
- increases the intestinal lactobacilli/bifidobacteria/beneficial bacteria
- promotes the maintenance of a good intestinal environment
- regulates/helps maintain good gastrointestinal condition
- maintains the intestine in good health
- helps balance the intestinal flora
- reduces harmful bacteria.

It is important to note that there are many other probiotic products marketed in Japan, which are not FOSHU. Animal and human studies have shown promising health promoting features in various targets, including immunity, allergy, cholesterol lowering, and *Helicobacter pylori* eradication, yet related health claims are still strictly prohibited in these cases due to lack of clinical trials and related studies (Shimizu, 2003; He and Benno, 2011).

7.3.1.3.1 *Regulations*

Food for Specified Health Uses: http://www.mhlw.go.jp/english/topics/foodsafety/fhc/02.html
Food with nutrient function claim: http://www.mhlw.go.jp/english/topics/foodsafety/fhc/01.html
Food Sanitation Law: http://www.tokio.polemb.net/files/Gospodarka/Handel/food-e.pdf

7.3.1.3.2 *Web pages*

Ministry of Health, Labour and Welfare. Available at: http://www.mhlw.go.jp/english/topics/foodsafety/fhc/index.html
Japan Health andd Nutrition Food Association. Available at: http://www.jhnfa.org/index.html
Japan Dairy Industry Association. Available at: http://www.jdia.or.jp/information/milk_know.html
Consumer Affairs Agency Food Labelling Division. Available at: http://www.caa.go.jp/en/index.html
National Institute of Health Sciences. Available at:
http://www.nihs.go.jp/english/index.html
National Institute of Health and Nutrition. Available at:
http://www0.nih.go.jp/eiken/english/index.html

7.3.2 Europe

Probiotics are consumed by Europeans in foodstuffs (food and food supplements) (Saxelin 2008). The legislation on foodstuffs in the 27 country states of the EU is not harmonized.

The principles concerning food safety and consumer protection are established in the legislation of the member states. However, EU has established general principles and requirements of food law with the aim of protecting human life and health and to integrate a food safety policy based on "farm to fork" approach. EU food law also aims to harmonize member states requirements in order to allow the free movement of food in EU. Food safety and general consumer protection is under competence of Directorate General for Health and Consumer (DG SANCO). For registration purposes, as already mention in Section 7.2.1, EU has developed the QPS list for microbial cultures, which does not need further safety determination.

Food and food supplements containing probiotics are covered by Regulation 178/2002/EC (which is the legal general framework) and Directive 2000/13/EC. EU Regulation 178/2002/EC defines food (or foodstuff) as "any substance or product, whether processed, partially processed or unprocessed, intended to be, or reasonably expected to be ingested by humans." The Directive 2002/46/EC relating to food supplements [which define as "foodstuffs the purpose of which is to supplement the normal diet and which are concentrated sources of nutrients (vitamins, and minerals) or other substances with a nutritional or physiological effect, alone or in combination, marketed in dose form, ..."] establishes harmonized rules for their labeling. Dose forms may be capsules, tablets, pastilles, pills, powders (in sachets) or liquids in measured doses, and so on. This legislation also aim to ensure that these products are safe and appropriately labeled so that consumers can make informed choices.

In EU, food labels may invoke nutrition claims, if they are listed in the annex of EC Regulation 1924/2006, and health claims, after approval by European Commission, according to the requirements set out in this Regulation. Any statement relating food and health may be interpreted as a claim and should be based on generally accepted scientific evidence and easily understood by consumers. Health claims are defined as any "claim that states, suggests or implies that a relationship exists between a food category, a food or one of its constituents and health." According to EC Regulation 1924/2006, health claims are the only ones that may be invoked by probiotic products. The last mentioned regulation established three types of health claims: (i) the reduction of disease risk; (ii) claims referring to children's development and health, (iii) other health claims than those referring to the reduction of disease risk and to children's development and health (c_1—role in the growth, development, and functions of the body; c_2—the psychological and behavioral functions; or c_3—relating to weight-control).

EFSA, established in 2002 as an independent body for risk assessment on food chain, is responsible for evaluating the scientific evidence that support health claims. Food-related general function health claims are assessed by the EFSA's Panel on Dietetic Products, Nutrition, and Allergies (NDA). Health claims for probiotics can be made under article 13 or 14 of EC Regulation 1924/2006 (Rijkers *et al.* 2011).

The three important areas the regulation pinpoints for assessment in health claims for each potentially probiotic strain are the following: (i) characterization of the strain or each of the strains in a probiotic mix, (ii) identification of the health relationship to benefit the general population or a defined part of it, and (iii) demonstration of health effects in a normal healthy target population. These three criteria form the essential basis for the establishment of potential human health claims for probiotic microorganisms (van Loveren *et al.*, 2012).

Until May 2012, none of the health claim applications for probiotic products submitted to EFSA had been accepted (http://ec.europa.eu/nuhclaims/ Accessed June 2012). Lack of adequate strain characterization or only partial characterization of strains in bacterial mixture, too general claimed health relationships without supportive evidence of beneficial clinical outcomes, claims oriented to subjects beyond the scope of the claims regulation, flaws in the studies designed to substantiate claims, or in the actual measurements are among the reasons for noneligible claims; recall that the regulation encloses claims that are designed for normal healthy populations or populations at risk of specific disorders (van Loveren *et al.*, 2012).

Alternatively, a probiotic product may encompass the legal European definition for medicinal product, but this will impose higher and more expensive requirements to applicants or manufactures. Nevertheless, due to special provisions or less stringent older legislations, several approved medicinal products that contain lactobacilli and/or bifidobacteria can still be found in many European countries.

7.3.2.1 Central Legislation

Directive 2001/83/EC of the European Parliament and of the Council of 6 November 2001 on the Community code relating to medicinal products for human use. (Medicinal products directive 2001)

Regulation (EC) No 178/2002 of the European Parliament and of the Council of 28 January 2002 laying down the general principles and requirements of food law, establishing the EFSA and laying down procedures in matters of food safety. (General Food Law, 2002)

Directive 2000/13/EC of the European Parliament and of the Council of 20 March 2000 on the approximation of the laws of the Member States relating to the labeling, presentation, and advertising of foodstuffs. (Food supplements labeling directive 2000)

Regulation (EC) No 1924/2006 of the European Parliament and of the Council of 20 December 2006 on nutrition and health claims made on foods. (Claim regulation 2006)

Regulation (EC) No 258/97 of the European Parliament and of the Council of 27 January 1997 concerning novel foods and novel food ingredients. (Novel food regulation 1997)

7.3.2.2 Web pages

http://eur-lex.europa.eu/ European Union legislation

http://www.emea.europa.eu/ema/ European Medicine Agency

http://www.efsa.europa.eu. EFSA

http://ec.europa.eu/dgs/health_consumer/index_en.htm Directorate General for Health and Consumer (DG SANCO)

7.3.3 United States of America

In the United States, probiotics are not defined as a regulatory product category; nevertheless, the FDA has issued draft guidance about complementary and alternative medicine products (FDA, 2006) wherein probiotics are referred saying that they may be regulated as foods, dietary supplements, or drugs under the Federal Food Drug and Cosmetic Act (Act). FDA is a regulatory, scientific, and public health agency that oversees food (except for meat and poultry), drugs, cosmetics, and other related products in the United States. Degnan (2008) stated that there are several regulatory categories that could be applied to products containing probiotics in the United States but four of which are fundamental: food (including food ingredients), dietary supplement, medical food, and drug (or biological product, FDA considers that if a probiotic is a drug, it is also a biological product). The classification of the products is primarily based on their intended use (largely determined by the claims invoked). Other factors such as type of formulation, route of administration, target consumers, and safety should also be considered (Hoffman *et al.* 2008).

Food means "articles used for food or drink for man and other animals" (section 201(f) of Act) and food ingredient may be food additives or GRAS substances. In a short definition, a food additive is a food component whose safety has to be demonstrated because it is not GRAS or was not already used in food prior to January 1, 1958.

A **dietary supplement** has four main characteristics: "supplement the diet," "intend for ingestion," contains or is a "dietary ingredient," and is not in "conventional food"(Degnan, 2008). Dietary supplements are a special category under the general umbrella of foods.

Medical food has a very narrow definition "a food which is formulated to be consumed or administered enterally under the supervision of a physician and that is intended for the specific dietary management of a disease or condition for which distinctive nutritional requirements, based on recognized scientific principles, are established by medical evaluation" in section 5(b) of the Orphan Drug Act (21 U.S.C. 360ee(b)(3)).

An article intended for diagnosis, cure, mitigation, treatment, or prevention of disease in man or other animals is a drug [the complete definition may be consulted in the section 201(g) (1) of the Act].

The regulatory categorization of probiotic product dictates the authorization requirements and evidentiary burdens to establish safety and to substantiate claims.

A probiotic product may need premarket authorization if it is a food additive or a drug (a biological product). In case of being a food additive, it is necessary to submit a food additive petition to Office of Food Additive Safety (OFAS) in the Center for Food Safety and Applied Nutrition (CFSAN) at FDA. This petition has four essential elements for the safety assessment: identity of the additive, probable exposure, evaluation of safety, and limitations of conditions of use. FDA recommends that manufacturers consult the FDA about food ingredient status (pre-petitions consultations).

If the probiotic product is considered a biologic product (a subset of drugs), a Biologics License Application is necessary (which includes applicant information, product/manufacturing information, pre-clinical studies, clinical studies, labeling) and the pertinent drug regulations, including applying for an Investigation New Drug Application, should be fulfilled.

A probiotic product categorized as a dietary supplement does not need a premarket approval, but the act requires that to market dietary supplements that contain "new dietary ingredients," manufacturers and distributors must previously notify FDA (it is necessary to wait at least 75 days after the filing date of the notification in order to market the product). Dietary Supplement Health and Education Act (DSHEA Act) of 1994, which significantly amends the Act, defines "new dietary ingredients" as a dietary ingredient that was not marketed in the United States before 15 October 1994. In a position paper, the International Probiotics Association, the European Food and Feed Cultures Association, and the International Food Additives Council state that "individual strains belonging to microbial species with a history of safe use as starter culture used for food fermentation or as a probiotic in food are not New Dietary Ingredients under the DSHEA Act;" on the contrary, each strain of microbial species without a history of safe use as food (including dietary supplements before 15 October 1994) must be evaluated individually and a premarket notification for a new dietary ingredient submitted to the FDA (http://internationalprobiotics.org/news/upload/pdf/11.pdf). There are three categories of claims that could be made for dietary supplements and foods: health claims, structure/function claims, and nutrient content claims. However, for food or dietary supplements containing probiotics, only the first and the second claim are relevant.

Health claims describe the relationship of a food, or ingredient to a disease or health-related condition. Legislation the 1990 Nutrition Labeling and Education Act (NLEA), the 1997 FDA Modernization Act, and the 2003 FDA Consumer Health Information for Better Nutrition

Initiative] considered three "kinds" of health claims: (1) NLEA Authorized Health Claims , (2) Heath Claims based on Authoritative Statements, and (3) Qualified Health Claims. In case of claims "type"1, the manufacturer must submit a health claim petition and FDA may authorize after an extensive review of the scientific evidence submitted in the petition. Claims of "type" 2, which are not applicable to dietary supplements, may be used on labels after successful notification to FDA on the basis of an "authoritative statement" from a scientific body of the U.S. Government or the National Academy of Sciences. If FDA found that there was not significant scientific agreement to authorize, a health claim may alternatively allow "qualified health claims based on less science evidence rather than just on the standard of significant scientific agreement, as long as the claims do not mislead the consumers"(CFSAN 2006).For this "type" of claims, the manufacturer must obtain the acquiescence of FDA, that as a matter of its enforcement discretion, they will accept the qualified health claim. According to usprobiotics.org, there are no authorized health claims for probiotics (usprobiotics.org, 2012).

Structure/function claims, which describe effects on normal functioning of the human body, have historically appeared on the labels of foodstuffs. These claims do not require a notification to FDA to be used in food, but the manufactures of dietary supplements must submit a notification no later than 30 days after marketing the product (FDA 2010).

As a medical food, a probiotic product does not need to undergo premarket review or approval by FDA, but it has to fulfil its very narrow definition and must comply with all applicable requirements for the manufacture of foods. Food additives regulations also apply to the ingredients used in medical foods (CFSAN 2007).

According to usprobiotics.org in the United States, most probiotic products are considered foods or dietary supplements and only few are marketed as medical foods.

7.3.3.1 Legislation

Federal Food Drug and Cosmetic Act of 1938
Public Health Service Act of 1944
Nutrition Labeling and Education Act of 1990
Dietary Supplement Health and Education Act of 1994
FDA Modernization Act of 1997

FDA Consumer Health Information for Better Nutrition Initiative: Task Force Final Report (2003)
FDA Food Safety Modernization Act of 2011

7.3.3.2 Web pages

http://www.fda.gov/ U.S. FDA
http://www.usprobiotics.org California Dairy Research Foundation
http://www.law.umaryland.edu/programs/health/events/probiotics/ University Maryland Francis King Carey School of Law

7.3.4 Latin America (Brazil)

In Latin America, Brazil was the first country to officially recognize functional foods in 1999 and subsequently issue specific legislation—"Food Functional Properties and/or Health Claims," including probiotics. In fact, Brazilian legislation does not define functional food (as Japan does), yet it does enable certain foods to claim specific functional health properties. In this sense, the Functional Property Claim of a food product is defined as a claim "concerning the metabolic or physiological role that the nutrient or non-nutrient has in growth, development, maintenance and/or other normal functions of the human organism" (Silveira *et al.*, 2009). Interestingly, one may claim a food to have "functional properties" and/or "health properties" claims approved by the Brazilian National Sanitary Surveillance Agency (ANVISA), yet it may not be considered as a functional food (Stringheta *et al.*, 2007; Silveira *et al.*, 2009). Recall that ANVISA in Brazil is in all similar to the FDA in the USA. Brazilian legislation establishes the basic guidelines for risk assessment and safety evaluation, analysis and verification of functional, and/or health properties claimed in labeling, as well as the conditions of registration for such foods in the main regulations listed at the end of this subchapter.

All these foods must also comply with general food legislation and they may never claim medicinal or therapeutic properties (Stringueta *et al.*, 2012).

Specifically for probiotics, ANVISA issued, in collaboration with the Health Ministry, at the beginning of 2002 the Executive Board Resolution (RDC) no. 2, 7 January 2002 (Brasil, 2002), which approved the Technical Rules for Bioactive and Isolated Probiotic Substances with Functional Properties or Health Claims; in this resolution, the guidelines required for safety assessment, registration and commercialization of bioactives, as well as probiotics claiming functional and/or health properties are placed. Therein, probiotics are defined as live microorganisms able to improve the microbial balance of the bowels, resulting in beneficial effects on people's health; bioactive substances were defined as nonnutrients that have specific metabolic or physiological actions (Brazil, 2002). It is compulsory that all probiotic products be registered and approved by health authority ANVISA before being placed on the market, as presented in Annex II of the RDC no. 27/2010. The registration of food with claims and the evaluation of new claims will be made by scientific evidence of effectiveness of these, given the criteria present in Resolution no. 18/99 and 19/99 (Stringueta *et al.*, 2012). In order to do so, the company needs to present a scientific-technical report containing a high number of specific details on the product (including description of the product, foreseen consumption, analytical methods to assess components object of claim, chemical composition with eventual molecular characterization, product formulation, usage conditions, and nutritional value and scientific evidences) together with the basic documents demanded by basic legislation to ANVISA for approval.

Several products, including probiotics, saw their claims being changed in the re-evaluation process promoted by ANVISA in 2005; such change had a better wording of claim as the main goal in order to improve consumer's understanding of product's functional properties (Brazil, 2011).

The list of approved claims in Brazil was updated in July 2008 and includes 10 probiotic strains (*Lactobacillus acidophilus, L. casei shirota, L. casei* var. *rhammosus, L. casei* var. *defensis, L. paracasei, Lactococcus lactis, Bifidobacterium bifidum, B. lactis, B. longum, Enterococcus faecium*). The approved claim's wording states: "The (indicates the microorganism species) (probiotic) contributes to the balance of intestinal flora. Its consumption should be associated with a balanced diet and healthy lifestyle." The specific requirements to uphold a claim associated with probiotics are listed in Table 7.3.

Table 7.3 Specific requirements established by ANVISA for approved claims concerning probiotic products

Parameter	Details
Minimum viable number	In the range 1×10^8–1×10^9 cfu for daily recommendation of product ready for consumption. Lower values may be accepted, if company proves its effectiveness.
Documentation on proof of efficacy	Report of the product analysis that prove the amount of the minimum viable microorganism until the end of shelf-life. Resistance test of the culture employed in product against the gastric acidity and bile salts.
Label/Claim	The amount of viable probiotics in cfu, contained in the daily recommendation intake in the product ready for consumption, must be declared on the label next to the claim.

Source: Adapted from Stringueta *et al.* (2012)

7.3.4.1 Legislation

- **Resolution no. 16**: Procedures for registration of food and/or new ingredients (Brazil, 1999d).
- **Resolution no. 17**: Risk assessment and food safety (Brazil, 1999e).
- **Ministerial Order 398/1999 and Resolution no. 18**: Basic guidelines for analysis and approval of claims for functional and/or health property mentioned on the labeling of the foods (Brazil 1999a, 1999b).
- **Resolution no. 19**: Procedures for registration of foods claiming functional and/or health properties (Brazil, 1999c).
- **Resolution RDC no. 2**: Technical Regulation of bioactive substances and isolated probiotics with claim for functional and/or health properties, annexed to that resolution (Brazil, 2002).
- **Resolution RDC no. 27:** Demonstrates about the categories of food and packaging, which are excepted or compulsory to sanitary registration, which apply to all types of food (Brazil, 2010).

7.4 Conclusions

The global regulatory situation related with probiotics is still undergoing development and change despite the tentative harmonization by all countries. It is clear from the different standpoints assumed by the different countries that probiotics are of importance in terms of health promotion and disease prevention among consumers. Nevertheless, there are still many challenges to overcome until a steady, harmonized, and overall regulatory framework is implemented worldwide to ensure the quality and safety for proper utilization of probiotics in different countries; in this context, regulatory bodies, food scientists, manufacturers, and even consumers need to brace forces in order to achieve such goal.

References

Amagase, H. (2008) Current marketplace for probiotics: a Japanese perspective. *Clin. Infect. Dis.*, **46**, S73–S75.

Brazil (1999a) Ministério da Saúde. Agência Nacional de Vigilância Sanitária. Portaria no 398, de 30 de abril de 1999. Regulamento Técnico que Estabelece as Diretrizes Básicas para Análise e Comprovação de Propriedades Funcionais e ou de Saúde Alegadas em Rotulagem de Alimentos. Diário Oficial da República Federativa do Brasil. Brasília, 03 maio, 1999. Available at: http://www.crn6.org.br/LEGISLACAO_%20ALIMENTACAO_E_%20NUTRICAO/portaria/Portaria%20ANVISA%20398-1999%20Rotulagem%20de%20alimentos.pdf. Accessed 24 september 2012.

Brazil (1999b) Ministério da Saúde. Agência Nacional de Vigilância Sanitária. Resolução no 18 de 30 de abril de 1999. Aprova o Regulamento Técnico que Estabelece as Diretrizes Básicas para Análise e Comprovação de Propriedades Funcionais e ou de Saúde Alegadas em Rotulagem de Alimentos. Diário Oficial da República Federativa do Brasil. Brasília, 03 nov. 1999. Available at: http://www.anvisa.gov.br/legis/resol/18_99.htm. Accessed 24 september 2012.

Brazil (1999c) Ministério da Saúde. Agência Nacional de Vigilância Sanitária. Resolução no 19, de 30 de abril de 1999. Aprova o Regulamento Técnico de Procedimentos para Registro de Alimento com Alegação de Propriedades Funcionais e ou de Saúde em sua Rotulagem. Diário Oficial da República Federativa do Brasil. Brasília, 10 dez. 1999. Available at: http://e-legis.bvs.br/leisref/public/showAct.php?id=110. Accessed 24 September 2012.

Brazil (1999d) Ministério da Saúde. Agência Nacional de Vigilância Sanitária. Resolução no 16, de 30 de abril de 1999. Aprova o Regulamento Técnico de Procedimentos para Registro de Alimentos e ou Novos Ingredientes. Diário Oficial da República Federativa do Brasil. Brasília, 03 dez. 1999. Available at: http:// e-legis.bvs.br/leisref/public/showAct.php?id=107. Accessed 24 September 2012.

Brazil (1999e) Ministério da Saúde. Agência Nacional de Vigilância Sanitária. Resolução no 17, de 30 de abril de 1999. Aprova o Regulamento Técnico que Estabelece as Diretrizes Básicas para Avaliação de Risco e Segurança dos Alimentos. Diário Oficial da República Federativa do Brasil. Brasília, 03 dez. 1999. Available at: http://e-legis.bvs.br/leisref/public/showAct.php?id=108. Accessed 24 September 2012.

Brazil (2002) Ministério da Saúde. Agência Nacional de Vigilância Sanitária. Resolução RDC no 2, de 7 de janeiro de 2002. Aprova o Regulamento Técnico de Substâncias Bioativas e Probióticos Isolados com Alegação de Propriedades Funcionais e ou de Saúde. Diário Oficial da República Federativa do Brasil. Brasília, 9 jan. 2002. Available at: http://e-legis.bvs.br/leisref/public/showAct.php?id=9059 &Word=. Accessed 24 September 2012.

Brazil (2010) Ministério da Saúde. Agência Nacional de Vigilância Sanitária. Resolução RDC no 27, de 06 de agosto de 2010. Dispõe sobre as categorias de alimentos e embalagens isentos e com obrigatoriedade de registro sanitário. Diário Oficial da República Federativa do Brasil. Brasília, 09 ago. 2010. Available at: http://bvsms.saude.gov.br/bvs/saudelegis/anvisa/2010/res0027_06_08_2010.html. Accessed 24 September 2012.

Brazil (2011) Ministério da Saúde. Agência Nacional de Vigilância Sanitária. Gestão 2005-2010. Principais Realizações, de 30 de março de 2011. Available at: http://portal.anvisa.gov.br/wps/wcm/connect/7122b3804745869c8feadf3fbc4c6735/Relatorio_5_anos_DEFINITIVO.pdf?MOD=AJPERES. Accessed 24 September 2012.

CFSAN (2006) *Guidance for Industry: FDA's Implementation of "Qualified Health Claims": Questions and Answers; Final Guidance.* FDA.

CFSAN (2007) *Guidance for Industry: Frequently Asked Questions About Medical Foods.* FDA.

Degnan, F. H. (2008) The US Food and Drug Administration and probiotics: regulatory categorization, *Clin. Infect. Dis.*, **46 Suppl 2**, S133–S136; discussion S144–S151.

EFSA (2010) Scientific Opinion on the maintenance of the list of QPS biological agents intentionally added to food and feed (2010 update).

EFSA J., 8(12), 1944 [56 pp.]. Available online: www.efsa.europa.eu/efsajournal.htm

EFSA (2011) Scientific Opinion on the safety and efficacy of Lactobacillus paracasei (DSM 16773) as a silage additive for all species, *EFSA J.*, **9**(2370), 1–11.

FDA (2006) *Complemantary and Alternative Medicine Products and Their Regulation by the Food Drug Administration* U.S. HHS, Rockville.

FDA (2010) Structure/Function Claims. Retrieved 18 June 2012, 2012, from http://www.fda.gov/Food/LabelingNutrition/LabelClaims/StructureFunctionClaims/default.htm.

He, F., and Benno, Y. (2011) Probiotics and health claims: a Japanese perspective. Chapter 8. In: *Probiotics and Health Claims*, Kneifel, W. & Salminen, S. (Eds). Blackwell Publishing Ltd, United Kingdom.

Henriksson, A., Borody, T., and Clancy, R. (2005) Probiotics under the regulatory microscope. *Expert Opin. Drug Saf.*, **4**, 1–9.

Hoffman, F.A., Heimbach, J.T., Sanders, M. E., and Hibberd, P. L. (2008) Executive summary: scientific and regulatory challenges of development of probiotics as foods and drugs, *Clin. Infect. Dis.*, **46 Suppl 2**, S53–S57.

ISAPP (2009) Probiotics: a consumer guide for making smart choices. [Online]. Available: http://www.isapp.net/docs/Consumer_Guidelines-probiotic.pdf [Accessed 9 August 2012].

Kaushik, N., and Kaushik, D. (2010) Functional foods: overview and global regulation, *Int. J. Pharma Recent Res.*, **2**(2), 47–52.

Lähteenmäki-Uutela, A. (2009) *Foodstuffs and Medicines as Legal Categories in the EU and China*. Faculty of Law. Turku, Turku. Ph.D.

Lähteenmäki-Uutela, A. (2011) Regulation of probiotics in China, *Probiotics and Health Claims*. W. Kneifel and S. Salminen. Wiley-Blackwell, Oxford, UK.

Patel, D., Y. Dufour, and Domigan, N. (2008) Functional food and nutraceutical registration processes in Japan and China: a diffusion of innovation perspective, *J. Pharm. Pharm. Sci.*, **11**(4), 1–11.

Rijkers, G.T., de Vos, W.M., Brummer, R. J., Morelli, L., Corthier, G., and Marteau P. (2011) Health benefits and health claims of probiotics: bridging science and marketing, *British J. Nutrition*, **106**(9), 1291–1296.

Sanders, M. E. and Marco, M. L. (2010) Food formats for effective delivery of probiotics. *Annual Rev. Food Sci. Technol.*, **1**, 65–85.

Saxelin, M. (2008) Probiotic formulations and applications, the current probiotics market, and changes in the marketplace: a European perspective, *Clin. Infect. Dis.*, **46 Suppl 2**, S76–S79; discussion S144–S151.

Silveira, T.F.V., Viana, C.M.M., and Mosegui, G.B.G. (2009) Brazilian legislation for functional foods and the interface with the legislation for other food and medicine classes: contradictions and omissions. *Physis Revista de Saúde Coletiva,* **19**, 1189–1202.

Shimizu, T. (2003) Health claims on functional foods: the Japanese regulations and an international comparison. *Nutrition Res. Rev.,***16**, 241–252.

Stringheta, P.A., Oliveira, T.T., Gomes, R.C., Amaral, M.P.H., Carvalho, A.F. and Vilela, M.A.P. (2007) Politicas de saúde e alegações de propriedades funcionais e de saúde para alimentos no Brasil. *Revista Brasileira de Ciências Farmacêuticas* **43(2)**,181–194.

Stringueta, P.C., Amaral, M.P.H, Brumano, L.P., Pereira, M.C.S.P., and Pinto, M.A.O. (2012) Public health policies and functional property claims for food in Brazil. Chapter 12 *In* Structure and function of food engineering. InTech (Ed), pp. 307–336.

usprobiotics.org. (2012). Regulatory Considerations. Accessed 19 June 2012, 2012, from http://www.usprobiotics.org/products.asp#products

van Loveren, H., Sanz, Y., and Salmine, S. (2012) Health claims in Europe: probiotics and prebiotics as case examples. *Annual Rev. Food Sci. Technol.,* **3**, 247–261.

Wassenaar, T.M., and Klein, G. (2008) Safety aspects and implications of regulation of probiotic bacteria in food and food Supplements. *J. Food Protection,* **71**, 1734–1741.

WHO (2012) 20 questions on genetically modified foods. Accessed 1 June 2012, 2012, from http://www.who.int/foodsafety/publications/biotech/20questions/en/

Index